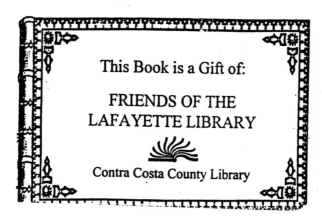

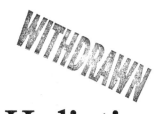

The American Holistic Medical Association Guide to Holistic Health

Healing Therapies for Optimal Wellness

Larry Trivieri, Jr.

and the American Holistic Medical Association

Foreword by Robert S. Ivker, D.O.

John Wiley & Sons, Inc.

New York • Chiche **3 1901 02924 2726** ngapore • Toronto

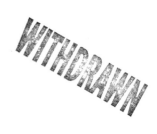

*To my parents, for their lifelong love and support
and the values they instilled in me by their example;
Paul Witte, friend among friends;
and Burton Goldberg, for opening the door.*

Contents

Acknowledgments

Though to the author it sometimes seemed otherwise, no book of this nature is written in a vacuum, and I am deeply indebted to all those who played a role in its creation. First and foremost, my thanks to my friends, Robert A. Anderson, M.D., Robert S. Ivker, D.O., and Michael C. Stern, D.C.; and to Todd Alan Bezilla, D.O., Kathleen K. Fry, M.D., Alan Gaby, M.D., Vasant Lad, B.A.M.S., David Molony, Ph.D, Steven Morris, N.D., Gary Oberg, M.D., and Candis Cantin Packard, all of whom graciously afforded me their time and expertise, greatly enhancing the worth of the chapters that follow.

I am also grateful to Thomas Dyja, who steadfastly stayed in the trenches on my behalf, ensuring that this project became a reality; and to Thomas Miller, my insightful and gracious editor, who first had the idea, and whose patience and understanding were much appreciated when my deadline was unavoidably missed due to unforeseen life events. Thanks, too, to my friend and fellow dreamer Paul Shaheen for initially bringing us together; and to Tim Berners-Lee, for inventing the World Wide Web, thereby immeasurably improving the lot of all authors everywhere.

As always, thanks too to my parents, my brothers and sisters: Daryl Andrea, Michelle, Karen, Laura, Michael, Cindy, Brian, Gina, Dianne, and Liz, and my wonderful nieces and nephews: Sonya, Bryan, Alyssa, Krystle, Brandon, Collin, Joseph, Michael, Eric, Joshua, Breana, Maria, Marisa, Skylar, and Gabriel. And of course, many thanks to my friends, particularly Paul and Jeanne Witte, Richard and Laurie Stark, Karen Defuria, Bob and Ellie Cohen, Ted Allen, Lynne Sable, Janet Roberts, Marc Rohrer, Marc Smith, Rich Stone, Marc Wilson, Frank Cranford, Nancy Morelle, Tana Acton, Paul Duran, Don Elefante, Jim Hagen, Cary Sullivan, Dan Zongrone, Dennis Rea, Lucille Kall, Moko, and Eyhraune Jau-Saune. If wealth is measured as family and friendship, I have an immeasurable fortune.

Finally, I would like to express my deep gratitude to my sister Liz, my brother-in-law Fabio Faro, and their children, Joshua and Breana, for demonstrating to me how miraculously the power of unconditional love can transform tragedy into triumph. Words cannot express the heroic dignity of their example.

Holistic Medicine

Primary Care for the Twenty-first Century

by Robert S. Ivker, D.O.

As Larry Trivieri makes abundantly clear in the pages that follow, the basic principles of holistic medicine are not new, having been around at least since the time of Hippocrates in the West, 2500 years ago, and even earlier in the Eastern healing traditions of Ayurvedic and traditional Chinese medicine. As you will also see, throughout history the healers and physicians who practiced the art and science of holistic medicine, all treated the *whole person*—body, mind, and spirit. This commonsense holistic focus has been largely ignored by most physicians during the past few hundred years. This has led to our current conventional system of disease care, which for all of its miraculous discoveries and highly effective treatment of acute and life-threatening illnesses and injuries, has become increasingly mechanistic and overly focused on the treatment of symptoms. As a result, the factors contributing to *causing* disease have not been adequately addressed, while more than 100 million Americans suffer from some form of chronic illness. Treatment of the whole person has focused on fixing the "broken part." This approach works quite well in mitigating or eliminating symptoms, but has resulted in our inability to prevent, cure (elimination of a physical problem), and/or heal (lessening of dis-ease with restoration of wholeness and balance) diseases of a chronic, multifactorial nature. Instead of meeting the needs of our patient population, we have created an overburdened health care system that costs the United States more than $1 trillion each year.

According to the most recent surveys, public frustration with physicians' inability to prevent or eliminate their suffering (or save their lives) from a variety of ailments—from cancer, AIDS, and heart disease, to sinusitis, arthritis, and backache—has led more than two-thirds of our population to seek alternative medical treatment, for which they spent $27 billion in 1997. Most of this expense was paid for out-of-pocket, since the majority of these treatments are not covered by health insurance. This powerful demonstration of interest in alternatives has helped to create the National Institutes of Health's Office of Complementary and Alternative Medicine, with its current research budget of $150 million. It has also spawned new terminology as we search for the best word to describe the new medicine. Beginning with *alternative*, we progressed to *complementary*, and now *integrative medicine* seems to be most popular. But the term that best describes this rapidly expanding field that extends beyond the scope of drugs and surgery is *holistic medicine*. This art and science of healing combines conventional and complementary therapies to prevent and treat disease, but its primary objective is to help create the experience of optimal, or *holistic*, health.

Far more than simply a set of new therapeutic options for treating chronic disease, the ancient baton of holistic medicine has been passed to the American Holistic Medical Association (AHMA), and, more recently, its sister organization, the American Board of Holistic Medicine (ABHM). It has become the responsibility of these two organizations to inspire and educate Americans, both laypeople and health practitioners alike, to make the commitment and assume greater responsibility for their own health. Since December 2000, the ABHM for the first time established board certification for M.D.'s and D.O.'s in holistic medicine, effectively setting a new standard for quality health care in America. The art, science, and practice of this brand of medicine is based upon the belief that *unconditional love* is life's most powerful medicine. Most physicians have been highly successful in the academic arena. But to practice holistic medicine, one must focus on expanding their heart's capacity to exceed that of the intellect. Holistic physicians, engaged in the "business of caring," guide their patients in a healing process of learning to nurture themselves physically, environmentally, mentally, emotionally, spiritually, and socially.

More than any other single volume, this book will help you to better understand the comprehensive scope of holistic medicine, making it an essential part of the medicine of the new millennium. It presents a wide array of therapies for treating disease and creating optimal health, while also explaining how each therapy originated and evolved, along with current research supporting each use. You'll learn what to expect during your treatment sessions and be provided with guidelines that will empower you to take greater responsibility for your own health.

You needn't be a physician or have medical training to heal yourself. All that's required is a commitment to nurture and have compassion for yourself, and to take the time, make the effort, and exert the discipline necessary to honor that commitment. Each of us has an "inner healer" residing in our hearts. We need only to listen to the guidance we receive from her on a regular basis. There are no shortcuts to realizing your full potential as a human being. It is truly a labor of love. I call it training to thrive, and it's still my full-time job. I invite you to make it yours, as well. The information Larry Trivieri shares will provide you with the foundation you need to get started.

> Robert S. Ivker, D.O.
> Past President of the American Holistic Medical
>   Association and author of *Sinus Survival, Thriving,*
>   and *The Self-Care Guide to Holistic Medicine*
> Littleton, Colorado

PART ONE

Holistic Health

Chapter 1

The History and Philosophy of Holistic Medicine

As we enter the twenty-first century, a revolution in health care is slowly yet inexorably taking place all around the world. What distinguishes this revolution from similar momentous changes sweeping through other fields of human endeavor is the fact that it is being sparked not so much by leaders in the health care field, but by burgeoning numbers of laypeople who are seeking more effective solutions to their health and wellness needs. The reason for that search is simple: despite a century of remarkable diagnostic and therapeutic advances in the field of conventional, or *allopathic*, medicine, chronic illness continues to spread at an alarming rate and is proving increasingly impervious to drugs and surgery. Just as important, more and more patients are looking for health care approaches that address their specific and unique traits and needs, rather than simply treating their symptoms. But perhaps the primary factor that accounts for the growing shift away from allopathic care is the fact that many patients with chronic conditions, such as chronic pain, anxiety, arthritis, headache, gastrointestinal disorders, addictions, fatigue, and lack of energy, simply are not getting better using the remedies prescribed by their conventional physicians. As a result, surveys show that as many as two-thirds of North Americans now use some form of complementary and/or alternative medicine in their quest to find the type of health care they desire. The solutions they are searching for are broad-based and comprehensive and are increasingly being found in the emerging new field of *holistic medicine.*

According to the American Holistic Medical Association (AHMA), holistic medicine is defined as the art and science of healing that addresses the whole person—body, mind, and spirit—by integrating conventional and alternative therapies to prevent and treat disease, and to promote optimal health. AHMA members recognize that both conventional and alternative therapies have their place and combine both in order to offer their patients a full range of treatment options tailored to each patient's specific needs. At the same time, holistic physicians emphasize personal responsibility and educate their patients about how to take care of themselves at all levels of their being.

Robert S. Ivker, D.O., past president of the AHMA, describes holistic or optimal health as "the unlimited and unimpeded free flow of life force energy throughout your body, mind, and spirit." Each of us has the capacity to nurture and to heal ourselves, but most of us have yet to tap into this wellspring of loving life energy. Holistic physicians recognize this fact and help their patients learn how to tap into this life force while simultaneously treating their disease conditions. "The result," Dr. Ivker says, "is that their patients learn to safely and effectively treat any physical, mental, and spiritual conditions that may be impeding the flow of this vital energy in their lives, so that they not only start to get better, they also begin to thrive and experience more energy and joy in being alive. When this happens, there is a sense of harmony and balance in the physical, environmental, mental, emotional, spiritual, and social aspects of their lives." Holistic medicine also emphasizes treating the *causes* of disease, not just its symptoms. This, coupled with its minimal toxic side effects and generally lower costs, explains why so many Americans are now choosing holistic medical approaches.

THE PRINCIPLES OF HOLISTIC MEDICINE

Holistic medicine's comprehensive definition of health is at odds with our predominant health care system, which is based almost entirely upon the diagnosis and treatment of disease symptoms. While conventional medicine is unsurpassed in treating acute life-threatening illness and injuries, its reliance on pharmaceutical drugs and surgery has left it largely a failure in terms of handling chronic conditions. As a result, over 100 million Americans now suffer from some type of chronic illness, driving the cost of health care in the United States above $1 trillion per year. Further compounding the problem is the fact that most conventionally trained physicians are taught little, if anything, about maintaining and enhancing health, or even preventing disease. Even within the fields of alternative and complementary medicine the primary focus is still on relieving symptoms and treating disease. Although holistic physicians also address their patients' immediate physical discomfort by using both alternative and conventional therapies, most of their time is spent determining the multiple underlying causes of their patients' ailments and helping them to correct the imbalances in their lives that are responsible for them. Throughout this process optimal health remains the chief objective.

Informing holistic physicians' approach to health care are twelve principles of holistic medicine that have been established by the board of trustees of the American Holistic Medical Association. Each of these principles is outlined below.

1. Holistic physicians embrace a variety of safe, effective diagnostic and treatment options. These include education for lifestyle changes and self-care; complementary diagnostic and treatment approaches; and conventional drugs and surgery. In diagnosing and treating disease, optimal outcomes are most often achieved by combining the best of both conventional and complementary medicine and teaching patients how to live a holistic lifestyle. The need for the synthesis of these options is reflected in the recent draft document for establishing curriculum guidelines for teaching complementary and integrative medical principles and applications to physicians in specialty training in family practice residencies. The committee of the Society of Teachers of Family Medicine, which developed these guidelines, believes this step to be essential for the 470 family practice training programs in the United States.

2. Searching for the underlying causes of disease is preferable to treating symptoms alone. This second principle of holistic medicine is bolstered by a 1987 study published in the *Journal of the American Medical Association (JAMA)*, in which researchers found that 40 percent of a large group of hypertensive patients maintained a normal blood pressure without drugs after losing an average of five pounds in body weight, reducing their sodium intake, and limiting alcohol consumption to one drink per day. Robert Anderson, M.D., is a founding member of the AHMA and president of its sister organization, the American Board of Holistic Medicine, the first organization to certify physicians in its practice. Dr. Anderson has observed that pursuing the answer to *why* patients have high blood pressure has resulted in 75 to 80 percent of patients being able to go off their medications, while the remaining 20 percent were able to reduce their dosage levels. "By losing weight, reducing sodium and alcohol intake, adopting a modest exercise program, paying attention to their attitude, and engaging in a regular program of deep relaxation or meditation, most patients can maintain a normal blood pressure without drugs," Dr. Anderson says. "Similar results can often also be achieved for most patients suffering with other forms of chronic illness. Moreover, many patients would prefer making such lifestyle changes rather than taking medications. The cost savings alone would make many consider this worthwhile, and surely it is the responsibility of the medical profession to look at these simplest solutions first."

3. *Holistic physicians expend as much effort in establishing what kind of patient has a disease as they do in establishing what kind of disease a patient has.* This hundred-year-old dictum from one of the revered fathers of American medicine, William Osler, M.D., emphasizes the multiple factors underlying the incidence and development of many diseases. In a group of women diagnosed with breast cancer, for instance, a recent study showed that the risk of recurrence of their cancer is nine times greater in women who are under high levels of stress compared to those whose stress levels are low. Failure to recognize the importance of stress and deal with it adequately greatly reduces the likelihood of a favorable outcome.

Further supporting this third principle is the fact that the internal healing capacity of the patient is the key to the presence or absence of disease. This basic medical truth was recognized in the late nineteenth century by Dr. Claude Bernard, the father of modern physiology, who pointed out that exposure to most bacteria, viruses, and toxins resulted in illness in only a portion of the population. Patient resistance to illness was, in his opinion, the consideration of first importance. A modern example of Bernard's tenet can be found in cases of tuberculosis. Recent research has revealed how lifestyle affects intrinsic resistance and immunity, and how it changes outcomes. Among the major lifestyle factors are attention to nutritional consumption, physical exercise, smoking, substance abuse, deeply held beliefs and attitudes, and protecting against accidents and trauma.

4. Prevention is preferable to treatment and is usually more cost-effective. The most cost-effective approach evokes the patient's own innate healing capacities. The conventional physicians' standard response to a diagnosis of chronic illness involves the prescribing of drugs. In cases of elevated blood pressure, these drugs include diuretics, beta-blockers, or angiotensin-converting-enzyme-inhibitors. While such drugs can often result in symptom relief, they do not alter the underlying causes of hypertension. But when unmanaged stress is recognized as a major contributing factor, a brief course in biofeedback/relaxation training greatly enhances a patient's ability to handle stress, reducing or normalizing blood pressure in the process. For patients who develop this skill, the benefits include improved immunity, faster reaction time, better hearing and pain tolerance, and a decrease in headaches, migraines, insomnia, ulcers, adrenaline, cortisone, cholesterol, and muscle tension. Similar results occur when both doctor and patient pay attention to diet and nutrition, since it takes five to seven times the normal amount of nutrition to build and repair as it does to maintain proper physiological function.

A physician who exemplifies the fourth principle of holistic medicine is Dean Ornish, M.D., who demonstrated that coronary artery disease can be reversed by instituting a combination of lifestyle changes. Two years after his pioneering research was published in *Lancet* in 1990, the Mutual of Omaha Insurance Company decided to cover the cost of his reeducation and training program for heart patients. Although expensive, it was a fraction of the cost of coronary artery surgery for just one patient out of an entire class of patients who followed Dr. Ornish's program.

5. Illness is viewed as a manifestation of a dysfunction of the whole person, not as an isolated event. Nonconventional healing systems in various parts of the world have recognized the importance of the whole person to a much greater extent than Western allopathic medicine. Traditional Chinese medicine, for instance, has for five thousand years recognized the importance of a balance of movement (a variety of martial arts), diet, herbal remedies, and the unimpeded flow of *qi*, or life force energy, as being essential for optimal health. The concept of the whole person has also been a core belief in Ayurveda, the traditional medicine of India and South Asia, for several thousand years.

The advantage of treating the whole person instead of an isolated disease is illustrated by comparing conventional and holistic approaches to treating cataracts, a common condition among elderly people in the United States. "Lens implant surgery is the largest single-issue medical expenditure for Medicare, and is the common approach undertaken by conventional physicians," Dr. Anderson explains. "Yet a cataract is much more than a disease of the eye. It is a manifestation of elevated free radical activity which has been developing in the body of the patient for many years due, at least in part, to decreased antioxidant levels." By incorporating better nutrition, exercise, smoking cessation, avoidance of extreme bright sunlight, and antioxidant supplementation into the treatment protocols of their patients, holistic physicians are able to reduce the risk of cataracts by as much as 70 percent.

6. *A major determining factor in the healing process is the quality of the relationship established between physician and patient, in which the patient is encouraged to take responsibility for his or her health.* The relationship between patient and physician is one of the most powerful influences on the eventual outcome of a medical disease or psychological condition. A high-quality relationship inspires willingness, confidence, and enthusiasm, and a sense of trust and satisfaction, all of which enhance healing. In a trusting relationship, a patient knows that the physician deeply cares and will focus his or her best effort on determining the cause of, and best treatment for, the patient's condition.

Participation in decision making, working cooperatively with one's physician and members of the health care team, and being highly informed about what is happening, all contribute to a heightened sense of autonomy on the part of the patient. Long-term studies in Europe have demonstrated much lower incidences of heart disease and cancer, for instance, in autonomous persons compared to more dependent people who allow their beliefs and attitudes to be determined by external factors. Members of the much healthier autonomous group espoused the belief that health is an "inside job," and were therefore more willing to do whatever was necessary to ensure their well-being.

7. *The ideal physician-patient relationship considers the needs, desires, awareness, and insight of the patient, as well as those of the physician.* "The beliefs, experience, and education of the patient will influence his or her desires and degrees of awareness regarding medical choices, and

also influence his or her physician," says Dr. Anderson. "If the physician and patient both believe in a given approach, it will be much more effective. This is an important point to consider, given that in many clinical situations a wide variety of choices are frequently present."

8. *Physicians significantly influence patients by their example.* A cartoon hanging on the wall of Dr. Anderson's waiting room shows a three-hundred-pound, cigar-smoking physician tilted back in his chair, asking a shivering, half-clad skinny patient across the desk, "Are you eating properly and getting plenty of exercise?" This ridiculous comparison has tickled thousands of his patients over the years. "In all walks of life, what we do speaks more loudly than what we say," Dr. Anderson points out. "Therefore, physicians need to be aware of the influence their actions can have on their patients, both positively and negatively, bearing in mind Hippocrates' injunction 'Physician, heal thyself.' At the same time, patients would do well to ask themselves if their health care providers are living the healthy lifestyle they expouse. If they're not, it may be time for the patient to consider seeking someone else to guide them in their health care needs."

9. *Illness, pain, and the dying process can be learning opportunities for both patients and physicians.* Dr. Anderson recalls the great shock of disbelief he experienced the first time a cancer patient in declining health said to him, "I'm glad I got my cancer." The patient was slowly losing her battle with breast cancer, yet as a result of her ordeal she had discovered some valuable life lessons. She had learned to appreciate every moment of her days: the incredible beauty of nature as she slowed her pace to pay attention; the wonder of moments of intimacy with her husband; her finite but previously unrecognized inner resources in dealing with the pain and fatigue of the cancer; the joy of plumbing the mysteries and meaning of life itself; and the ability to use her experience in helping others in similar circumstances. "She taught me that the quality of life in our brief span of life is perhaps our most important consideration," Dr. Anderson says. "After my experience with her, at least half a dozen other cancer patients have shared with me the same sentiments. All have learned things about themselves that overshadowed even their desire to prolong their lives." When both patients and physicians are able to recognize the healing potential inherent in pain, disease, and dying, miraculous resolutions in their lives can occur. And if death proves inevitable, it usually comes more peacefully and with greater acceptance on the part of everyone involved. On the other hand, sometimes the

recognition of the gifts and lessons involved during the disease process can mobilize our innate healing abilities, even to the point of spontaneous remission.

10. Holistic physicians encourage their patients to evoke the healing power of love, hope, humor, and enthusiasm, and to release the toxic consequences of hostility, shame, greed, depression, and prolonged fear, anger, and grief. Extensive research documents the detrimental effects of hostility, depression, and anxiety in chronic disease conditions such as heart disease, cancer, stroke, and autoimmune diseases like rheumatoid arthritis, to name just a few. One study, for example, found that among a group of patients undergoing angioplasty for threatening coronary artery disease, the risk for restenosis (the recurrent closing down of the artery) was 250 percent greater in patients found to have high levels of hostility, compared to patients with low hostility levels. Another study of two thousand male employees of Western Electric, all of whom were initially free of heart disease, found that the rate of coronary heart disease over a ten-year period was 32 percent greater among those whose psychological tests showed great hostility. A third study found that when volunteers were asked to recall the last time they became extremely angry, measurements of their hearts' pumping ability decreased 12 percent in only fifteen minutes. Such studies clearly reveal that negative emotions and attitudes are toxic to the physical, mental, and emotional function of us all.

On the positive side, the therapeutic benefits of humor and laughter have also been repeatedly shown. One study, for instance, showed that volunteers who viewed humorous videotapes strengthened their immune systems within thirty minutes. According to Dr. Anderson, children laugh an average of four hundred times a day; adults only fifteen times a day. "No doubt that is one reason that adults are far more prone to chronic illness than children are," he says.

11. Unconditional love is life's most powerful medicine. Holistic physicians strive to adopt an attitude of unconditional love for patients, themselves, and other practitioners. "Unconditional love, released through the act of forgiveness, is the most important tool for self-empowerment, development of positive attitudes, and optimism, all of which contribute to better therapeutic outcomes," Dr. Anderson says. A growing number of studies demonstrate the healing power of love and intimacy.

12. Optimal health is much more than the absence of sickness. It is the conscious pursuit of the highest qualities of the physical, environmental, mental, emotional, spiritual, and social aspects of the human experience. The principal emphasis of Western medicine has been intervention in disease processes, primarily through the use of drugs or surgery. Holistic medicine adds a twofold question to this conventional approach: What has caused the patient's condition to develop, and what can be done to help him or her reverse that cause? In addition, what fundamental changes can the patient undertake to limit further degeneration, reverse the degenerative process, cure the disease, and pursue optimal health with the highest-quality physical, environmental, mental, emotional, spiritual, and social experience of life itself?

"In nearly every instance in which an individual commits to a significant change in diet, exercise, or other health practice, there is an incremental improvement in their state of health, even at an advanced age," Dr. Anderson reports. Illustrating his point is the case of one of his patients, a sixty-four-year-old woman who developed widespread ovarian cancer. Surgery removed the bulk of the tumor, but significant amounts of the cancer remained. She refused chemotherapy. Respecting her choices, Dr. Anderson responded to her request that he help her to get well. Together they developed a comprehensive strategy to enhance her immunity, evoke her determination and will, improve all aspects of her lifestyle, and enhance her spiritual life, including forgiving a large number of people. One of her life's greatest pleasures was attending opera. As part of her recovery, she saved her money to fulfill a lifelong dream and was able to hear some of the greatest stars of opera perform for three nights at La Scala in Milan, Italy. Later, surgery showed her cancer to be totally gone. She eventually died of unrelated causes after eight years of enjoyable, satisfying life, having accomplished what she wanted to do in this lifetime, while overcoming an aggressive cancer that could have taken her life a year after its discovery.

HOLISTIC AND CONVENTIONAL MEDICINE: A COMPARISON

It is holistic medicine's focus on optimal wellness that most clearly distinguishes it from conventional medicine. The strengths and weaknesses of both systems are summarized in the following table, created by Dr. Ivker.

Holistic Medicine	Conventional Medicine
Philosophy	
Based on the integration of allopathic (M.D.), osteopathic (D.O.), naturopathic (N.D.), energy, and ethnomedicine	Based on allopathic medicine
Primary Objective of Care	
To promote optimal health, and as a by-product, to prevent and treat disease	To cure or mitigate disease
Primary Method of Care	
Empower patients to heal themselves by addressing the causes of their disease and facilitating lifestyle changes	Focus on the elimination of physical symptoms
Diagnosis	
Evaluate the whole person through holistic medical history, holistic health score sheet, physical exam, lab data	Evaluate the body with history, physical exam, lab data
Primary Care Treatment Options	
Love applied to body, mind, and spirit through diet, exercise, environmental measures, attitudinal and behavioral modifications, relationship and spiritual counseling, bioenergy enhancement	Drugs and surgery
Secondary Care Treatment Options	
Botanical (herbal) medicine, homeopathy, acupuncture, manual medicine, biomolecular therapies, physical therapy, drugs, and surgery	Diet, exercise, physical therapy, and stress management
Weaknesses	
Shortage of holistic physicians and training programs; time-intensive, requiring a commitment to a healing process, not a quick fix	Ineffective in preventing and curing chronic disease; expensive
Strengths	
Teaches patients to take responsibility for their own health, and in so doing is cost-effective in treating both acute and chronic illness; therapeutic in preventing and treating chronic disease; essential in creating optimal health	Highly effective in treating both acute and life-threatening illness and injuries

(Courtesy of Robert S. Ivker, D.O. Used with permission.)

HISTORICAL PRECEDENTS

The underlying concepts of holistic medicine are not new. In actuality, they represent a return to medical principles that have shaped our understanding of health and illness for thousands of years in both Eastern and Western cultures. In the East, the idea that each of us is a being of body, mind, and spirit has played an integral role in shaping the traditions of Chinese and Ayurvedic medicine, both of which are thousands of years old. In the West, the idea that health is directly related to a state of harmonious balance, both within oneself and with the outer world, also extends back thousands of years, and was a major tenet in the teachings of Hippocrates, the father of Western medicine.

Disease, from the perspective of both the Eastern and Western medical traditions, was recognized as a consequence of disharmony, or living "out of tune" with the natural order of things. Among the conditions that both cultures recognized as being crucial to health were a healthy diet, proper hygiene, exercise, a calm mental and emotional state, home and work environments conducive to well-being, and a recognition of a natural life force, or spirit, that pervades and sustains all life. Similar tenets can also be found in the healing traditions of ancient Africans, Native Americans, and other indigenous cultures. Teaching patients how to live in harmony with themselves and their environment by emphasizing each of the areas above was the primary goal of the healers and physicians within these cultures. Over time, however, they lost sight of much of what they had learned in these areas, especially after the discoveries of Pasteur and the advent of "germ theory." Since then, modern medicine has becoming increasingly one-sided in its focus, seeking out ever more powerful drugs to treat bacteria, viruses, fungi, and other microorganisms, while focusing on body parts and specialization to the point where the individual being treated is altogether forgotten.

Recognition of this fact led world-renowned neurosurgeon C. Norman Shealy, M.D., Ph.D., to found the American Holistic Medical Association in 1978, in order to provide a "common community" for physicians committed to treating the "whole person" according to the philosophy of holistic medicine. Since its inception, the AHMA has emphasized the principle that "drugs and surgery are often the treatment of necessity and of choice in acute illness, and often inadequate in significant healing for those with chronic illness." In order to better serve their patients, AHMA members also emphasize nutrition, exercise, various bodywork therapies, energy medicine, mind/body medicine, "and, above all, an emphasis on spirituality." In so doing, they are leading the way toward a new system of health care that combines the best of both modern allopathic medicine and the far older or more holistic medical systems around the world.

BODY, MIND, AND SOUL:
A MULTILEVEL APPROACH TO WELLNESS

According to Dr. Ivker, true holistic health can be achieved only when there is harmony and balance in body, mind, and spirit.

> Each of these three levels of health contain two components. Being healthy in body means not only being physically healthy, but also creating a healthy environment, both at home and where you work. Mental health comprises the quality of our thoughts and emotions, and also our attitudes and beliefs about ourselves. And being healthy in spirit means being connected both spiritually and socially to the flow of life force energy. A weakness in any one of these areas will eventually lead to a decline in all areas, and ultimately result in disease. As holistic physicians, our primary job is to help our patients recognize this fact and guide them towards healing whichever areas of their lives are out of balance. As a specialist in the holistic treatment of sinusitis and other respiratory conditions, for instance, I've found that many of my patients have problems with unresolved anger. Helping them learn how to express their anger safely and appropriately can make a big difference with their sinus problems, and often is the key factor in curing their condition.

Dr. Ivker further describes each of these six components as follows:

1. Physical health is a condition of high energy and vitality. Hallmarks of physical health include strong immune function; the absence of, or high adaptability to, physical pain and disability; a body that is strong and flexible with good aerobic capacity; and a healthy libido.
2. Environmental health is the state of being in harmony with your environment. It is experienced as a sense of "groundedness" and awareness of nature's rhythms, breathing healthy air, drinking pure water, eating nutritious food, and respect for your home, earth, and all of its creatures.
3. Mental health is experienced as contentment and peace of mind. Hallmarks of mental health are a sense of humor and optimism.

Financial well-being, having a job that is fulfilling, and living your life according to your vision of what is right for you all contribute to a healthy mental state.

4. Emotional health is reflected in self-acceptance and high self-esteem. Being emotionally healthy means being able to accept and express all of your feelings, whether painful or joyful. Playfulness and the regular experience of "peak" functioning or "being in the zone" are other healthy emotional traits.

5. Spiritual health is the experience of unconditional love and the absence of fear. Feelings of gratitude and being connected to God or Spirit exemplify this state, as does having a sense of purpose, trusting your intuition, and being open to change. Prayer, meditation, and the regular observance of the Sabbath or other spiritual ritual all contribute to our spiritual well-being.

6. Social health is a condition of deep, committed relationships and the ability to forgive. Social health is best demonstrated by an ability to be intimate with your spouse or partner, family members, and close friends. Selflessness and altruism are natural consequences of being socially healthy and connected, as is having a sense of belonging to your community.

In addition to the factors above, optimal health also depends on the healthy functioning of the body's interdependent systems. According to Joseph Pizzorno, N.D., founding president of Bastyr University and author of *Total Wellness*, chief among the body's intrinsic healing systems are the immune system (including the lymphatic system), the detoxification system, the inflammatory system, the metabolic system, the regulatory system, and the rejuvenation system. As Dr. Pizzorno points out, these systems "must work effectively for each of us to establish and maintain total wellness." In addition, only by understanding and correcting whatever imbalances may be present in these systems can we reestablish normal function and create lasting optimal health. As Dr. Pizzorno writes, "It is easy to prescribe a whole-foods diet, more exercise, less pollution, and less stress for everyone, but such generic prescriptions do not recognize the unique needs of each individual." Recognizing such individual needs and creating a wellness program to match them is the goal of holistic medicine.

In designing a wellness program for their patients, holistic physicians also recognize and honor the principle of *homeostasis*, which refers to the body's wondrous capacity to maintain and repair itself by supporting the equilibrium within the various body systems. When we are healthy, this homeostatic process occurs automatically so that if we cut ourselves, for example, the healing process begins immediately. But when our body systems are overtaxed or out of balance, this self-regulatory process becomes impeded. Restoring homeostatic function, therefore, is one of the primary goals of holistic physicians when treating disease, and is one of the ways that their approach to health care differs from their conventional counterparts.

When a person becomes ill, homeostasis manifests itself in the form of symptoms. Holistic physicians recognize that these symptoms are signs that the body is homeostatically trying to restore proper function. Instead of trying to suppress such symptoms through the use of drugs, holistic physicians seek to assist the body in ridding itself of whatever infectious agents may be present so that it can restore itself. Only in cases where the symptoms are life-threatening or tremendously painful will they consider interrupting this process. Otherwise, they monitor the situation and use whatever measures are most advisable and most appropriate for each patient in order to help the process run its course. This means making sure that the patient's needs are being met on all levels—body, mind, and spirit. The resultant healing crisis may be uncomfortable, but when it is over, typically the patient will experience a new level of wellness. "Many times, too, patients will have a new understanding about themselves," Dr. Ivker points out, "since in our society it is often only when we are forced to rest that we take the time to reconnect with ourselves and discover what our inner guidance is trying to tell us."

Symptoms of the body's homeostatic response to disease include fever, inflammation, vomiting, and diarrhea, all of which will usually run their course within a few days without the need for outside intervention. All too often, however, both patient and physician will seek to arrest such symptoms prematurely. When this happens, many times the initial symptom will disappear, only to be replaced later with a different symptom that is more severe, as the body creates a stronger "message" in order to get our attention. But if such messages aren't heeded, the symptom picture can progressively worsen and ultimately become chronic.

THE PATH TO HEALTH

As the following chapters make clear, the field of holistic medicine encompasses a wide range of modalities and treatment options. From the holistic perspective, however, all such therapies are based on a philosophy informed by the following principles:

1. All patients should be empowered by accepting responsibility for at least part of the task of their recovery and future well-being.
2. Sound nutrition is a core requirement for health, as is a lifestyle that is balanced and provides appropriate amounts of exercise and rest.
3. Harmony within our environment, being socially connected, and mental, emotional, and spiritual stability are all essential factors for optimal health.
4. True health care treats the person, not his or her presenting symptoms, recognizing that each of us has specific individual and biochemical needs.

The road to health is a journey that each of us must travel according to who and what we are uniquely. It is also a road that must address our entire being—body, mind, and spirit—and assist our bodies' interdependent systems to function properly while honoring the principle of homeostasis. Because holistic medicine understands and respects these concepts, it continues to increase in popularity and offers the promise of most effectively treating our many chronic health conditions.

CHAPTER 2

The Holistic
Self-Care Program

Holistic medicine's primary emphasis is on achieving and maintaining optimum wellness. To a large degree, holistic practitioners accomplish this by teaching their patients principles of *self-care* and *prevention*. This chapter provides basic guidelines for creating and maintaining health from the perspective of the whole person—body, mind, and spirit. While not intended as a substitute for professional care, the principles and exercises that follow can be used to cultivate greater vitality and balance in your life.

BODY

Health of the body means being well both *physically* and *environmentally*. Healthy people tend to bounce out of bed each day refreshed from a good night's sleep, eager to be about the challenges of the day ahead. Not only do they have high levels of energy, they also tend to be happier and more successful and to have fuller and deeper relationships with their spouses, partners, families, friends, and coworkers. They are also in harmony with their environment, both at home and at work. Achieving this optimum state of physical health involves an ongoing commitment to three factors: diet and nutrition, exercise, and environmental awareness (safeguarding against toxins and allergenic substances at home and work, including hidden allergies that can sap energy). By becoming familiar with these factors and following the guidelines below, you can improve your health and increase your resistance to disease.

Diet and Nutrition

Diet. The importance of proper diet in relationship to health was stressed as long as twenty-five hundred years ago, when Hippocrates, the father of Western medicine, proclaimed his famous dictum "Let thy food be thy medicine and thy medicine be thy food." In the twelfth century, famed physician Moses Maimonides echoed Hippocrates with the instruction "No illness which can be treated by diet should be treated by any other means." This emphasis on diet is known in holistic medicine as nutritional medicine (see Chapter 3). Unfortunately, today's conventional medical schools and universities offer little training in diet and nutrition. Consequently, many allopathic physicians, unless they have studied nutrition on their own, are incapable of recommending a diet and nutritional program that meets the specific needs of each patient. Fortunately, this trend is beginning to change, but simply recognizing the importance of diet is not enough. It is also necessary to know what types of foods to eat according to our unique biochemical needs. Despite the glut of books on the best-seller lists each year telling us otherwise, there is no such thing as an "ideal diet" that is suited to everyone. No matter how healthy a diet may be overall, invariably a certain percentage of people who try it will experience little or no benefit, while some people will actually become less healthy because of it. Before beginning a specific dietary regimen, there are two things you should do to ensure that it will work for you: determine your biochemical nutritional needs, and determine whether you are allergic to the foods you are eating.

As the research of Peter D'Adamo, N.D., author of *Eat Right for Your Type*, suggests, various genetic factors, including blood type, determine what kind of diet is optimally suited for each person. Matching one's diet to one's genetic heritage and body type is also the basis of the *dosha* system of Ayurvedic medicine, which states that there are three primary body types, *vata*, *pitta*, and *kapha*, and that for good health we should eat according to which dosha, or dosha combination, we belong to.

Knowing which type of diet you are suited for and following it can make a dramatic difference in your health. If you suspect your current diet is not serving you, seek out a physician trained in nutrition, or a certified clinical nutritionist. Naturopathic physicians and many chiropractors can also offer dietary and nutritional guidance, as can practitioners of Ayurvedic and traditional Chinese medicine. (See the relevant chapters in Part 2 for more information about these therapies.)

The concept of food allergy remains controversial among conventional physicians but is recognized by holistic practitioners as an important aspect of proper diet. Nor is the concept new. Hippocrates, for instance, discerned that milk could trigger hives and gastrointestinal upset. Despite the fact that food allergies are becoming increasingly common, they remain one of the most misdiagnosed conditions. Ironically, people who suffer from food allergies often crave the very foods that are harmful for them. People who are allergic to wheat, for example, will often have pasta or bread throughout the week and feel deprived if they don't. Common food allergens are milk and dairy products, wheat, corn, tomato products, peanuts, chocolate, and shellfish, as well as food additives, dyes, and preservatives. If you suspect you suffer from food allergies, consult a practitioner of environmental medicine (see Chapter 4).

The key to healthy eating can be summarized in two words: *whole foods*. Whole foods are unprocessed and unadulterated, and free of hydrogenated oils, sweeteners, additives, or preservatives. These include all fresh and organic fruits and vegetables; complex carbohydrates (such as whole grains, starchy vegetables, and legumes); seeds and nuts; free-range meats and poultry; fish; and dairy products such as milk, yogurt, and cheese (use sparingly and avoid altogether if you are lactose-intolerant). Healthy fats and oils should also be included as a dietary staple. Good food sources include olives, avocados, wheat germ, seeds, and nuts, while healthy oils include olive, safflower, sesame, sunflower, canola, wheat germ, and flaxseed (do not use for cooking). Fiber is another important component of a healthy diet. Besides fruits and vegetables, good sources of fiber include brown rice, whole wheat, and rolled oats.

All of the above food types provide an abundant supply of the necessary vitamins, minerals, amino acids, and essential fatty acids necessary for good health. Eating at least five to seven servings of fresh fruits and vegetables per day will also provide you with a rich source of enzymes, which help digestion and assimilation. You can easily accomplish this by making salads or steaming or sautéing a variety of vegetables, and by snacking on fruits between meals. Alkaline-rich fruits and vegetables also help to maintain the body's proper pH level, something that many researchers point to as playing a crucial role in resisting disease.

Also be sure to drink adequate amounts of filtered water throughout the day, rather than coffee, nonherbal tea, soda, and commercial fruit juices (which are usually laced with artificial sweeteners). Sufficient water intake is extremely important for good health, because water is the medium through which all bodily functions occur. Instead of the more common recommendation of eight 8-ounce glasses of water a day, many holistic physicians recommend that we drink half (healthy but sedentary individuals) to two-thirds (active individuals) of an ounce of water for every pound that we weigh. This means that a healthy, sedentary adult who weighs 160 pounds should drink about 80 ounces of water a day, while his more active counterpart should drink up to 112 ounces. People whose diets are already high in raw, fresh fruits and vegetables may need less water intake, however, since such foods are 85 to 90 percent water. Herbal teas and natural fruit juices that are free of sugar are also acceptable water substitutes.

In addition to the recommendations above, none of the following ingredients belong in a healthy, whole foods diet: sugar; salt; saturated (animal) fats and hydrogenated oils (found in margarine, cooking fats, packaged foods, commercial cereals, and many brands of peanut butter); and refined carbohydrates (white bread, biscuits, cakes, white rice, pastas made from white flour, and other processed foods). Caffeine and alcohol can also have a negative impact on your health and should be used only in moderation (200 mg or less of caffeine, and no more than one glass of wine or beer per day).

✿ FOOD COMBINING ✿

Many health practitioners recommend the principle of food combining in addition to a healthy whole foods diet, for optimal health. A number of books, such as *Fit for Life*, have been written on this subject, but the basic rules are as follows: Fruits are best eaten alone away from meals. Proteins and carbohydrates should not be combined, because the body can only digest them one at a time, not together. (This eliminates not only a meal of steak and potatoes, but also a tuna fish sandwich.) Proteins and nonstarchy vegetables are fine together, as are carbohydrates and vegetables. And water should be consumed at least twenty minutes before eating, especially before protein meals, to avoid diluting the digestive juices necessary for the proper breakdown of food. Adherents of food combining also advocate that each mouthful of food be thoroughly chewed before it is swallowed, making it far easier to digest. Although much skepticism surrounds the theory of food combining, even among holistic practitioners, many people report improved health and the disappearance of disease symptoms after adopting such a program. ✿

The quality of the foods you eat determines the quality of the "fuel" available to your body as it performs its countless functions. A healthy diet can dramatically increase your energy level over time and is the primary preventive measure you can take to safeguard against disease. On the other hand, it is not necessary to become a fanatic about the foods you eat. For most people who are already in a reasonably good state of health, eating healthy 80 percent of the time, while satisfying a sweet tooth or craving for pizza the other 20 percent, is a good rule of thumb. If you are not used to eating whole foods, you may experience initial symptoms of headache, fatigue, and increased trips to the bathroom as you transition to a healthier diet. Such symptoms are simply signs that your body is finally feeling well enough to throw off toxins long stored in your tissues. Usually, they will pass within a few days as your improved eating habits start to take hold. If they persist or become too uncomfortable, it may mean that you are trying to do too much too soon. Increased water intake can often help during this time by flushing toxins out of the bloodstream. Be sure to get adequate rest as well.

Nutritional Supplementation. The stress of daily life, environmental pollution, and the diminished trace mineral content in the soil in which our foods are grown mean that for most people a healthy diet alone is not enough to ensure health. For this reason, holistic physicians recommend nutritional supplements as part of a daily health regimen. Once again, individual body chemistry plays a role in determining the proper dosages.

Every person requires the same nutrients for proper physiological functioning, but the amount of each nutrient needed by each of us varies greatly, because of differences in our genetic predispositions, stress levels, the environments in which we live and work, and lifestyles (active or sedentary). People who smoke, drink alcohol, or suffer from illness or allergies all have greater nutritional needs, as do pregnant women. To get the best results from nutritional supplementation, you should consult with a nutritionally oriented health practitioner. In the meantime, the list below, created by Drs. Robert Ivker and Robert Anderson, provides a suggested dosage range for the most common antioxidant vitamins and minerals that most people can use as part of their daily routine for maintaining their health.

Vitamin C (as polyascorbate)—1,000 to 2,000 mg 3 times per day
Beta-carotene—25,000 IU 1 to 2 times per day
Vitamin E—400 IU 1 to 2 times per day
B-complex vitamins-—50 to 100 mg of each B vitamin per day

Folic acid—400 to 800 mcg per day
Selenium—100 to 200 mcg per day
Zinc picolinate—20 to 40 mg per day
Calcium citrate or apatite—1,000 mg per day
Magnesium citrate or aspartate—500 mg per day
Chromium polynicotinate (ChromeMate[R])—200 mcg per day
Manganese—10 to 15 mg per day
Copper—2 mg per day
Iron—10 to 18 mg per day.

"People who are exposed to higher levels of stress and increased exposure to pollutants, or who are not feeling well or experiencing diminished sleep, should use the higher doses," Dr. Ivker advises. "Otherwise, take at least the minimum dose of each nutrient every day, preferably with your meals." A number of formulas on the market contain all of these ingredients, making it easier to adopt such a program. Dr. Ivker also recommends that people take one or two tablespoons of flaxseed oil daily, either on salads or mixed with an equal amount of low-fat cottage cheese, in order to receive a good supply of essential fatty acids, particularly omega-3 fatty acids.

Exercise

According to Dr. Ivker, regular exercise can contribute more to optimal physical health than any other factor, with the possible exception of diet. Adopting an exercise program at least three times a week can improve your energy level, aid in digestion, increase circulation, promote restful sleep, decrease stress, increase self-esteem, raise HDL (good) cholesterol levels, increase longevity, enhance mental function, and decrease depression and anxiety. "Ideally, an exercise program should incorporate a mix of activities that increase your aerobic capacity, while at the same time enhancing strength and flexibility," Dr. Ivker says. "A routine geared solely towards strength conditioning, for instance, does little to increase aerobic capacity and can even diminish flexibility, so it's a good idea to add a stretching routine and an aerobic workout on alternate days to get the full benefits of an effective exercise practice."

Aerobic Exercise. Aerobic exercise refers to any form of exercise that requires increased oxygen intake in order to supply energy to the muscles via the mechanism of fat and carbohydrate metabolism. Such exercise over time produces many benefits to the cardiovascular system and delivers oxygen throughout the body, resulting in greater cardiac efficiency, lower blood pressure, and a slower heart rate, along with an overall feeling of well-being.

There are a variety of aerobic exercises to choose from. Among them are hiking, swimming, bicycling, and jumping rope. Jogging is another popular form of aerobic exercise, although care should be taken to stretch before and after you jog, to wear good running shoes to support your arches and ankles, and to avoid the heavy impact of hard surfaces. Many sports also provide a good aerobic workout, such as racquetball, handball, basketball, and tennis. You can also try treadmills, rowing machines, or the StairMaster.

An increasingly popular aerobic exercise among health enthusiasts is rebounding, which can be performed at home on a mini-trampoline (available at most sports stores). Rebounding takes only fifteen to twenty minutes a day, and as little as ten minutes of vigorous rebounding has been shown to offer the same benefits as an hour of jogging, without the accompanying joint and ligament strain. Rebounding is also considered the best single form of exercise for keeping the lymphatic system healthy, which in turn boosts immune function.

Far and away the safest and easiest form of aerobic exercise is brisk walking. Walking two miles at a brisk pace burns almost as many calories as jogging, as well as offering other similar health benefits. Swinging your arms when you walk will burn up to an additional 10 percent more calories and can also provide an upper-body workout.

The key to any successful aerobic routine is to follow it consistently, which is easier to do if you select an activity that you enjoy. If you are not in the habit of exercising, consult your physician before beginning. You might also want to seek instruction from an aerobics instructor, who can help you determine and maintain you target heart rate (60 to 85 percent of your age subtracted from 220). If possible, exercise outdoors when convenient, since fresh air and sunshine provide greater health benefits than a workout indoors. Also make sure that you exercise at least half an hour before meals, or two and a half hours after you eat, to avoid indigestion. Be careful about beginning any aerobic activity in the midst of an emotional crisis, especially one involving feelings of anger, as doing so can trigger a heart attack.

Strength Conditioning. There are three types of strength conditioning: calisthenics, strength conditioning with aids, and strength conditioning in combination with aerobics. Calisthenics include sit-ups, push-ups, jumping jacks, and swimming. Strength conditioning with aids involves working out with free weights and weight machines, while strength conditioning in combination with aerobics refers to various forms of interval training, which can be accomplished through running, bicycling, or jumping rope.

The most popular form of strength conditioning in America is weight training. If you have never trained with weights before, it is advisable to consult with a trainer, who can help design a weight training program tailored to your needs and abilities. A typical routine is to use weights two or three times a week, alternating with aerobics and stretching exercises.

Building and maintaining muscle strength is an essential part of good overall physical health, and strength conditioning is an excellent way of doing so. It isn't necessary to lift a lot of weight to get results, however. In fact, to tone muscle you will get better results using less weight and performing more repetitions. But if you want to bulk up, you will need to increase the amount of weight you use and do fewer reps. Wear a weight belt during weight training to keep the spine aligned, and exhale as you exert effort. Working with a spotter when using free weights is also advisable, in order to avoid injury.

Flexibility Exercises. Maintaining a limber, flexible body is another essential component of optimal physical health. Flexibility enhances overall physical performance by allowing the various muscle groups to operate at peak efficiency, maintains good posture, and decreases the chance of injury. Improved circulation and increased tendon and ligament health are other benefits of having muscles that are strong and flexible.

The most common way to promote flexibility is to stretch. Stretching exercises are best performed before and after other types of exercise, after five minutes or more of movement, which improves circulation and makes stretching easier. As you stretch, you should feel tension in the muscle or muscle group you are stretching, but not to the point of pain. Breathe into the stretch as you perform it. This both elongates the muscle further and relaxes it, enabling you to hold the stretch for thirty seconds. Repeat each stretch two or more times, which will increase your range. Over time, a few minutes of daily stretching will result in a noticeable improvement in how you feel.

Yoga is another popular form of stretching, which both improves flexibility and increases muscle strength. Proper breathing is essential to all forms of yoga and, in addition to enhancing flexibility, also results in improved concentration and mental and emotional well-being. There are many forms of yoga, with *hatha yoga* being the most popular form in the West. Yoga is increasingly being recognized by researchers as an optimum form of overall exercise, since it combines aerobics and strength conditioning with stretching to provide a total body workout. Ideally, it is best to spend a few months receiving instruction from a qualified yoga teacher in order to learn the proper way to perform each yoga pose, or *asana*. Yoga is discussed in greater detail in Chapter 14.

A variety of bodywork techniques, such as Rolfing and the Feldenkrais Method, also promote increased flexibility and greater body awareness and physiological function. These are described in Chapter 9.

🌿 GET ENOUGH SLEEP 🌿

According to Joseph Pizzorno, N.D., a leading holistic physician and founding president of Bastyr University, one of the most important aspects of ensuring optimal health is adequate sleep. "It's while we are sleeping that the body's regenerative processes are at work," Dr. Pizzorno explains. "But in our society today, adequate sleep is becoming lost. We are averaging almost two hours less sleep a night than we got one hundred years ago. And even when we are getting the sleep, we aren't sleeping as deeply. We're sleeping later at night and bypassing the normal circadian rhythm that's created by nature."

Dr. Pizzorno's claims are borne out by the fact that 60 million Americans suffer from insomnia. Lack of sleep results in depressed immune function, increased susceptibility to disease, stress, diminished mental acuity, depression and anxiety, poor job performance, and increased risk of accidents. While commonly prescribed sleeping pills can provide benefit in cases of insomnia and other sleep problems, they can also be fraught with side effects and possibly lead to dependency. A more holistic approach to promoting proper sleep is to establish a regular bedtime each night in order to reattune yourself to nature's circadian rhythms, which research shows has a definite counterpart in the human body, both neurologically and within the endocrine system. To improve your sleeping habits, consider retiring no later than 10 P.M. and establishing an early wake-up time of 6 to 7 A.M. every day, regardless of when you go to bed. If additional help is needed, consult with a holistic physician, who can help you determine and alleviate whatever other factors may be interfering with your ability to get a good night's rest. 🌿

Environmental Awareness

Living in an environment free of environmental toxins and pollutants, breathing good-quality air, and drinking pure, clean water are essential for good health. Unfortunately, these essentials are becoming scarce commodities in today's world. A variety of self-care measures are available that you can employ preventively and therapeutically to protect yourself from harmful chemicals and pollutants.

According to Dr. Ivker, an internationally recognized specialist in the holistic treatment of respiratory conditions, one of the most important aspects of environmental health is clean, fresh air. "Sixty percent of all Americans live in areas where the air quality is unhealthy, according to EPA standards," he points out. "In addition, many new, air-conditioned buildings suffer from 'sick building syndrome,' and are breeding grounds for airborne bacteria and fungi." To counteract such factors, Dr. Ivker recommends supplementing with antioxidants, following a healthy, whole foods diet, and drinking plenty of pure, filtered water to flush out toxins in your system. "It's also helpful to create a setting of indoor plants in your home and at work," he says. "Plants oxygenate the air, create more moisture, which makes for healthier breathing, and some plants also filter out carbon monoxide and organic chemicals. Plus, they add beauty and can increase feelings of well-being." More important, Dr. Ivker also recommends using a humidifier and especially a negative ion generator, which functions as an efficient air cleaner.

Using natural products that emit no pollutants is another important step anyone can take to reduce indoor environmental pollution. Such products include wood, cotton, and metals, as opposed to synthetic particle board, plastics, and polyester. Other environmental self-care measures include avoiding secondhand smoke (if you smoke, get help to quit), using efficient furnace filters at home, reducing the use of coal- and wood-burning fireplaces and stoves, replacing commercial cleaning agents with nontoxic products (available in most health food stores), regularly cleaning carpets and rugs to prevent mold and bacteria build-up, keeping the bedroom window open during sleep to ensure a stream of fresh air, maintaining proper ventilation at home and at work, taking regular breaks away from your computer, and spending regular periods of time outdoors in a natural, unpolluted setting.

MIND

Holistic physicians view mental health as a condition of peace of mind, contentment, and positive beliefs and attitudes. These mental and emotional aspects are interrelated and fall under the province of mind-body medicine (see Chapter 5). While competent professional care may be required for people suffering from depression, bipolar disorder (manic depression), or chronic, unresolved grief, sorrow, or anger, a number of self-care measures are available for creating a more positive mental and emotional outlook. Among them are affirmations, breathwork, journaling, and conscious laughter. Working with one or more of these methods will help you become more aware of your thoughts, emotions, and beliefs in a way that will enhance your ability to meet your personal and professional goals, and experience improved levels of energy and greater well-being.

Affirmations

Most people's predominant beliefs are handed down to them as children by their parents, teachers, and other influential adults. The thoughts and ideas they heard expressed helped to shape their own world view, and for the most part remained with them as they grew into adulthood. Usually this process occurs unconsciously, and often with limiting consequences during adulthood, if the beliefs remain unexamined. By becoming conscious of our beliefs, we gain the power to change or eliminate those that no longer serve us, replacing them with those that do. Working with affirmations is one way of accomplishing this.

Affirmations are positive messages that you repeat to yourself either verbally or in writing in order to produce a specific outcome. Over time, they affect the unconscious by "reprogramming" it with the thought patterns you consciously select to influence your behavior. In the process, they can unleash and stimulate healing energies in all areas of your life.

The greatest challenge in working with affirmations is to suspend judgment long enough to allow them to produce the results you desire. In addition, it helps to feel your affirmations as you recite or write them, since this brings more energy to the experience. Make the process as vivid and real as possible.

The following guidelines are recommended for anyone interested in beginning an affirmation program:

1. Always state your affirmation in the present tense and keep it positive.
2. Keep your affirmations short and simple, no longer than two brief sentences.
3. Write or verbalize each affirmation ten to twenty times each day.
4. Whenever you find yourself thinking or hearing a habitual negative message, counteract it by focusing on your affirmation.
5. Schedule a regular time each day to do your affirmations to add momentum to what you are trying to achieve until it becomes a positive, effortless habit.
6. Repeat your affirmations in the first, second, and third person, using your name in each variation. First-person affirmations address any mental conditioning you have given yourself, while affirmations in the second and third person help to release the conditioning you may have accepted from others. In each case, write out or repeat the affirmation ten times.
7. Make a commitment to practice your affirmations for at least sixty days or well beyond the time you begin experiencing the results you desire.
8. Visualize your affirmations by closing your eyes and imagining what the affirmation looks and feels like as you say or write it. Try to engage as many of your senses as possible.

An additional affirmation technique, developed by Leonard Orr, the founder of Rebirthing (see following page) makes use of a "response column." According to Orr, who has worked with affirmations for over four decades, this technique will help you become more aware of unconscious limiting thoughts and beliefs. The exercise is performed as follows: Draw a line down the middle of a piece of paper. On the left-hand column, write out the affirmation you are working with. On the right-hand column, immediately write the response that occurs to you without judging it. For example, if you desire more energy, your affirmation might be "I have abundant energy throughout the day," while your initial response might be "It's all I can do to get out of bed in the morning!" Note your response, then write your affirmation again, followed by your next response. Do this at least ten times, twice a day, until your response becomes neutral or you truly feel in agreement with your affirmation. In this way, over time, you will be dredging up and releasing the various limiting, negative beliefs you've unconsciously been holding on to, and replacing them with thoughts and images that better serve you.

Breathwork

We can live for weeks without food, and days without water, but if we stop breathing for more than a few minutes, we die. Yet most people breathe inefficiently and unconsciously, breathing shallowly through the chest and depriving themselves of the many benefits proper breathing can provide. These benefits are not only physical. Proper breathing also relieves stress, enhances feelings of well-being, and promotes clearer thinking. According to Leonard Orr, who has taught Rebirthing to thousands of people for the last four decades, learning to breathe fully and consciously can also heal the parts of ourselves that are wounded, rejected, or disowned, restoring them to wholeness.

Rebirthing, or "conscious connected breathing," is perhaps the most popular form of modern breathwork techniques, all of which focus on breathing in a manner that moves energy through the body and connects you with suppressed emotions and limiting beliefs in order to heal them. Most forms of breathwork employ connected breathing, meaning that each inhalation and exhalation is connected and occurs without pausing, unlike unconscious breathing, in which there is typically a gap between the inhale and the exhale. The rate of respiration varies; sometimes it is rapid; sometimes it is deep, slow, and full. Because of the emotional release that can result from such techniques, it is advisable to learn them under the direction of a skilled breath therapist. The following exercise, however, can be safely performed by anyone to relieve stress and increase energy.

Sit straight and in a relaxed manner, placing your palms on your chest and belly. Now breathe as you normally do. Most likely when you inhaled your hand covering your chest moved, while your other hand did not. In this exercise, you are going to reverse this pattern by breathing in through your stomach area. Keeping your hands in the same position, inhale once more, this time directing your breath in and out through your belly. Don't strain, and remember to breathe fully, without pausing between the inhale and exhale. At first, this exercise may feel odd and even difficult, but with practice it will become easier. The goal is to breathe freely and deeply only through the belly, so that your chest does not rise. (Keeping your hands in position will help you monitor your progress.)

Breathing in this manner on a regular basis is a very effective way to relieve stress, improve energy, curtail anxiety and depression, and enhance digestion. Try to breathe in this manner for at least twenty minutes each day, and whenever you feel tired, tense, or irritable.

THE RELATIONSHIP BETWEEN
❦ TOUCH AND MENTAL HEALTH ❦

For centuries touch has been an essential component of many healing traditions, including the biblical practice of "laying on of hands." Touch is also one of the most powerful means of conveying and receiving love. The United States, however, in comparison to other parts of the world, is, in Dr. Ivker's words, a "touch-averse" society. "In order to be optimally healthy," he recommends, "we need to consciously make touch a more frequent occurrence in our lives, recognizing that touch is a gift we can give ourselves and each other every day."

Two of the easiest ways of learning how to accept touch are *self-touch* and *hugging*. Self-touch can be as simple as giving yourself a foot massage or kneading your shoulders. Focus on what you are doing and be attentive. Self-touch can also promote calm and help you become centered during times of stress. Gently cradling your face in your hands for a few minutes with your eyes closed, for example, can restore your energy after time spent sitting at a desk or computer.

Hugging and being hugged is another simple, yet powerful way of relieving stress and enhancing well-being. "To truly benefit from giving and receiving a hug, it pays to be more conscious," Dr. Ivker says, pointing out that many people are uncomfortable with physical closeness and unconsciously pull away from a hug before it is completed. "Make a practice of giving and receiving several hugs each day with your family and friends," he advises. "Holding hands or a friendly pat on the back are also ways to give and receive the benefits of touch. Petting and holding household pets can bring similar benefits, as well." ❦

Journaling

Also known as "expressive writing," journaling is an easy yet powerful way to keep track of your personal experiences, while also allowing you to develop new insights and solutions to your problems, discover unconscious beliefs that may be limiting your growth, and appreciate all for which you currently feel grateful. People who make a daily habit of writing entries in their journals report a deeper understanding of themselves and often become better able to achieve their goals, including health. For many people, journaling becomes a productive form of therapy that can lead to a new understanding of how and why they act the way they do. In the process, they often become more aware of their beliefs and discover how to change those that don't serve them. Journaling is also valuable for people who have difficulty expressing their emotions. In their journals they have the opportunity to write out and resolve what they are feeling, without having to worry about others judging them.

The most common form of journaling is keeping a diary. What follow are three other forms of journaling you can use to create more vitality and personal satisfaction in your life.

The Gratitude Journal. This type of journaling is best performed at the end of the day, prior to going to bed. Its purpose is to help you better appreciate all that you have to be grateful for each and every day of your life. No matter how unfortunate you may feel at any given time, if you honestly examine your life you can always find reasons to be grateful, even when you are sick. By focusing on these positive factors, you can stimulate your immune system to operate more efficiently.

To keep a gratitude journal, write down each night all the events of the day that caused you to feel happy, even those you may not have noticed when they happened. Don't rush this exercise. Take time to really examine your day and make a list of all the people and events that made you happy, allowing yourself to reexperience that happiness as you write about it. Over time, this exercise can substantially improve your mood, self-esteem, and confidence levels, boosting your physical well-being in the process.

The Stream-of-Conciousness Morning Journal. This method of journaling was popularized by Julia Cameron, author of *The Artist's Way.* She suggests that upon arising each morning, you fill up three pages of paper, writing down whatever thoughts come into your head. Don't edit yourself, just write all the thoughts that occur to you. Cameron and other advocates of this method claim that this exercise helps people rid themselves of "mental debris," allowing them to become better able to focus on, and accomplish, their goals during the rest of the day.

A variation of this technique is to write for fifteen minutes and then read over what you wrote, underlining any thoughts that you find negative. Then rewrite each of them as a positive affirmation (see "Affirmations" earlier in this chapter). For example, if you wrote, "I'm feeling tired and I wish I didn't have to get up and go to work," your rewrite might read, "I am naturally energetic and enjoy my job." Do this for each sentence you underlined. At first, you may feel resistance during this process, yet over time you will discover how performing it helps you create the reality you prefer for yourself.

The Illness Dialogue. Illness often has a mental or emotional component that isn't readily apparent. This form of journaling helps to uncover the "hidden" meaning or message of your illness so that you can better understand the causes behind your symptoms. Often, once these psychological causes are understood and accepted, the illness itself also resolves.

Perform this exercise by asking yourself the following question: "If this illness (or pain) could speak, what would it say?" Then write down the first impression that comes to you. Once again, don't edit yourself. Write down whatever occurs to you, even if it seems ludicrous or upsetting. Then read your response and ask yourself the first question that presents itself. Then write down your next response. Repeat the process until no further questions occur to you or until you feel that you have the answer that can help you. Most likely you will need to repeat this exercise for a few days or more before your questions are resolved, but the rewards of doing so can be well worth it.

Conscious Laughter

Modern science is now beginning to validate the adage "Laughter is the best medicine." One of the most famous examples illustrating this point is that of Norman Cousins, who wrote of recovering from a potentially crippling arthritic condition after spending hours watching Marx Brothers movies and reruns of *Candid Camera* while taking megadoses of vitamin C. Laughing regularly caused his pain to diminish, until eventually his illness disappeared altogether. More recently, the work of Patch Adams, M.D., founder of the Gesundheit Institute in Arlington, Virginia, has spurred increased interest in laughter's therapeutic effects.

Hearty laughter offers many of the same benefits as gentle exercise. Laughing exercises the facial muscles, shoulders, diaphragm, and abdomen. Laughter also decreases anxiety and stress and can improve our outlook on life, which is very useful when we get sick. Research shows that laughter may also boost endorphin levels, increase circulation, and enhance immune activity.

All of us laugh at certain times throughout each day, but we can increase laughter's benefits by consciously choosing to laugh more often. Doing so requires commitment and a willingness to cultivate a sense of optimism and humor, however. Like any skill, learning to become a conscious laugher takes practice, but when you find yourself laughing throughout the day, you can be sure that you are becoming healthier in every area of your life.

SPIRIT

Spiritual health, while often the most overlooked aspect of healing, is actually the ultimate goal of holistic medicine and leads to a heightened awareness of the Divine Spirit referred to by all religions. "It isn't important what name you give it," Dr. Ivker points out. "What matters is that you come to know and attune yourself to its guidance in all areas of your daily life. Doing so will reduce your feelings of fear and provide you with a greater capacity for loving yourself and others unconditionally. It will also help you reconnect to your special talents and gifts and use them to fulfill your life's purpose."

In addition to being aware of the role Spirit plays in your life, being spiritually healthy also means being intimately connected to your spouse or partner, family, friends, and community, resulting in social health, as well. "Spiritual and social health are interconnected, since it is through our committed relationships that we find the greatest opportunities for spiritual growth and for learning how to receive and impart unconditional love," Dr. Ivker says.

In addition to the observance of spiritual and religious traditions, working with spiritual counselors and participating in support groups are common methods of creating spiritual and social health, as are the opportunities afforded us through our friendships, marriage, intimate relationships, and parenting. A variety of self-care approaches, including prayer, meditation, gratitude, and spending time within nature, can further deepen your awareness of yourself as a spiritual, socially connected being, and are increasingly being recommended by conventional and holistic physicians alike.

Prayer

Prayer is the most common form of spiritual practice performed by most Americans, and the majority of people who pray report a greater sense of well-being than those who don't. Harvard researcher and mind-body medicine expert Herbert Benson, M.D., author of *The Relaxation Response*, has found that regular prayer or the repetition of spiritual phrases such as "Shalom" or "Hail Mary" triggers relaxation and reduces stress.

There are many effective ways to pray, both for yourself and for others. Many people find great benefit using the prayers from their religious upbringing. Others make prayer a time of personal conversation with God, stating their need or concern and asking for divine intervention. Others find taking a mindful walk in a place of natural beauty to be a form of prayerful worship. Simply taking the time to acknowledge all you have to be grateful for and giving thanks can be effective as well. Choose the form of prayer that feels most comfortable for you, then establish a regular routine of repeating your prayers daily.

Meditation

Meditation has been scientifically researched for decades and has been proven to have physiological benefits. Besides its physical benefits, which include stress relief, improved immune and cardiovascular function, relaxation, and decreased pain, the regular practice of meditation can lead to new insights about life issues (often resulting in the healing of past emotional trauma), heightened creativity, inspiration, greater compassion for others, and a stronger connection to one's own inner guidance.

There are a wide variety of meditative techniques to choose from and, as with prayer, choosing the one that you are most comfortable with will provide the greatest benefit. Meditation can be performed while sitting, lying down, or while walking or jogging. Some people also prefer singing or chanting a word or phrase that has spiritual significance to them. What all meditative techniques have in common is conscious breathing (see "Breathwork" earlier in this chapter) and a focus on what is happening in each present moment, until the mind becomes empty of thoughts, judgments, and past and future concerns.

A simple way to meditate is to sit comfortably erect with your eyes closed, while paying attention to your breathing. Observe yourself inhaling and exhaling, allowing whatever thoughts you have to pass you by. In the beginning of your practice, you will find your mind wandering. Each time this occurs, gently refocus on your breath. To improve your concentration, you can also silently repeat a word, or mantra, such as love, peace, or Jesus. Eventually, you will experience longer periods of silence between each thought, although it may take months before this occurs. Be patient and don't force matters. Try to sit for ten to twenty minutes once or twice a day, but if you find yourself too distracted or pressed for time, end your session, instead of sitting restlessly. With commitment and consistent practice, the benefits of meditation will become apparent to you.

Gratitude

Dr. Robert Anderson describes gratitude as the Great Attitude. "Gratitude produces feelings of joy and self-acceptance, and is an attitude that anyone can choose to have, just as we can choose to see the glass half full or half empty," Dr. Anderson says. "Being grateful for what you have, instead of worrying about what you lack, enables you to let go of negative thoughts and attitudes more easily. This can be difficult at times, especially if you are feeling a great deal of fear or anger, but if you make the effort to release these painful emotions and choose to be grateful, instead, positive benefits can be achieved."

One method of cultivating feelings of gratitude is keeping a gratitude journal. A variation of this technique is to close your eyes before bed and mentally review your day, taking an inventory of all the things that happened for which you feel grateful, silently giving thanks for them. "By making gratitude a regular part of your daily experience, you set the stage for living more deeply connected to spirit," Dr. Anderson says. "In the process, your life will be transformed into an increasingly joyous adventure."

Spending Time in Nature

The most visible manifestation of spirit is nature, where we most fully encounter and interact with life's primal energies in the form of earth, water, fire, and air. Taking a walk in a park or hiking through the woods is an easy and practical way of reconnecting with nature, as are gardening, bike riding in the country, and camping and boating trips. By making it a habit to spend regular amounts of time outdoors within a natural setting, you enable yourself to better appreciate the rhythms of life, including your own. As Dr. Ivker points out, "We need to recognize that cities and other industrialized areas can prevent us from living a life of balance. Spending time in nature helps restore that balance, while also deepening our connection with Spirit."

Spending time near the water can also be a spiritually healthy experience, due to water's higher concentration of negative ions, which can contribute to feelings of well-being. Swimming in the ocean, lakes, or rivers is a great way to benefit from this life-enhancing energy. Soaking in a mineral hot spring can provide therapeutic benefits for a variety of ailments, as well.

Exposure to fire around a campground or before a fireplace can also have health benefits, according to Leonard Orr, who has found that fire cleanses the bioenergy field of negative energies and can be a powerful aid in curing physical disease. Orr recommends spending a few hours each day before fire for people who want to experience such benefits. Fire is also an important component of the vision quests undertaken by Native Americans to connect with the Great Spirit and discover their life purpose.

Of all nature's elements, perhaps the closest expression of Spirit is the air. Clean, fresh air is essential to health on all levels, and practicing conscious breathing as outlined above is a potent self-care method for restoring energy and making you more aware of the power of Spirit as it flows through you.

Regular exposure to each of these four elements can help you become more conscious of how Spirit's loving intelligence sustains the world, while more deeply recognizing your place within it.

All of the principles and practices outlined above can lead to a significant improvement in your physical, mental and spiritual well-being once you make them part of your regular health routine. Rather than try to adopt them all at once, it is best if you choose one or two areas to work on until you feel comfortable enough to incorporate more. Doing so will help you create momentum and lessen the likelihood of failure and discouragement. At times, however, self-care alone will not be enough to meet the challenges of disease or other life challenges. During such times, the services of a skilled health practitioner should be sought. Within the field of holistic medicine a variety of therapies are available to assist you on your healing journey. In Part Two, we will examine the most common of them and explore how and why they work.

The Major Therapies
of Holistic Medicine

CHAPTER 3

Nutritional Medicine

Nutritional medicine is a cornerstone of holistic medicine. It involves the use of a diet of healthy foods matched to patients' biochemical individuality, along with the judicious use of nutrient supplements to help maintain optimal physical and psychological health. Holistic physicians have long emphasized the importance of healthy eating and nutritional supplementation in relationship to overall health, and addressing their patients' dietary and nutrient status plays an integral part in their treatment of disease, both preventively and therapeutically. The importance of proper diet and overall nutrition is often overlooked by conventional physicians, however, who receive very little education about nutrition during their medical training. "The principle that what you eat has a major influence on your health is so simple and logical that it is surprising that the medical profession has had such a difficult time grasping it," says Alan Gaby, M.D., past president of the American Holistic Medical Association and a leading authority on nutritional medicine. "Unfortunately today, the average doctor, despite having taken the Hippocratic oath, still rejects Hippocrates' famous dictum 'Let your food be your medicine and let your medicine be your food,' even though research continues to show that degenerative diseases are caused, at least in part, by our modern diet."

Like all holistic physicians, Dr. Gaby routinely advises his patients to adopt a healthier diet, regardless of their medical complaints. He instructs his patients to avoid "junk foods" and to increase their consumption of whole grains, fresh fruits and vegetables, nuts, seeds, beans, and other unprocessed foods. "The majority of my patients who follow this advice find that their health improves in some way," Dr. Gaby reports. "They experience increased energy, improved sleep, better bowel and bladder function, and find they are more alert and productive. They also suffer from fewer headaches, anxiety, depression, and fluid retention, and find that their joints don't hurt as much. In many cases, this is confirmed by laboratory tests, which show improvement in such areas as their serum cholesterol, triglycerides, liver enzymes, and uric acid levels."

While a shift to a healthier diet can improve health in and of itself, in many cases nutritional supplementation is also needed, due to a variety of factors, such as environmental pollutants, the stresses of daily life, and modern farming and food packaging methods that further deplete the nutrient content of our foods. Holistic physicians focus on both improving their patients' diets and devising a nutritional supplementation program to meet their specific nutrient needs, as determined by a variety of testing methods. The primary supplements used by holistic physicians are vitamins, minerals, amino acids, and essential fatty acids.

❦ FAST FACTS ❦

An estimated 80 percent of all Americans are said to be suffering from some form of malnutrition (nutrient deficiencies).

Poor diet and nutrient deficiencies have been linked to a wide variety of chronic disease conditions, including heart disease and cancer, our nation's two most prevalent killers. Conversely, healthy eating habits have been shown to prevent or help reverse most diseases of a chronic nature. Sixty percent of all cancers, for instance, can be prevented by good diet and proper nutrition.

High-fiber diets have been found to significantly reduce the risk of certain cancers (especially of the colon and rectum), coronary heart disease, and hypertension; lower cholesterol and triglyceride levels; help stabilize diabetes; and minimize the incidence of hemorrhoids, ulcerative colitis, gallbladder disease, and diverticulitis. Yet the average American diet supplies only 25 to 33 percent of the amount of fiber necessary for optimum health.

Excessive weight can contribute to many forms of illness, including adult-onset diabetes, yet as a nation we are continuing to grow fatter. Currently, 22 percent of all Americans are obese, and over 30 percent are overweight, due in large part to poor eating habits and lack of exercise.

Included as part of the standard American diet are six substances known to pose health risks: sugar, salt, refined carbohydrates, unhealthy fats, and excessive amounts of caffeine and alcohol. The average American eats 150 pounds of sugar each year, or the equivalent of over 40 teaspoons a day, and daily drinks a minimum of two and a half cups of coffee.

Most Americans are also unknowingly chronically dehydrated, due to their failure to consume enough pure water each day, relying instead on coffee, soda, and commercially prepared, nutritionally lacking, juices and teas.

The mineral content of soil used to grow today's crops is on average one-sixth of what it was fifty years ago, due to commercial farming methods, resulting in devitalized produce. Additional commercial farm production methods, along with shipping and storage procedures, further deprive crops of their nutrient value.

An estimated 50 million Americans are lactose-intolerant (sensitive or allergic to dairy products), many of them unknowingly.

Due to biochemical individuality, the amounts of specific nutrients required for health can vary as much as 700 percent from person to person. 🌿

HISTORY OF NUTRITIONAL MEDICINE

The relationship between diet and optimal health has been understood by healers throughout recorded history. Although it is well known that Hippocrates regarded food as a primary form of medicine 2,500 years ago, his teachings on the subject were predated by the ancient Egyptians millennia earlier. Perhaps the oldest known evidence of man's understanding of proper diet are Egyptian pictographs from approximately 5000 B.C. which clearly point out the link between food and health. Egyptian papyrus records from 1500 B.C. also show that the Egyptians employed specific foods to treat assorted disease conditions. Diet has also been an integral element of Ayurvedic and traditional Chinese medicine (see Chapters 12 and 13) since their inception thousands of years ago.

Following Hippocrates, dietary recommendations continued to be made throughout subsequent centuries by such healers as Galen, Maimonides, and Paracelsus, but true scientific understanding of diet did not occur until the eighteenth century, beginning with the work of French physicist René de Reaumur, who is credited with conducting the initial research on digestive chemistry. Later in that same century, the chemist

Antoine Laurent Lavoisier built upon Reaumur's work and, prior to being guillotined during the French Revolution, provided the scientific foundation for the study of how the body metabolizes food to create energy. The first person to show a direct link between disease and the lack of a specific nutrient, however, was James Lind, a physician in the British navy, who discovered that sailors on long voyages without rations containing citrus fruits developed bleeding gums, rough skin, poor muscle tension, and slow-healing wounds, all symptoms characteristic of scurvy. In 1757, in one of the first controlled medical experiments, Lind demonstrated that when sailors were supplied with lemons, limes, and oranges, scurvy could be prevented. As a result of his findings, Captain James Cook made it mandatory for every English sailor to be supplied with rations of lemons and limes, enabling them to sail around the world scurvy-free, as well as supplying them with the nickname limeys. Today, it is well known that scurvy is caused by vitamin C deficiency.

Throughout the nineteenth century, naturopathic physicians (see Chapter 10) also began their use of dietary therapy, along with fasting methods, to cleanse the body and stimulate its ability to heal. During the same century, further scientific discoveries established a link between other nutrients and various illnesses. In 1838, for instance, the Swedish chemist Baron Jons Jakob Berzelius discovered the link between iron and hemoglobin production, leading to the use of iron-rich foods to treat anemia. In 1897, Dutch physician Christiaan Eijkman proved that an element in unpolished rice was essential to proper functioning of the nervous system and carbohydrate metabolism, and that a deficiency in that ingredient could cause beriberi and other diseases. In 1929, his research resulted in his sharing the Nobel Prize for physiology or medicine with British biochemist Sir Frederick Gowland Hopkins.

The beginning of the twentieth century heralded a new understanding of nutrition, beginning with Hopkins's work, which was pivotal in determining that nutritional factors besides proteins, carbohydrates, lipids (fats), and sodium were required in order to sustain life. Hopkins's research pioneered the study of vitamins and later resulted in his discovery of the amino acid L-tryptophane and the essential role it played in various life processes. It was Polish-American biochemist Casimir Funk who actually named the nutritional factors Hopkins was researching, by coining the term *vitamine*, which was later changed to the more familiar *vitamin*. In 1911, building on Eijkman's research, Funk isolated the pure chemical from yeast and rice polishings that later became known as vitamin B_1, or thiamine, and his research an other food factors contributed to modern science's better understanding of vitamin deficiency.

In 1913, American biochemist Elmer McCollum discovered the first vitamin, which was designated vitamin A precisely for that reason. Another important twentieth-century nutritional researcher was the Hungarian-American biochemist Albert von Szent-Gyorgi, who was awarded the Nobel Prize for physiology or medicine in 1937 for his discovery of vitamin C and his research into its role as a catalyst in cellular oxidation.

By the mid-1900s, researchers had isolated and identified more than forty nutrients essential to health, and in 1940 the Food and Nutrition Board of the National Research Council of the National Academy of Sciences established Recommended Daily Allowances (RDAs) for many of them. (RDAs are now referred to as Reference Daily Intakes, or RDIs.) As a result of such research, scientists and physicians alike gained a new understanding of how diet affects biochemistry, and by the 1960s, growing numbers of physicians began to use dietary and nutritional measures to treat a variety of disease conditions. Around the same time, two-time Nobel laureate Linus Pauling, Ph.D., one of the most accomplished biochemists and molecular biologists who ever lived, became a staunch advocate of taking vitamin C in large doses, both as a preventive and a therapeutic measure for the common cold. Pauling firmly believed that daily supplementation of vitamins in optimum amounts, in addition to following a healthy diet, was the most important step that anyone could take to live a long and healthy live, and by following his own advice, he lived productively for ninety-three years. Dr. Pauling also coined the term *orthomolecular medicine* to describe the use of vitamins, minerals, and amino acids, and other nutrients in optimum dosages to treat disease.

Another important researcher in the history of nutritional medicine is Denham Harman, M.D., who in 1956 pioneered the free-radical theory of aging. Based on Denham's research, scientists now know that cell damage caused by free radicals (toxic singlet oxygen molecules) not only accelerates the aging process, but also contributes to numerous disease conditions, including cancer and cardiovascular disease. Harman and other researchers have also shown that the oxidizing effects of free-radical activity can be minimized or reversed by antioxidant nutrients such as vitamins C and E, and today antioxidant multivitamin/mineral supplements are widely recommended by conventional and holistic physicians alike.

HOLISTIC GUIDELINES FOR HEALTHY EATING

Because of biochemical individuality, no single diet is ideally suited to everyone, which explains why some people thrive on a vegetarian lifestyle, while others require a regular intake of animal food products in order to stay healthy. Holistic physicians recognize that a number of factors, including blood type, heredity, metabolism, environment, stress, and predispositions to food allergy and sensitivity, can influence health and nutrition, and therefore take the time to properly address each patient's specific nutritional requirements. Overall, however, the following dietary principles can help most people maintain and improve their health.

Eat health-promoting foods. "The most basic principle of good nutrition is to consume a wide variety of health-promoting foods, and to avoid or minimize your intake of foods that are known or suspected of causing adverse effects," Dr. Gaby says. Among the health-promoting foods Dr. Gaby recommends are whole grains, fresh fruits and vegetables, nuts, seeds, legumes, and moderate amounts of low-fat animal foods, such as eggs, fish, poultry, and beef. Whenever possible, he also advises choosing foods that are raised organically, as well as drinking adequate amounts of pure, unpolluted water, while drinking alcohol only in moderation.

Avoid refined carbohydrates. Refined, processed carbohydrates are devoid of nutrients and can contribute to a wide range of chronic disease conditions. The most prevalent form of refined carbohydrate in the average American diet is refined sugar, which includes not only table sugar, but also sucrose, fructose, glucose, dextrose, and corn syrup, all of which are common food additives in processed foods. White bread and white rice should also be avoided. According to Dr. Gaby, such refined grains account for 30 percent of the caloric content of the standard American diet, and they lack the nutrient and fiber of grains that are whole and unprocessed.

Eliminate unhealthy fats. Contrary to popular belief, a certain amount of fat is necessary for optimum health. One of the keys to healthy eating lies in ensuring that the foods you eat contain adequate amounts of healthy fats (essential fatty acids) and are free of unhealthy fats. Among the unhealthiest fats are trans-fatty acids, which are extremely rare in whole foods, but quite common in margarine and commercially processed, hydrogenated vegetable oils, which are used as additives in many types of processed foods, including most commercial breakfast cereals. Polyunsaturated oils heated to a high temperature, as when they are used for deep-frying, are another source of unhealthy fat. "When the polyunsaturated fatty acids found in most vegetable oils are heated in the presence of oxygen, some of them are converted to toxic compounds called lipid peroxides," Dr. Gaby explains. "Consuming excessive amounts of lipid peroxides can cause free-radical damage." In place of trans-fatty acids and polyunsaturated vegetable oils, Dr. Gaby recommends using oils rich in omega-6 and omega-3 essential fatty acids. Goods sources of omega-6 include sunflower, safflower, and soybean oils, while flaxseed and fish oils are rich in omega-3.

Minimize or eliminate caffeine. Caffeine is another staple of the standard American diet and is contained not only in coffee, but also in non-herbal teas, chocolate candies, and sodas such as Coca-Cola and Pepsi. "Because caffeine consumption is so widespread, many of us overlook the fact that it is an addictive and potentially toxic chemical that has profound effects on human physiology," Dr. Gaby says. Among the conditions caffeine can contribute to are adrenal exhaustion, anxiety, insomnia, hypertension, headache, gastrointestinal disorders, fatigue, and osteoporosis.

Beware of food additives. "Modern processed foods contain so many chemical additives that it is impossible to determine all the effects they have on our bodies," Dr. Gaby says. Among the additives common in commercially produced food are artificial colorings and food dyes, sulfites, sodium benzoate, artificial sweeteners (aspartame), pesticides, and hormones and antibiotic residues in animal foods, all of which have been linked to numerous health problems. For this reason, Dr. Gaby recommends eating organic, fresh, unprocessed foods when they are available.

Determine food allergies and sensitivities. Many people unknowingly suffer from hidden or "masked" allergies or sensitivities to certain foods they eat. Typically, these foods comprise a regular part of the diet of people with food allergies or sensitivities. "Food allergies and sensitivities are difficult to identify because they are often delayed, sometimes for as long as several days after an individual eats an offending food, and because they don't necessarily occur every time the food is eaten," Dr. Gaby explains. Food allergies are estimated to affect as many as 60 million people in the United States. (For more on food allergies and how to deal with them, see Chapter 4, "Environmental Medicine." For additional dietary guidelines, see the diet section in Chapter 2.)

❧ ORTHOMOLECULAR MEDICINE ❧

Orthomolecular medicine, sometimes referred to as orthomolecular psychiatry for its ability to treat a variety of psychiatric disorders, is a specialized form of nutritional medicine that involves treating disease conditions with nutrients that occur naturally in the body. The term *orthomolecular*, which means "pertaining to the right molecule," was coined in 1968 by two-time Nobel laureate Linus Pauling, Ph.D., who described orthomolecular medicine as "the preservation of good health and the prevention and treatment of disease by varying the concentrations in the human body of the molecules of substances that are normally present, many of them required for life, such as vitamins, essential amino acids, essential fats, and minerals."

Orthomolecular medicine is often erroneously referred to as "megavitamin therapy." While high doses of vitamins and other nutrients are sometimes employed by practitioners of orthomolecular medicine, administered intravenously in certain situations, its emphasis is not on megadoses per se, but on providing patients with the proper amounts of nutrients that each of them individually requires. Its basic premise is that long-term health is best established by following a healthy diet and providing the body with the nutrients it needs to function optimally, while correcting faulty biochemistry. In 1987, well-known orthomolecular physician Richard Kunin, M.D., outlined the basic principles of orthomolecular medicine as follows:

Nutrition is a primary aspect of medical diagnosis and treatment, and nutrient-related disorders are usually curable once nutritional balance is achieved.

Due to biochemical individuality, universal Recommended Daily Allowance (RDA) values are unreliable nutrient guides, since many people require amounts of certain nutrients much higher than the suggested RDAs, due to such factors as genetics and the environments in which they live.

Conventional blood tests do not always provide an accurate assessment of the levels of nutrients in body tissues.

Both environmental pollution and food adulteration are inescapable facts of modern life and must be taken into consideration by physicians when treating their patients.

While drugs may be appropriate in the treatment of certain disease conditions, physicians must always be aware of their potential health risks and side effects.

Hope is indispensable, both as an ally to physicians and as an absolute right of their patients.

The roots of orthomolecular medicine date back to the 1920s, when physicians first began to use vitamins and minerals to treat various disease conditions. During that time, for instance, it was learned that vitamin A could help prevent childhood deaths caused by infectious illness, and that magnesium supplementation could arrest arrhythmia (irregular heartbeat). During the 1950s, the first real scientific support for nutritional therapy's value began to be established, thanks to the work of Abram Hoffer, M.D., and Humphrey Osmond, M.D., who were able to successfully treat schizophrenics by administering high doses of niacin (vitamin B_3), as well as vitamin C and other nutrients. Their studies revealed that when niacin was used in conjunction with standard psychiatric care, the recovery rate among their schizophrenic patients during a one-year period was twice that achieved by conventional care alone. As a follow-up to their work, Dr. Pauling worked with over a thousand schizophrenics for two years using high doses of nutrients. At the end of that period, 60 percent of the patients were either completely recovered or experienced a significant improvement in their symptoms. Subsequent studies using orthomolecular medicine to treat schizophrenia have shown recovery rates as high as 90 percent. Besides being more effective than conventional care, the orthomolecular approach has been shown to be shorter in duration, cheaper, and requiring less professional supervision.

Today, the number of disease conditions for which orthomolecular medicine offers benefits continues to expand. In addition to being effective for a variety of psychiatric disorders, it is also useful as a treatment for allergies, arthritis, autism, backache, psoriasis, and senility. As the link between nutrition and disease continues to be better understood, orthomolecular medicine's applications are apt to increase, as well. ❧

HOW NUTRITIONAL MEDICINE WORKS

Nutritional medicine works both preventively and therapeutically to ensure that patients are following the diet and receiving an adequate supply of nutrients appropriate to their individual needs. Practitioners of nutritional medicine also screen their patients for food allergies and sensitivities, and assess their digestive capacity in order to optimize the proper assimilation of the foods their patients eat. Eating well, along with proper nutrient supplementation, is an essential step in achieving and maintaining optimal health and safeguarding against illness. When illness is already present, nutritional medicine can play an important role in reversing disease conditions by supplying the body with the nutrients it needs to heal. Nutrients fall into three primary categories: macronutrients, vitamins, and minerals. What follows is an overview of the nutrients in each category, and their health-giving properties.

Macronutrients

The macronutrients are organic compounds and are classified as proteins, carbohydrates, or lipids (fats). Among their many functions, macronutrients serve as the body's source of energy.

Proteins, which account for 20 to 25 percent of a person's body weight, are second only to water in terms of the body's overall composition. In addition to the carbon, oxygen, and hydrogen molecules that occur in all forms of macronutrients, proteins also contain nitrogen and are essential for growth and maintaining the health of body tissue. They are also the primary building blocks for the body's muscles, internal organs, skin, hair, eyes, and nails, and play an integral role in the formation of immune system antibodies. Proteins are essential for the growth, maintenance, and repair of body tissues, as well as the production of various body substances, such as antibodies, enzymes, hemoglobin, hormones, and nerve chemicals. Proteins also help maintain the body's acid-alkaline (pH) balance, as well as regulating the amount of fluid within the cells and preserving normal sodium and potassium balance. When the body's fat and carbohydrate stores are low, the body also draws on dietary protein to maintain energy levels. When dietary protein isn't available, the body will break down tissue proteins, although this will eventually result in energy depletion and disease if dietary protein is not replenished. Food sources of complete proteins include meats, cheese, eggs, fish, milk, and poultry, while grains, legumes, nuts, seeds, and various vegetables contain partial protein sources.

Proteins consist of various combinations of twenty-five amino acids. In addition to serving as the building blocks for all proteins in the body, amino acids are also involved in a variety of vital biological processes, including energy production, bone and muscle growth, tissue repair (wound healing), and the formation of the brain's neurotransmitters. Eight amino acids have been classified as essential, due to the fact that the body cannot produce them on its own. Essential amino acids, therefore, must be supplied through the foods we eat. The eight essential amino acids are isoleucine, leucine, lysine, methionine, phenylalanine, threonine, tryptophan, and valine. When all eight of these amino acids are supplied to the body in adequate amounts, it is able to synthesize the other seventeen amino acids required for other biological processes. Three of these seventeen amino acids, arginine, histidine, and taurine, are considered semiessential, since they are vital for growth during infancy, childhood, and adolescence, and also during pregnancy. The remaining amino acids are alanine, aspartic acid, carnitine, cysteine, gamma-aminobutyric acid (GABA), glutamine, glutathione, glycine, homocysteine, hydroxyproline, ornithine, proline, serine, and tyrosine. Although these amino acids are considered nonessential, they can be vital during times of extreme illness and can help offset the effects of a poor diet.

Note: Although dietary protein is essential for optimum health, most Americans consume far more protein per day than they need, particularly from animal foods. Excessive consumption of animal foods, especially meats, has been associated with a number of degenerative conditions, including cancer and cardiovascular illness.

Carbohydrates are another class of macronutrients and serve as the body's primary source of energy. Carbohydrates are also vital to proper function of the nervous system, muscles, and internal organs. In addition, they help regulate fat and protein metabolism, as well as promoting the body's use of fats and proteins to fight infection, grow body tissue, and lubricate the joints. Whole, or unrefined, carbohydrates are also high in fiber, which aids the body in eliminating toxins via the colon. Carbohydrate foods include fruits, vegetables, grains, legumes, and tubers.

There are three categories of carbohydrates: sugars, starches, and fibers. Sugars occur in two forms: simple, or monosaccharides, and multiple, or disaccharides. Simple sugars are primarily found in fruits and honey, and include glucose, fructose, and galactose. Multiple sugars, which commonly occur as table and malt sugar, include maltose and sucrose. Lactose, or milk sugar, is another form of disaccharide. Foods high in either simple or multiple sugars can cause rapid shifts in glucose levels in the blood, which can contribute to a number of disease conditions. For this reason, holistic physicians recommend avoiding sugar carbohydrates, with the exception of fresh fruits.

Starches, also known as complex carbohydrates or polysaccharides, are considered the healthiest form of carbohydrates, since they contribute to more balanced blood sugar levels, as well as sustained energy. The best food sources of complex carbohydrates are potatoes, root vegetables, corn, wheat, rice, and other whole grains.

Fibers, while supplying the body with little caloric energy, play an important role in maintaining proper gastrointestinal function and elimination. The average American diet is notoriously lacking in fiber, however, which is the main reason why each year in the United States billions of dollars are spent on laxatives to deal with constipation. Because fibers are undigestible, they absorb water and bind toxins in the gastrointestinal tract. Certain fibers also help reduce fat absorption and lower cholesterol levels. Common food fibers include cellulose, contained in the skins of fruits and vegetables and in the outer hulls of grains; psyllium seed husks; carrageen; guar gum; pectin; and agar and alginate, both of which are derived from seaweed.

Lipids (fats) are the final class of macronutrients. In addition to acting as insulation for the body, fats play an essential role in the transport of fat-soluble vitamins and, as part of cell membranes and fatty tissues, protect internal organs from the effects of trauma and shifts in temperature. The body also uses lipids as energy reserves, burning fats when more energy is needed than the diet supplies. Lipids aid in the digestion and assimilation of other nutrients, as well. On average, lipids comprise from 10 to over 30 percent of an adult person's total body weight.

Lipids in the body are primarily in the form of triglycerides, which make up approximately 95 percent of the lipid content in foods. Triglycerides are the only form of fat that provides the body with caloric energy. Triglyceride fatty acids are either saturated or unsaturated, with unsaturated fatty acids being either monounsaturated or polyunsaturated. Saturated fatty acids are primarily derived from animal sources (including butter, cheese, and yogurt) and are also found in margarine, lard, and coconut and palm oils. Unsaturated fatty acids are derived from plants, with monounsaturated fatty acids occurring in avocados, as well as olive, almond, and canola oil. Corn, cottonseed, peanut, safflower, sesame, and soybean oils are all good sources of polyunsaturated fatty acids.

Three types of polyunsaturated fatty acids—linoleic, linolenic, and arachidonic acids—cannot normally be manufactured in the body and are therefore classified as essential fatty acids (EFAs). EFAs are essential for proper growth and for protecting the skin and other body tissues through lubrication. Linoleic and arachidonic fatty acids are known as omega-6, while linolenic fatty acids are called omega-3 oils.

Phospholipids are another form of lipids and play a vital role in maintaining membrane structure. The most common phospholipid is lecithin. Other forms of phospholipids are phosphatidyl choline, phosphatidyl inositol, phosphatidyl anolamine, phosphatidyl serine, and sphingomyelin. Among the functions of phospholipids are maintaining the health of the brain, supplying brain cells with vital nutrients, and protecting nerve cells.

The third class of lipids is known as sterols. These include cholesterol, plant sterols (phytosterols), and certain steroid hormones. Cholesterol is manufactured in all body tissues except those of the brain and is a component of bile acids and salts, and a precursor of vitamin D and the body's sex hormones. It is most highly concentrated in the liver, blood, and brain and nerve tissue and is found in all animal tissue. Without adequate supplies of cholesterol, the body would not be able to properly form cells of the brain and nervous system, nor would these cells be able to function correctly. However, excessive amounts of cholesterol, especially when it becomes oxidized, have been linked to heart disease, stroke, and atherosclerosis.

Most health practitioners agree that no more than 20 to 30 percent of one's diet should consist of calories derived from lipids, with 10 to 15 percent being essential. The fat content of the average American diet is over 40 percent, however.

THE POTENTIAL INADEQUACY OF ❦ REFERENCE DAILY INTAKES (RDIs) ❦

Since 1940, the United States government has provided suggested levels of essential nutrients based on the recommendations of government-sponsored scientists and other nutritional experts. Formerly known as Recommended Daily Allowances (RDAs), these suggested levels are now called Reference Daily Intakes (RDIs) and are intended as guidelines to help Americans meet their nutritional needs. However, most holistic practitioners of nutritional medicine find little value in the RDIs, since they are based only on the levels of nutrients required to prevent deficiency, rather than achieving and maintaining optimal health. In addition, they fail to take into account each person's specific nutritional needs, which can vary substantially depending on such factors as biochemical individuality, level of wellness, stress, and exposure to environmental pollutants.

While meeting the RDIs' nutritional standards is enough to prevent conditions caused by severe nutritional deficiencies, such as rickets or scurvy, growing numbers of physicians and nutritional researchers now recognize that the RDI levels for nutrients are often inadequate for avoiding the wide range of diseases caused, at least in part, by less severe nutritional deficiencies. Their view is supported by a fifteen-year study conducted by Emmanuel Cheraskin, M.D., D.M.D., and other researchers at the University of Alabama, the results of which were published in 1994. Conducted in six different geographical regions across the United States, the study involved 13,500 people who were each given a variety of physiological medical tests, along with a comprehensive analysis of their diet, and asked to complete a detailed health questionnaire. The study found that regardless of their location, the participants who exhibited the highest levels of optimal health all received a daily intake of nutrients from diet and supplementation that was usually at least ten times higher than suggested RDI levels. Based on this evidence, Dr. Cheraskin and his colleagues suggested an alternative to the RDIs known as Suggested Optimal Nutrient Allowances (SONAs). Today, SONAs are used as guidelines by many holistic physicians as an alternative to RDIs, due to the increased success they are achieving with their patients by doing so. Nonetheless, they also still take care to meet each patient's unique nutritional needs rather than relying on a standard formula for everyone. ❦

Vitamins

Vitamins play a vital role in human nutrition and, for the most part, cannot be manufactured by the body. Although many people take vitamins in hopes of improving their energy levels, of themselves vitamins are not energy sources. Instead, vitamins are essential for properly regulating the body's metabolic reactions and biochemical processes. When vitamins are deficient in the diet, these various biological functions are impeded, resulting in suboptimal health and a variety of disease conditions specifically related to nutrient imbalances. There are two classifications of vitamins, those that are fat-soluble and those that are water-soluble.

Fat-soluble vitamins are stored in body tissues and can therefore be drawn upon when they are not obtained daily from the diet. Because they are not easily excreted, however, excessive intake of fat-soluble vitamins can cause toxicity. The fat-soluble vitamins are vitamins A, D, E, and K and the carotenoids.

Vitamin A was the first vitamin to be discovered and officially named, hence its letter *A*. Vitamin A is not a single substance, but a group of nutrients that include retinol, retinal, and the carotenoids. Retinol and retinal are both known as preformed vitamin A and are found in a variety of animal foods, especially liver. Butter, cream, egg yolk, fish oils, and whole and fortified nonfat milk are all good sources of preformed vitamin A. Orange fruits and green, leafy, and yellow vegetables are all rich sources of various precursor carotenoids, particularly beta-carotene, which the body converts to vitamin A.

Vitamin A is important for a variety of body functions, including eyesight, healthy teeth and skin, bone growth, cell differentiation, and tissue repair. Vitamin A also plays an important role in maintaining proper function of the cornea, lungs, mucus membranes, the lining of the gastrointestinal tract, and the bladder and urinary tract. It also acts as an antioxidant, helps prevent infectious disease, and is needed for the production of various antitumor compounds in the body.

Vitamin A stores are diminished by both stress and illness, as well as alcohol consumption, which also interferes with its absorption. One of the first signs of vitamin A deficiency is night blindness. Other signs of deficiency include suboptimum bone and tooth formation, eye inflammation, impaired immune response, weight loss, and keratinosis, a condition resulting in hardened pigmented deposits around hair follicles and the body's upper and lower extremities.

Vitamin D occurs in ten forms, D_1–D_{10}. The two most important forms are D_2 and D_3. The best food sources of vitamin D are cod liver and fish liver oils, butter, egg yolk, liver, vitamin D–fortified milk, and oily fish such as herring, mackerel, sardines, and salmon. The body can also manufacture vitamin D in the skin when it comes in contact with the sun's ultraviolet rays. People who live in areas of smog or infrequent sunlight, as well as strict vegetarians, should consider daily supplementing with 400 IUs of vitamin D.

Vitamin D is essential for the absorption of calcium and for regulating the metabolism of calcium and phosphorus, both of which are integral components of healthy bones and teeth. It also aids in regulating the nervous system and maintaining cardiovascular health and normal blood clotting and is an important nutrient for childhood growth. Because of its ability to aid in the calcification process, vitamin D can also be useful for maintaining bone health during menopause.

In childhood, the primary sign of vitamin D deficiency is rickets, while in adults, lack of the vitamin can result in softening of the bones (osteomalacia). Tetany (a form of muscle spasm), hearing loss, nearsightedness, psoriasis, celiac disease, and osteoporosis can also result from vitamin D deficiency.

Vitamin E refers to a group of substances known as tocopherols. The most active form of vitamin E is d-alpha tocopherol, which is also the form that is most prevalent in nature. The primary food sources of vitamin E are seed and vegetable oils, especially safflower oil. Other food sources include wheat germ, wheat germ oil, nuts, green leafy vegetables, whole grains, butter, and egg yolk.

Vitamin E acts as a potent antioxidant and works synergistically with other antioxidants like vitamin C and selenium to minimize the effects of free-radical damage and as an antitumor agent. It also enhances the health properties of vitamin A, with the two vitamins working together to reduce cholesterol and fat accumulation. Currently, vitamin E is also being investigated for its potential antiaging properties, and has been shown to reduce the risk of atherosclerosis. In addition, it is an important nutrient for the nervous, reproductive, and skeletal systems, as well as for muscle tissue and red blood cells and corpuscles. Applied topically, it is useful for treating burns, wounds, abrasions, lesions, and dry skin.

Even though vitamin E is more easily excreted from the body than other fat-soluble vitamins, signs of deficiency are less obvious than other nutrient deficiencies, and therefore more difficult to detect. Adding to this difficulty is the fact that vitamin E deficiency can manifest itself in a variety of ways. One possible indication of deficiency is decreased red blood cell levels due to damaged cell membranes.

Vitamin K also occurs in various forms: K_1 (phylloquinone) and K_2 (menaquinone), both of which occur naturally, and K_3 (menadione), a synthetic version that is twice as active biologically and is administered only to people who have difficulty using the natural forms because of conditions such as reduced bile secretion. Approximately half of the body's vitamin K needs are met by the biosynthesis of various bacteria in the intestines. Food sources of vitamin K include dark green leafy vegetables, kelp, alfalfa, egg yolk, yogurt, fish liver oils, and legumes, as well as safflower oil and blackstrap molasses.

Vitamin K's primary function in the body is to assist in normal blood clotting, especially in the synthesis of various proteins involved in the coagulation process. Since the body is able to manufacture its own supply of vitamin K, deficiencies are rare, although they can be compounded by impaired intestinal absorption, overuse of antibiotics (which destroy healthy intestinal bacteria), and poor liver function or liver disease. Symptoms of deficiency include abnormal bleeding or hemorrhaging, and miscarriage due to abnormal blood loss.

Carotenoids refer to over five hundred substances that naturally occur in fruits and vegetables. Some fifty carotenoids act as precursors to vitamin A, with beta-carotene being the best known and most prevalent. More recently, lycopene has become another popular carotenoid because of its various healing properties. The best food sources of carotenoids are yellow and dark green vegetables, orange fruits, tomatoes, watermelons, and cherries.

Carotenoids primarily act as antioxidants in the body and are also capable of minimizing the formation of abnormal and precancerous cells and preventing age-related vision problems. Some researchers also speculate that carotenoids can improve immune function by stimulating immune antibodies, lymphocytes, and natural killer and T-helper cells. Symptoms of carotenoid deficiency include diminished immune function, free-radical damage, and increased susceptibility to various cancers and cardiovascular illness.

Vitamins that are water-soluble include all B-complex vitamins (thiamine, riboflavin, niacin, pantothenic acid, pyridoxine, folic acid, cobalamin, biotin, and choline), vitamin C, and bioflavonoids (vitamin P). In contrast to fat-soluble vitamins, water-soluble vitamins are more easily destroyed by cooking and storage and are more readily excreted by the body and therefore require daily replenishment through the diet. With the exception of vitamin B_6, this also makes them less toxic in high doses.

Thiamine (B_1) plays a key role in the health of the heart, the nervous system, the muscle tissue, and the blood cells and is essential for metabolizing glucose in the cells to produce energy. Thiamine also aids in converting carbohydrates into fats that the body uses as energy reserves. Research suggests that thiamine is also potentially useful for mental function and for minimizing nutritional imbalances caused by too much alcohol consumption. Like all B vitamins, thiamine works best when taken as part of a complete B-complex supplement.

Thiamine is found in all plant and animal foods but is especially available in pork, organ meats, seafood, eggs, milk, pulses (seaweed), and wheat germ, barley, brown rice, and other whole grains. Despite this fact, cases of thiamine deficiency are quite common, due to exposure to stress, cigarettes, and regular alcohol consumption. Long-term thiamine deficiency can cause beriberi. Early signs of deficiency include fatigue, muscle weakness, constipation and other gastrointestinal disorders, confusion, depression, and memory loss.

Riboflavin (B₂) plays an important role in the body's production of energy, acts as an antioxidant, and promotes cell growth. It also works synergistically with various enzymes to help the body metabolize proteins, carbohydrates, and fats. Healthy skin, hair, and nails all depend on adequate amounts of riboflavin, as does good vision.

One of the best food sources of riboflavin is brewer's yeast. Organ meats, milks, eggs, cheese, green leafy vegetables, millet, wild rice, legumes, and oily fish such as mackerel and trout are other good sources. Riboflavin is also produced by intestinal bacteria. Sunlight destroys riboflavin, as do stress and alcohol consumption, and some health experts say riboflavin deficiencies are more common than any other nutrient deficiency, especially among the elderly, people with poor eating habits, and alcoholics. Deficiency symptoms include mouth and tongue sores, eye fatigue and redness, sensitivity to light, hair loss, digestive problems, dermatitis, and general fatigue.

Niacin (B₃) occurs in two forms, niacinamide and nicotinic acid, and is important for the overall health of the nervous system and the brain. Niacin also plays a vital role in the synthesis of sex hormones, enhances circulation, assists in energy production, and aids the body in flushing out toxins. Niacin can also be useful in reducing cholesterol and other body fats, and as a protective agent for the heart.

The body manufactures niacin when it has an adequate supply of the amino acid tryptophan, along with enough iron and vitamins B_1, B_2, B_6, and C to assist in the conversion process. The richest food sources of niacin are organ meats, fish, poultry, peanuts, legumes, eggs, milk, and cheese. Long-term niacin deficiency can result in pellagra, which affects every cell in the body and can lead to symptoms of dementia, diarrhea, and dermatitis. Other signs of deficiency include skin sensitivity to light, gastrointestinal disorders, fatigue, headache, insomnia, irritability, memory loss, and emotional problems.

Pantothenic acid (B₅) is sometimes known as the antistress vitamin for its ability to assist the adrenal cortex in producing cortisone and other hormones in response to stress. It also helps brain and neuromuscular function by converting the amino acid choline into the neurotransmitter acetylcholine, contributes to the overall health of the nervous system, and improves energy. Normal growth functions of the body are also supported by pantothenic acid, and some research indicates that it is a protective nutrient for the heart and useful for reducing cholesterol.

Pantothenic acid is widely available in most foods, with brewer's yeast, organ meats, eggs, brown rice, whole grain cereals, cheese, sweet potatoes, cauliflower, and molasses all being good sources. The body also converts intestinal flora to pantothenic acid. With the exception of people who subsist on an entirely refined "junk foods" diet, deficiency of pantothenic acid is extremely unlikely.

Pyridoxine (B₆) plays many roles in the body and is essential for the proper absorption of vitamin B_{12}, protein synthesis, and over sixty enzymatic functions. It is also vital for the production of white blood cells and immune system antibodies. In addition, it helps regulate the body's sodium-potassium balance, which in turn helps regulate the body fluid balance and nerve, heart, and musculoskeletal function. The release of glycogen from the liver in muscles is also enhanced by adequate pyridoxine supply, making for greater levels of energy. Pyridoxine is an important nutrient for women, as well, especially during pregnancy, pre-menstruation, and menopause.

Although pyridoxine is common in many food sources, few foods contain it in high amounts. It is also easily destroyed during cooking and improper storage. Wheat germ, meat, fish, poultry, eggs, whole grain cereals, soybeans, potatoes, cauliflower, cabbage, and bananas are some of the best sources of pyridoxine.

Since pyridoxine plays an essential role in numerous body functions, lack of this vitamin can result in a wide variety of deficiency symptoms, beginning with impaired amino acid metabolism and decreases in neurotransmitter and hemoglobin production. Anemia, fatigue, nerve-related disorders, insomnia, skin problems, headache, concentration problems, nausea, and muscle cramps or spasms are other possible signs of pyridoxine deficiency.

Folic acid (B₉), also known as folacin or folate, aids in the production of red blood cells and helps metabolize protein by aiding in various amino acid conversions. It also plays a vital role in cell division, making it an important nutrient during times of growth, including pregnancy. Folic acid is also required by the body to properly use sugars and is involved in the production of neurotransmitters.

The richest food sources of folic acid are dark green vegetables, such as spinach, asparagus, and kale. Other good sources are brewer's yeast, wheat germ, nuts, eggs, and organ meats. Excessive heat and overcooking destroy folic acid, which is why it is important to consume adequate amounts of raw vegetables that contain it. Under conditions of good intestinal health, the body can also manufacture folic acid from intestinal bacteria.

Folic acid deficiency is quite common, due to such factors as poor diet, illness, malabsorption, stress, and alcohol and drug abuse. Deficiency symptoms include anemia, fatigue, diarrhea, gastrointestinal disorders, headache, irritability, palpitations, and overall weakness.

Cobalamin (B$_{12}$) is considered the most complex vitamin due to the fact that it is the only vitamin that also contains essential minerals, particularly cobalt, which is necessary for the manufacture of cobalamin in the intestines. Cobalamin is required for the formation of protein from amino acids and also aids in the metabolism of proteins, carbohydrates, and fats. It is also necessary for proper metabolism of nerve tissue and overall maintenance of the nervous system and aids in the formation of red blood cells. Because of its ability to enhance the body's ability to utilize macronutrients and iron, as well as the role it plays in the synthesis of DNA and RNA, cobalamin can also improve energy levels.

Cobalamin is not found in significant amounts in plants and can be depleted by stress, aging, exposure to light, and the excessive use of antacids and laxatives. The best animal food sources for cobalamin include beef, pork, organ meats, fish, eggs, milk, and yogurt. As a result, vegetarians who avoid dairy products are often deficient in cobalamin unless they take it in supplement form.

Long-term lack of cobalamin can result in pernicious anemia. Other deficiency symptoms include dizziness, fatigue, gastrointestinal disorders, hypotension (low blood pressure), memory problems, moodiness, numbness, and vision problems.

Biotin, sometimes referred to as vitamin H despite the fact that it is not a true vitamin per se, works as a cofactor with other B-complex vitamins to break down and metabolize fats and to synthesize fatty acids. Biotin can also minimize symptoms of zinc deficiency.

The best food sources of biotin include liver, brewer's yeast, nuts, milk, and egg yolk. Raw eggs eaten in large amounts can deplete biotin absorption, however, due to their avidin content. (Avidin is inactivated by cooking.) Excessive alcohol and use of antibiotics can also impair biotin absorption and destroy biotin stores.

Symptoms of biotin deficiency include appetite loss, depression, fatigue, hair loss (especially among teenagers), muscle pain, and skin problems.

Choline helps the body utilize fat and is an essential component of acetylcholine, a neurotransmitter that plays a crucial role in brain function. Choline also enhances liver and gallbladder function, helps maintain the myelin sheaths (nerve fiber coverings), and is combined in the body with glycerol and phosphate to create lecithin, an important fat and cholesterol emulsifier.

Good food sources of choline include brewer's yeast, wheat germ, soybean lecithin, egg yolks, peanuts, fish, and organ meats. There are no specific signs of choline deficiency, although lack of the nutrient can result in impaired fat metabolism, loss of cell membrane integrity, and damage to the myelin sheaths.

Vitamin C (ascorbic acid) serves many functions in the body. Its importance was popularized by Linus Pauling, as discussed earlier in this chapter. One of the least stable vitamins, vitamin C cannot be manufactured in the body and, among food sources, is found only in fruits and vegetables. In addition to acting as a potent antioxidant and immune system enhancer, vitamin C is essential for the formation of collagen, which acts as the basis for the body's connective tissue. As a result, vitamin C contributes to the overall health of blood vessels, capillary walls, cartilage, joint linings, ligaments, vertebrae, bones, teeth, and skin, and plays a vital role in wound healing. It also aids in the metabolism of amino acids and cholesterol, and in the synthesis of hormones, and helps the body cope with the effects of stress. In addition, vitamin C's detoxification properties make it useful for protecting the body against heavy metal toxicity, environmental pollutants, and nicotine poisoning. It is also effective in fighting bacterial and viral infections and acts as a natural histamine, making it useful for dealing with allergies.

The best food sources of vitamin C include citrus fruits, rosehips, cherries, cantaloupe, papaya, strawberries, red and green peppers, parsley, and dark green and leafy vegetables.

Because vitamin C is not readily stored in the body, it must be supplied daily through the diet or supplementation. The most famous sign of vitamin C deficiency is scurvy, a disease that is extremely rare today. Other deficiency symptoms include anemia, reduced resistance to infections, increased tendency toward bruising, slow wound healing, bleeding gums, and mouth ulcers.

Bioflavonoids are water-soluble nutrients that act as cofactors with vitamin C and commonly occur in the same food sources. Like vitamin C, bioflavonoids were discovered by Albert Szent-Gyorgi (see "History" above) in the 1930s. The best-known bioflavonoids include catechin, citrin, flavonals, flavones, hesperidin, quercitin, and rutin. Together, they are sometimes referred to as vitamin P, for their ability to increase permeability factor, meaning they enhance the ability of other nutrients, oxygen, and carbon dioxide to pass through capillary walls. Their other main function lies in increasing capillary strength and integrity, thereby helping to prevent them from hemorrhaging. Bioflavonoids also improve the body's absorption of vitamin C and therefore play a role in the formation and maintenance of collagen.

The best food sources of bioflavonoids are the same as those for vitamin C. Bioflavonoid deficiency is rare, although a lack of this nutrient group can diminish the body's ability to use vitamin C, thus contributing to increased bruising and slower wound healing.

Minerals

Minerals are found in the body's fluids and tissues and make up approximately 4 percent of the body's total weight. Working in conjunction with vitamins, enzymes, hormones, and other substances, minerals play an important role in numerous biological functions, including the growth and maintenance of bones and teeth, muscle contraction, nerve transmission, blood formation, energy production, fluid regulation, macronutrient metabolism, acid-alkaline balance (pH), and various other enzymatic reactions.

Nutrient minerals are classified according to how much of the body's total weight they comprise. Macrominerals comprise at least 0.01 percent of body weight, while trace or microminerals constitute less than 0.01 percent. An adequate supply of both macro- and trace minerals is equally important for optimal health, however. Macrominerals include calcium, chloride, magnesium, phosphorus, potassium, and sodium, while trace minerals include chromium, cobalt, copper, iodine, iron, manganese, molybdenum, selenium, sulfur, and zinc.

Calcium is the most plentiful mineral in the human body, with approximately 99 percent of it occurring in bone tissue, and the remaining 1 percent being used for a variety of other functions, including blood clotting, muscle contraction, and nerve function. Healthy teeth and bones both depend on an adequate calcium supply, and calcium also contributes to healthy skin, helps regulate cardiovascular function and blood pressure levels, aids in the metabolism of iron, and is required for proper cell division.

Calcium must be supplied daily to the body through the diet or supplementation. The best food sources of calcium include milk, yogurt, cheese, cottage cheese, dark green leafy vegetables, broccoli, turnip and collard greens, salmon, sardines, canned fish, almonds, and brazil nuts. The standard American diet is estimated to supply only one-third of our daily calcium needs.

Signs of calcium deficiency include bone and skeletal problems (most notably osteoporosis and fracture), anxiety, brittle nails, depression, insomnia, muscle cramps and twitching, and diminished nerve function. Calcium is best supplemented as part of a multivitamin/multimineral formula.

Note: Excessive amounts of calcium over time can lead to kidney stones and soft tissue calcification, and possibly contribute to atherosclerosis.

Chloride is an essential part of hydrochloric acid (HCl), a vital stomach digestive acid, and also plays a role in regulating the body's acid balance. It is also useful in helping the liver eliminate toxins and for transporting carbon dioxide to the lungs for excretion. Among the best food sources of chloride are common table salt, sea salt, seaweeds, celery, lettuce, and tomatoes. The standard American diet contains more than enough chloride due to its high salt content.

Chloride loss can easily occur following bouts of diarrhea or vomiting, as well as periods of profuse perspiration. Overall, however, chloride deficiencies are rare, with the most common symptoms being acid-base imbalances and excess alkalinity of body fluids.

Magnesium acts as a muscle relaxant in the body and is involved in hundreds of enzymatic reactions. Approximately 65 percent of the body's magnesium supply is contained in the bones and teeth, with the second-highest concentration occurring in the muscles. The remaining magnesium supply is found in the blood and other body fluids.

In addition to its ability to relax smooth and skeletal muscles, magnesium is an important nutrient for the heart, especially in preventing spasms of the coronary arteries, which can cause heart attacks. It is also needed for energy production, the maintenance and repair of cells, healthy cell division, proper nerve transmission, hormone regulation, and the metabolism of proteins and nucleic acids.

Food sources of magnesium are primarily plants rich in chlorophyll, particularly dark green vegetables. Nuts, seeds, legumes, tofu, wheat germ, millet, brown rice, apricot, and avocado are other good sources.

Magnesium deficiency is more common than many physicians realize, because of factors such as poor diet, overcooking, deficient soil, and the overuse of alcohol. Deficiency symptoms include depression, fatigue, gastrointestinal disorders, high blood pressure, irregular heartbeat, memory problems, mood swings, impaired motor skills, muscle spasm, nausea, and tetany.

Phosphorus ranks second behind calcium as the body's most abundant mineral. It is found in every cell of the body but primarily (approximately 85 percent) in the bones and teeth. In addition to contributing to bone and teeth structure, phosphorus helps form DNA and RNA, catalyzes B-complex vitamins, is involved in cellular communication and numerous enzymatic reactions, and helps produce energy and increase endurance.

The best food sources of phosphorus are protein foods, such as meats, fish, poultry, eggs, milk, and cheese. Other good sources include nuts, seeds, wheat germ, whole grains, and brewer's yeast. The standard American diet can be overly high in its phosphorus content, especially with regard to soda, which can contain up to 500 mg of phosphorus per serving and create calcium-phosphorus imbalance.

Because phosphorus is contained in all animal foods, phosphorus deficiency is rare. Overuse of antacids, excessive calcium intake, and lack of vitamin D can all result in phosphorus deficiency, however. Signs of deficiency include anxiety, arthritis, impaired bone growth, irritability, and weakness.

Potassium, along with chloride and sodium, is an electrolyte, or essential body salt, that conducts electric current throughout the body. Approximately 98 percent of the body's potassium supply is contained inside the walls of the cells, where it regulates water and acid-base balance. It is vital to cellular integrity and fluid balance and plays an important role in nerve function. It also helps metabolize proteins and carbohydrates, aids in energy production, and helps regulate heartbeat.

Optimum food sources of potassium are fresh fruits and vegetables, with bananas being a particularly rich source. Whole grains, seeds, nuts, wheat germ, salmon, and sardines are also good food sources.

Potassium deficiencies are fairly common, particularly among older people and people suffering from chronic disease. Diarrhea, diabetes, fasting, and the overuse of diuretics and laxatives all contribute to potassium loss. Deficiency symptoms include arrhythmia, depression, fatigue, high blood pressure, hyperglycemia, impaired growth, mood swings, and unhealthy changes in the nervous system.

Sodium is also present in all of the body's cells, as well as in the blood and other body fluids. Approximately 60 percent of the body's sodium content is contained in extracellular (outside the cells) fluids, with 10 percent found inside the cells, and the remainder occurring in the bones.

Like potassium, sodium helps maintain the body's fluid balance within and without the cells, thereby regulating the body's acid-base balance. It also helps transport carbon dioxide and plays a role in muscle contraction and nerve transmission. In addition, sodium is involved in the production of hydrochloric acid and helps transport amino acids into the bloodstream to all the cells of the body.

Nearly all foods contain some sodium, with seafood, beef, and poultry containing particularly high amounts. The primary dietary source of sodium is table salt, and sodium is also present in significant amounts in most canned and processed foods.

Chronic sodium deficiency is rare, although sodium loss can occur because of diarrhea, vomiting, profuse perspiration due to exercise and other strenuous activity, and the overuse of diuretics. Problems related to excessive sodium intake are far more common among people who eat the standard American diet, and can lead to high blood pressure and premenstrual syndrome, among other conditions. Deficiency symptoms include dehydration, low blood pressure, muscle cramping and twitching, and muscle weakness.

Chromium is an essential component of glucose tolerance factor (GTF), which enhances insulin function, making it vital for proper carbohydrate metabolism and for regulating blood sugar levels. By improving how glucose is transported into the cells, chromium and GTF are also important for energy production. Research suggests that chromium may also be useful for regulating body cholesterol levels.

One of the best food sources of chromium is brewer's yeast. Other food sources include whole grain breads and cereals, wheat germ, eggs, meats, and shellfish. Chromium deficiency is quite common, especially in the United States, due to mineral-depleted soils and and overreliance on refined and processed foods. In addition, many people have problems absorbing chromium, particularly as they age. Deficiency symptoms include diabetes-like blood sugar problems caused by a reduction in peripheral tissue sensitivity to glucose. Anxiety, fatigue, and impaired cholesterol metabolism are also associated with a lack of chromium in the diet.

Cobalt, in addition to being a component of cobalamin (vitamin B_{12}), plays an essential role in the production of red blood cells and is involved in a number of enzymatic reactions. Adequate vitamin B_{12} intake normally provides sufficient amounts of cobalt to the body. Food sources include beet greens, cabbage, figs, legumes, lettuce, liver, and fish and sea vegetables. Cobalt deficiencies are similar to those caused by a lack of B_{12}, including anemia and nerve damage.

Copper is present in all body tissues but is particularly concentrated in the liver and brain. It aids in the manufacture of collagen and hemoglobin and, along with iron, is necessary for the synthesis of oxygen in red blood cells. It also acts as an antioxidant, increases iron absorption, and serves as a catalyst for a variety of enzymatic reactions.

The best food sources of copper include dark green leafy vegetables, eggs, organ meats, poultry, nuts, shellfish, and whole grain breads and cereals. Although dangerous copper deficiencies are rare, less serious copper deficiencies are more common. Symptoms include anemia, dermatitis, diarrhea, edema, fatigue, impaired collagen production, labored respiration, and tissue and blood vessel damage.

Iodine is essential for healthy thyroid function because of its role in the production of thyroid hormones. It helps regulate metabolism and energy production in the body, as well as cellular oxidation. Since thyroid hormones play a role in all body functions, iodine is of vital importance to overall health, yet iodine deficiency is estimated to affect at least 200 million people worldwide, due in part to depleted soil conditions.

The best food sources of iodine are iodized salt, followed by seafood and seaweed. Deficiency symptoms include fatigue, goiter, hypothyroidism, decreased libido, impaired mental functioning, impaired metabolism, and weight gain.

Iron is present in all the cells of the body, usually in combination with protein. Iron's primary function is the manufacture of hemoglobin, which is integral to the transport of oxygen throughout the body. Iron is also essential for healthy immune function and energy production. Research suggests it may additionally play a role in protecting cells and tissues from damage due to oxidation.

Among the best food sources of iron are beef, brewer's yeast, kelp, molasses, organ meats, dark green leafy vegetables, legumes, oysters, and sardines. In supplement form, it is best taken with vitamin C, which aids in its assimilation.

Women, especially during their childbearing years, require more iron than men, particularly during pregnancy and menstruation. Approximately 10 percent of all women in the Western world are estimated to be iron-deficient. Children and the elderly are also more prone to iron deficiency. Deficiency symptoms include iron-deficiency anemia, dizziness, fatigue, headache, learning disabilities, lowered immunity, and impaired sleep.

Manganese supports a variety of enzymatic reactions in the body and is essential for proper brain function and the overall health of the nervous system. It also helps metabolize proteins and carbohydrates and is required for cholesterol and fatty-acid synthesis, as well as collagen formation. The best food sources of manganese are green leafy vegetables (especially spinach), nuts, organ meats, and whole grain breads and cereals.

Manganese deficiency in humans is rare. Deficiency symptoms include dizziness, hearing problems, and weakness.

Molybdenum, along with copper, is necessary for the body's proper utilization of iron and aids in metabolizing carbohydrates. It also helps the body detoxify potentially toxic sulfites commonly used to preserve food. Molybdenum deficiency is rare and is primarily caused by eating foods grown in molybdenum-deficient soils or a diet high in refined and processed foods. Deficiency symptoms include anemia and a greater risk of dental caries. Excessive molybdenum intake can also result in various symptoms, including goutlike symptoms and elevated levels of uric acid.

Selenium in recent decades has become recognized as an important antioxidant capable of performing many of the same antioxidant functions as vitamin E, including protecting cellular membranes from free-radical damage, and minimizing the risk of cardiovascular disease. In addition, selenium aids liver function, assists in the manufacture of proteins, helps neutralize heavy metals and other toxic substances, and acts as an anticarcinogen.

The best food sources of selenium include brewer's yeast, wheat bran and wheat germ, Brazil nuts, organ meats, and seafood. A number of plant foods, such as broccoli, onions, and tomatoes, can also be good sources, depending on the soil content in which they are grown.

Symptoms of selenium deficiency can mimic those of a lack of vitamin E, and a selenium deficiency can also result in an increased risk of cancer, cardiovascular disease, high blood pressure, and stroke.

Sulfur occurs in all cells and body tissues, especially those high in protein content. It is a necessary nutrient for collagen formation and is involved in the synthesis of protein. In addition, sulfur helps maintain the health of hair, skin, and nails. It also plays a role in a number of enzymatic reactions and contributes to the process of cellular respiration.

The best food sources of sulfur are those high in protein, such as eggs, fish, legumes, meat, milk, and poultry. Plant food sources include Brussels sprouts, cabbage, garlic, onions, and turnips.

No deficiency symptoms for sulfur have been established.

Zinc is one of the most important mineral nutrients and is necessary for the proper function of over two hundred enzymatic reactions in the body. It also acts as a potent antioxidant and detoxifier and is essential for growth and development, healthy body tissues, regulation of insulin, proper immune function, and in men, the health of the prostate gland. In addition, zinc plays a vital role in cellular membrane structure and function and helps maintain adequate levels of vitamin A in the body.

The best food sources of zinc include herring, shellfish (especially oysters), egg yolk, milk, and beef and other meats. Whole grain breads and cereals, nuts, and brewer's yeast are other food sources. Zinc deficiency is quite common, with vegetarians having a particularly high risk unless they consume adequate amounts of whole grains and other non-animal foods containing zinc.

Symptoms of zinc deficiency include impaired energy production and protein synthesis and suboptimal formation of collagen. Other symptoms include dermatitis, fatigue, greater risk of environmental sensitivity, hair loss, impaired immune function, diminished libido, and greater risk of prostatic conditions.

Note: Zinc can interfere with copper absorption, therefore zinc and copper supplements should be taken separately from each other.

CONDITIONS THAT BENEFIT FROM NUTRITIONAL MEDICINE

Holistic physicians recognize that the problematic symptoms of nearly all chronic illnesses, both physiological and psychological, can be alleviated once patients upgrade to a healthier diet and receive nutrients adequate to their needs. They also employ diet and nutrition preventively, both to ensure against disease and to help their patients achieve optimal health. Thousands of scientific studies support the use of nutrients for achieving and maintaining health. "The rationale for using nutritional medicine extends beyond the rather obvious fact that refined, processed foods grown on depleted soil are low in vitamins and minerals," Dr. Gaby says. "Even people who consume the most nutritious diets, particularly people suffering from illness, can often benefit from nutritional medicine."

Among the reasons that nutritional medicine can benefit so many people, according to Dr. Gaby, is its ability to:

compensate for a weak digestive system
overcome defects in the transportation of nutrients in body tissues
compensate for genetic deficiencies, including genetically abnormal enzymes
overcome the effects of environmental pollution
correct nutritional deficiencies caused by prescription drugs

make use of direct chemical or pharmacological effects of specific nutrients, such as vitamin C, vitamin B_{12}, and magnesium

Nutritional medicine offers many preventive and therapeutic benefits for most disease conditions, as well. What follows is a sampling of specific nutrients and the disease conditions for which research has shown them to be beneficial.

Vitamin A: acne, alcoholism, anorexia, birth defects (preventive), cancer, Crohn's disease, cystic fibrosis, ear infections, eczema, immune dysfunction (infectious disease), infant mortality, infertility, kidney stones, measles, peptic ulcer, stroke, vision problems (conjunctivitis, eye inflammation, night blindness, etc.), wound healing, ulcerative colitis.

Vitamin B_1 (thiamine): alcoholism, Alzheimer's disease, ataxia, cardiovascular disease, coronary disease, cirrhosis (and other forms of liver disease), age-related dementia and depression, epilepsy, fatigue, memory impairment due to alcohol abuse or aging, stress.

Vitamin B_2 (riboflavin): alcoholism, anemia, depression, migraine, sickle cell disease.

Vitamin B_3 (niacin): alcoholism, anxiety, atherosclerosis, coronary artery disease, diabetes, hyperlipidemia, hypertension, ischemic heart disease, pellagra, schizophrenia.

Vitamin B_5 (pantothenic acid): alcoholism, birth defects (preventive).

Vitamin B_6 (pyridoxine): anemia, asthma, behavioral and mood disorders, cardiovascular disease, carpal tunnel syndrome, coronary heart disease, diabetes, immune dysfunction, premenstrual syndrome (PMS).

Vitamin B_9 (folic acid): anemia, arthritis, birth defects, cancer (preventive), cardiovascular disease, cervical dysplasia, coronary heart disease, gingivitis, kidney disease, multiple sclerosis.

Vitamin B_{12} (cobalamin): anemia, dementia, hepatitis, mouth ulcers (aphthae), multiple sclerosis, sleep disorders.

Vitamin C: alcoholism, angina, arthritis, asthma, cancer, cardiovascular disease, cataracts, cervical dysplasia, common cold, coronary heart disease, Crohn's disease, diabetes, ear infections, eczema, fatigue, gallstones, glaucoma, gout, hepatitis, herpes simplex, high cholesterol, immune dysfunction, infertility, irritable bowel syndrome, lupus, macular degeneration, migraine, obesity, Paget's disease (skeletal disease), pancreatitis, Parkinson's disease, periodontal disease, premature aging, psoriasis, respiratory conditions, schizophrenia, shingles, sickle cell anemia, stroke, tetanus, ulcerative colitis, wound healing.

Calcium: anemia, calcium pancreatitis, colorectal cancer (preventive), dental conditions, hip fracture, hypertension, osteoporosis, urinary tract infections.

Carotenoids: atherosclerosis (preventive), cancer, high cholesterol, immune dysfunction, cataracts, macular degeneration related to aging.

Choline: headache, head injury, hemiplegia (paralysis due to stroke), memory loss, neurological dysfunction, seizure, stroke, tardive dyskinesia (involuntary muscle movement).

Chromium: cardiovascular disease, diabetes, high cholesterol, obesity.

Copper: arthritis, atherosclerosis (preventive), brain and nerve dysfunctions, Crohn's disease, diabetes, high cholesterol, impaired immunity, infertility, lupus.

Vitamin D: cancer, kidney stones, osteoporosis, psoriasis.

Vitamin E: alcoholism, Alzheimer's disease, anemia, arthritis, ataxia, brain injury, cancer, canker sores, cataracts, cervical dysplasia, Crohn's disease, cystic fibrosis, diabetes, epilepsy, hearing loss, hepatitis, herpes simplex, hypertension, immune dysfunction, kidney disease, leg cramps, lupus, multiple sclerosis, neurological conditions, osteoarthritis, Parkinson's disease, peripheral neuropathy, premature aging, PMS, pulmonary conditions, respiratory conditions, recurrent infection, stress, tardive dyskinesia, thyroid conditions, tuberculosis, ulcerative colitis, wound healing.

Iron: anemia, canker sores, fatigue, infertility, low birth weight and premature births, recurrent infections, ulcerative colitis.

Magnesium: angina, attention deficit hyperactivity disorder (ADHD), asthma, atherosclerosis, birth defects (preventive), cardiovascular disease, chronic fatigue syndrome, diabetes, epilepsy, gastrointestinal conditions, hypertension, kidney stones, migraine, nausea, mood problems, muscle tremor, osteoporosis, PMS, respiratory conditions, ulcerative colitis.

Manganese: diabetes, epilepsy, osteoporosis.

Omega-3 fatty acids: arthritis, cancer, cardiovascular disease, coronary heart disease, diabetes.

Potassium: atherosclerosis, hypertension, water retention.

Selenium: acne, atherosclerosis (preventive), cancer, cardiovascular disease, cervical dysplasia, herpes simplex, high cholesterol, impaired immune function, infertility, lupus, macular degeneration, osteo- and rheumatoid arthritis, recurrent infections, shingles.

Zinc: acne, ADHD, atherosclerosis (preventive), birth defects (preventive), benign prostate hyperplasia (BPH), canker sores, Crohn's disease, diabetes, ear infections, eczema, herpes simplex, impaired immune function, infertility, lupus, macular degeneration, osteoporosis, peptic ulcer, recurrent infection, rheumatoid arthritis, ulcerative colitis.

Caution: The above sampling of nutrients is not intended as a self-care guide for treating disease. If you suffer from a serious disease condition, seek professional medical attention.

HEALING HEART DISEASE:
❦ A CASE HISTORY ❦

The health results that can be achieved when patients receive the proper amount of nutrients specific to their needs is often remarkable, as the following case history involving one of Dr. Gaby's patients illustrates.

The patient in question was a seventy-nine-year-old rabbi who came to Dr. Gaby after suffering four heart attacks that left his heart badly damaged and in the final stages of congestive heart failure. "This necessitated his having to spend most of the previous year in the hospital, since his health was going relentlessly downhill," Dr. Gaby explains. "Like many patients with congestive heart failure, he also suffered from dramatic weight loss, dropping from 171 to 113 pounds, leaving him severely emaciated. His cardiac ejection fraction, the percentage of blood ejected into circulation with each beat of the heart, was only 19 percent and barely enough to keep him alive. As a result, he was confined to bed and required supplemental oxygen much of the time. To make matters worse, his peripheral circulation had deteriorated so badly that six of his toes had become gangrenous. As his condition progressed, even maximum doses of morphine taken every three hours could barely alleviate the severe pain in his toes."

Prior to seeing Dr. Gaby, the rabbi had been evaluated by two cardiologists, both of whom had recommended that his legs be amputated above the knees in order to prevent bacteria from his gangrenous tissue from entering his bloodstream and killing him. But even with the operation, they believed that he only had another month at best to live. It was after refusing their advice that the rabbi first came to Dr. Gaby seeking nutritional therapy. Because of the severity of his condition, Dr. Gaby began his treatment by using orthomolecular medicine (see "Orthomolecular Medicine" earlier in this chapter). "I gave him intravenous injections of magnesium, B-complex vitamins, and trace minerals, as well as large oral doses of vitamins C and E, plus folic acid and certain other nutrients," Dr. Gaby says.

Within six weeks, the rabbi began to improve dramatically. "His pain diminished, he no longer required supplemental oxygen, and his cardiac ejection fraction nearly doubled to 36 percent," Dr. Gaby reports. As Dr. Gaby's treatment continued, the gangrenous tissue around the rabbi's toes sloughed off, to be replaced by pink, healthy tissue. He also began to regain weight, a feat his cardiologists had considered impossible, given the severity of his condition prior to consulting with Dr. Gaby. "Both of his cardiologists were so convinced that his weight loss was irreversible that when the rabbi started to regain weight, they told him it was because his lungs were filling up with fluid," Dr. Gaby says. "But over the next twelve months, he continued to gain 34 additional pounds of healthy tissue and muscle, with his lungs remaining clear of fluid throughout that time. He was also able to keep his legs, and his heart remained reasonably healthy for the rest of his life." With additional maintenance nutritional treatment, the rabbi greatly exceeded his doctors' estimates of survival by living for another eight years.

"Although nutritional medicine doesn't always achieve such dramatic results as this," Dr. Gaby says, summarizing the rabbi's case, "it's common for individuals suffering from a wide range of disease conditions to gain relief from their symptoms from nutritional medicine and other holistic measures, even after conventional methods have been exhausted and failed." ❧

GUIDELINES FOR USING NUTRITIONAL MEDICINE

While the therapeutic use of diet and nutritional supplements is generally safe and, in many cases, can be adapted as part of an overall self-care regimen, for best results it is advisable to seek the professional assistance of a holistic physician or nutritional therapist to ensure that your nutrient needs are optimally met. The following guidelines can assist you in receiving the fullest benefit from a dietary and nutritional program.

For best results, eat healthily. No amount of nutritional supplementation can take the place of a diet of nutrient-dense foods. To ensure good health, follow the dietary recommendations provided earlier in this chapter in "Holistic Guidelines for Healthy Eating," as well as in Chapter 2. Also take care not to overcook your foods, since high temperature can destroy even the healthiest foods' nutrient content.

Read the label. Since not all brands of nutritional supplements are the same in terms of quality, efficacy, and price, it is important to know the quality of the brand you are buying. By reading the label of the supplements you purchase, you can determine their dosage range and whether the supplements also contain fillers, binders, and other additives of no nutritional value, and to which you might be allergic or sensitive, such as sugars or gluten. (Generally safe additives include alginic acid, cellulose, calcium or magnesium stearate, dicalcium phosphate, gum acacia, and silica.) Labels usually also contain instructions for how nutrients should best be consumed to optimize their effectiveness. Reputable companies typically list all ingredients in their nutritional formulas and, upon request, are usually willing to also provide further information regarding their efficacy.

Know when and how to take your supplements. As a general rule, vitamin and mineral supplements are best taken during meals or fifteen minutes before or after eating, in order to enhance their assimilation. This is especially true of fat-soluble vitamins, which ideally should also be taken during the meal of the day with the highest fat content. Overall, however, most vitamin and mineral supplements are best taken with the first meal of the day.

Amino acid supplements, on the other hand, are best taken at least an hour before or after meals. To promote their absorption, take them with fruit juice. In addition, single amino acids should be supplemented with a complete amino acid formula for best results.

Similarly, single B vitamins should be consumed only with a total B-complex supplement, while minerals are best taken as part of a complete multivitamin/mineral formula.

When using high dosages of vitamin C and B-complex vitamins, take them in divided doses throughout the day, rather than all at one time.

Beware of "megadosing." Certain nutrients, including all fat-soluble vitamins and certain minerals and B-complex vitamins, can be toxic in high doses. To avoid the risk of toxicity, avoid taking high doses of nutrients unless you do so under the guidance of a physician trained in their use.

Pay attention to any reactions following supplementation. If you experience nausea or other side effects after taking supplements, immediately discontinue their use. In many cases, such reactions are due to excessive dosages or symptoms of detoxification provoked by supplementation and will cease once supplementation is discontinued. But if symptoms persist, seek medical attention.

Consult with your physician before mixing supplements with medication. While most supplements taken in moderate doses are generally safe, certain nutrients can be contraindicated when used with prescribed medications. Iron tablets, for instance, should not be taken when using antibiotics. To ensure safety, always consult with a nutritionally oriented physician prior to beginning any supplementation program.

Be consistent. Irregular use of nutritional supplements provides little or no benefit, since the benefits of diet and proper nutrition are cumulative and accrue over time. By following a daily supplement routine, you can ensure that your body regularly receives the nutritional support it requires to properly perform its many functions.

FUTURE OF NUTRITIONAL MEDICINE

Today, the amount of research devoted to investigating the roles diet and nutritional supplementation can play in preventing and reversing disease, as well as extending longevity and creating optimal health, is greater than ever before. As a result, increasing numbers of conventional physicians are joining their holistic counterparts in recommending dietary and nutritional approaches to their patients. Moreover, an expanding sector of the lay population in the United States, as well as abroad, is now recognizing the value proper nutrition has for overall health, as evidenced by the steady increase in consumer purchases of nutritional supplements in recent years, almost all of which were paid for out-of-pocket. Based on such trends, it seems certain that nutritional medicine will increasingly become a centerpiece of both conventional and holistic health care throughout the twenty-first century.

RESOURCES

To learn more about the role diet and nutrition can play in health, contact the following organizations.

American College of Nutrition
722 Robert E. Lee Drive
Wilmington, Delaware 28480

Phone: (252) 452-1222
Web site: *www.am-coll-nutr.org*

American Aging Association (AGE)
The Sally Balin Medical Center
110 Chelsey Drive
Media, Pennsylvania 19063
Phone: (610) 627-2626
Fax: (610) 565-9747
E-mail: ameraging@aol.com
Web site: *www.globalimpression.com*
(AGE was founded by, and carries on the research of, Dr. Denham
 Harman.)

Council for Responsible Nutrition
1875 Eye Street, NW, Suite 400
Washington, D.C. 20006
Phone: (202) 872-1488
Fax: (202) 872-9594
E-mail: webmaster@crnusa.org
Web site: *www.crnusa.org*

Council for Science in the Public Interest
1875 Connecticut Avenue NW, Suite 300
Washington, D.C. 20009
Phone: (202) 332-9110
Fax: (202) 265-4954

RECOMMENDED READING

Bland, Jeffrey, with Sara Benum. *Genetic Nutritioneering.* Keats Publishing, 1999.
Garrison, Robert, and Elizabeth Somer. *The Nutrition Desk Reference.* 3d ed. Keats Publishing, 1997.
Holford, Patrick. *The Optimum Nutrition Bible.* The Crossing Press, 1999.
Pearson, Durk, and Sandy Shaw. *Life Extension.* Warner Books, 1982.
Werbach, Melvyn. *Nutritional Influences on Illness.* Third Line Press, 1992.
Wright, Jonathan, and Alan Gaby. *The Patient's Book of Natural Healing.* Prima Publishing, 1999.

CHAPTER 4

Environmental Medicine

Environmental medicine is a significantly expanded outgrowth of the pioneering work of Theron G. Randolph, M.D. Gary R. Oberg, M.D., F.A.A.P., F.A.A.E.M., describes it as "the health care strategy for the future, dedicated to the diagnosis, treatment, and prevention of environmentally triggered illnesses (ETI). Environmentally triggered illnesses are health problems that result from adverse interactions between a person and the environment and diet. This approach provides powerful insights and tools to improve the quality and cost-effectiveness of health care and is effective because it is proactive, cause-oriented, patient-centered, individualized, and preventive."

Dr. Oberg, a physician practicing in Crystal Lake, Illinois, is a leading educator in the field of environmental medicine and the chairman of the American Academy of Environmental Medicine (AAEM)'s Committee on Continuing Medical Education. The AAEM is a not-for-profit professional medical organization devoted to educating physicians and other health care professionals in the diagnosis, treatment, and prevention of diseases caused by environmental factors and the diet. There is also an American Board of Environmental Medicine (ABEM) that provides board certification for medical doctors (M.D.'s) and osteopaths (D.O.'s) who wish to become certified as experts in this approach. A variety of other health practitioners interested in applying this approach to their professions also attend the AAEM's educational courses, according to Dr. Oberg. These include dentists, naturopaths, chiropractors, nurses and nurse practitioners, clinical nutritionists, psychologists, social workers, and Ph.D.'s in various disciplines, among others. A number of them also join AAEM as associate members of the Academy, he says.

The range of illnesses that have been linked to the environment and diet is extensive and growing. These include many common pediatric diseases; eye, ear, nose, and throat conditions; skin conditions; autoimmune diseases; certain forms of mental illness; and symptoms in the body's cardiovascular, respiratory, endocrine, gastrointestinal, nervous, genitourinary, and musculoskeletal systems. According to Dr. Oberg, conventional medicine fails to fully address how environmental and dietary factors can contribute to such chronic disease conditions:

> The current medical model has assumed for many years that good health is the natural ongoing homeostatic state of the human body. The environment is seen as an essentially benign place that generally has little effect on health, and the diet is viewed simply as a passive source of fuels for the body's inherently stable metabolic functions. When physicians look for the cause of a chronic disease, this same assumption is applied. The potential roles of the environment and diet may be superficially acknowledged, but usually their importance to chronic disease is neither appreciated nor effectively accommodated in actual practice.
>
> Unfortunately, for the past several decades, there has been a rapidly increasing growth in the incidence of more complex and chronic diseases in our population that is directly due to environmental and dietary factors. Under the current medical model, treatment for these diseases has resulted in rapidly escalating costs, accompanied by a decrease in treatment response rates, and mounting dissatisfaction with the quality of life resulting from such care. Such treatment failures seem to result when too much emphasis is placed on the nature of the disease and just treating symptoms. Not enough attention is given to the causes and why the disease developed in the first place. Environmental medicine is a new, more comprehensive, cause-oriented model that was formed to correct this situation. The purpose of our field is to provide an entire medical health care paradigm that is patient-centered, preventive, proactive, and designed to discover the specific causes of each patient's illness and then correct the dysfunctions found in their various biological systems and their mechanisms.

❦ FAST FACTS ❦

Food allergy and sensitivity is one of the most commonly mis- or undiagnosed medical conditions in the United States. An estimated 10 to 30 percent of the population suffers from this form of environmentally triggered illness. Of this number, approximately 95 percent have not been properly identified and treated. Food allergies and sensitivities annually result in 3.4 million lost workdays in the United States, at an estimated cost of $639 million. Overall, Americans spend $2 billion each year on various forms of allergy treatments.

Furthermore, the average American spends 90 percent of each day indoors, breathing air that, according to the Environmental Protection Agency (EPA), can be as much as 100 times more polluted than outdoor air. According to the EPA, 60 percent of all Americans live in areas where poor air quality is a health risk.

An estimated 20,000 different types of pesticides are currently in use, with over 4 billion pounds used worldwide each year. Fifty percent of all pesticide use (2 billion pounds) occurs in the United States, resulting in related health care costs estimated at $780 million annually. Worldwide, 25 million people succumb to pesticide poisoning each year.

According to the EPA, 98 pesticides, and over 600 other chemicals, have been detected in U.S. drinking water since 1984. More than 400 toxic chemicals have also been identified in human tissue.

There are an estimated 80,000 chemicals regularly in use today, with an additional 1,000 to 2,000 chemicals added to this list each year. Only 3 percent of them have been tested to determine whether they are toxic or carcinogenic.

In 1998, the United States released approximately 500 billion tons of toxic chemicals into the environment. ❦

HISTORY OF ENVIRONMENTAL MEDICINE

The knowledge that both diet and the environment can affect health has been a basic tenet of a number of holistic therapies for centuries. Both Ayurveda and traditional Chinese medicine (see Chapters 12 and 13) have recognized the relationship between health and dietary and environmental factors since their inception thousands of years ago, and a patient's environment and diet are also taken into consideration by homeopathic physicians (see Chapter 11) when selecting patient remedies. Environmental medicine itself, however, is a thoroughly twentieth-century development that originated with, and has evolved in response to, the modern-day proliferation of chemicals in nearly all aspects of life, as well as modern farming and food production methods that have contributed to the average American's typically devitalized diet.

The founder of environmental medicine was Theron G. Randolph, M.D., a preeminent allergy specialist from Chicago, who also taught medicine at four medical schools, including Northwestern University, where he served as professor of Allergy and Immunology. Beginning in the 1940s, Dr. Randolph began to suspect that a wide range of his patients' disease conditions were due to allergies or sensitivities to the foods they ate regularly. To test his hypothesis, Dr. Randolph had his patients abstain from eating suspect foods for four days or more before reintroducing them into their diet. Through this method, Dr. Randolph discovered that offending foods could trigger a host of chronic diseases, including gastrointestinal disorders, respiratory disease, arthritis, depression, anxiety, headache, eczema, fatigue, and hyperactivity. Further experimentation on Dr. Randolph's part revealed that even small amounts of foods that others could tolerate without symptoms could cause illness in susceptible individuals. As a result, he pioneered a number of methods to test for food allergies.

In the 1950s, he started to investigate how chemical compounds, such as pesticides, solvents, food additives, natural gas, and car exhaust, were also capable of triggering chronic illness, and he was the first person to describe the concept of chemical sensitivity. Based on his findings, in 1962 Dr. Randolph published *Human Ecology and Susceptibility to the Chemical Environment*, the first textbook devoted to the subject of environmental medicine. Shortly afterwards, in 1965, a group of physicians influenced by Dr. Randolph's work formed the organization that eventually became the American Academy of Environmental Medicine (AAEM). Since its inception, the AAEM has continued its mission of educating physicians (primarily M.D.'s and D.O.'s) in the most effective ways of diagnosing, treating, and preventing environmentally triggered illness, as well as educating the public about how their diet and environment may be adversely affecting their health. In recent years, the AAEM has expanded Dr. Randolph's concepts to encompass the roles of all of the body's specific systems as they interact with one another and with the environment and diet.

DO YOU SUFFER FROM ENVIRONMENTALLY ❧ TRIGGERED ILLNESS? ❧

According to most practitioners of holistic medicine, the incidence of environmentally triggered illness (ETI) is much higher than is commonly believed. Part of the reason that ETI is so often undetected lies in the fact that a great many patients are unaware that they have ETI as the cause of their symptoms, or are unable to identify the substance, or substances, causing their symptoms. In addition, many physicians frequently miss the fact that ETI is the cause of many of their patients' chronic complaints. Substances that can cause ETI generally fall into one of several categories and include any substance or situation that has the potential to disrupt normal biological functions in a susceptible individual.

Biologically derived substances include *microorganisms:* bacteria, viruses, fungi, prions, and their by-products; *parasites:* amoebae, worms, and protozoa; *foods:* animals, plants, fungi, and their by-products; *organic inhalants:* dusts, molds, danders, and pollens of all types; and *chemicals:* inorganic and organic, natural and man-made. Other stressors include nutritional excesses and deficiencies, trauma, psychological stresses of all types, and physical phenomena such as heat, cold, humidity, barometric pressures, vibration, ionizing and non-ionizing radiation, and electromagnetic fields.

The following physical symptoms are often seen with an ETI: dark circles, swelling, or wrinkles under the eyes; runny or stuffy nose; postnasal drip; excessive mucus; watery eyes and/or blurred vision; ringing of the ears; recurrent ear infections; sinusitis; sore throats, hoarseness or chronic coughing; coated tongue; chest congestion; heart palpitations; vascular headaches; gagging; mucus or undigested food in the stool; nausea; vomiting; diarrhea; constipation; bloating after meals; flatulence; abdominal pains or cramping; extreme thirst; anal or vaginal itch; hives or rashes; dermatitis; brittle nails and hair; dry skin; dandruff; skin pallor; joint pain; frequent or urgent urination; symptoms of PMS; and obesity or weight fluctuations during the course of the day.

Psychological or neurological symptoms of ETI can manifest as unnatural or persistent fatigue or drowsiness, anxiety or panic attacks; depression, crying jags; aggressive behavior; irritability; mental dullness, concentration problems, or confusion; lethargy; excessive daydreaming; restlessness; poor work habits; slurred speech; diminished enthusiasm for life; faintness; dizziness; sleepiness soon after a meal; insomnia; and restless sleep.

If you suffer chronically from any of the above symptoms, you may have some form of an ETI. For definitive diagnosis and treatment, contact a member physician of the American Academy of Environmental Medicine (see the "Resources" section at the end of this chapter). 🌿

HOW ENVIRONMENTAL MEDICINE WORKS

"The model of environmental medicine recognizes that the human body is constantly coping with its dynamic environment via various innate and complex interrelated biological systems and their mechanisms that are designed to maintain overall homeodynamic functioning," Dr. Oberg explains. "The functions of these mechanisms are reversible, and their ongoing adjustments are unique to each individual and change continually over time. From the perspective of environmental medicine, substances in one's diet and the environment are viewed as potential stressors which are capable of destabilizing these homeodynamic functions, thereby causing disease." Dr. Oberg prefers the term *homeodynamic functioning* to the more commonly used *homeostasis* "because it reflects the fact that maintenance of optimal health is an active process rather than a passive one, and requires a continuous ongoing expenditure of metabolic energy. Homeodynamic functioning is a fundamental, inborn propensity of life itself. The mechanisms of all biological systems are designed to maintain ongoing stability of their functions despite constantly varying exposures to stressors from diet and the environment."

The Governing Principles of Environmental Medicine

In each patient, the ongoing manifestations of his or her environmentally triggered illness depend largely upon the dynamic interactions among the seven fundamental biological principles that govern ETI. These principles are biochemical individuality, individual susceptibility, the total load, the level of adaptation, the bipolarity of responses, the spreading phenomena, and the switch phenomena.

Biochemical individuality recognizes that each individual is unique, both in terms of his or her genetic makeup, and his or her acquired nutritional status. "Each individual has a unique genetic endowment that profoundly affects the function of each and every organ system and its biological mechanisms," Dr. Oberg explains. "Additionally, each person has a unique combination of nutrient fuels present in his or her body that is determined by the adequacy of his or her ongoing diet. Moreover, both the clinical expression of each person's genetic programming, and the quality of his or her nutritional status vary dynamically over time in a manner that is unique to each individual." This principle explains why one individual may experience health problems following exposure to a small amount of a specific triggering agent, such as formaldehyde, and another person has no reaction at all to the same amount of the same substance. This principle underscores why environmental medicine requires customizing the diagnosis and treatment of each individual.

Individual susceptibility recognizes that in a group of patients who are all susceptible to the same stressor, each will have a unique clinical response to the stressor. For example, if two people are both sensitive to a mold, one may react with a runny nose, while the other may become hyperactive or fatigued. Also, in a group of patients who all share the same clinical symptom, each will have a unique set of stressors that can trigger that symptom. For example, if two patients have asthma, one may wheeze from dust while the other wheezes from wheat products.

The total load refers to the sum total at any given point in time of all an individual's exposures to all of the stressors, both external and internal, to which that person is individually susceptible. "The categories of possible stressors that are part of a person's daily total load include all biological, chemical, social, psychological, and spiritual stressors, all physical phenomena, and trauma," Dr. Oberg says. Each individual's total load is unique and is in a continuous state of flux over time. As a result, ETI-related reactions and symptoms can vary, as well.

The level of adaptation refers to the body's attempts to maintain healthy homeodynamic functioning in the face of changing environmental conditions and stressors. "Upon exposure to a stressor, an individual will respond within a range of several dynamically reversible stages, ranging from a state of nonsusceptibility to irreversible end-stage system damage or even organ failure," Dr. Oberg says. "The stage of adaptation that a person is in will determine his or her clinical response to a stressor at that time."

There are three stages of adaptation within the model of environmental medicine. The first stage has two substages *preadapted*, in which there is no previous exposure to a stressor, and *nonadapted alarm*, which refers to the first-time response to a stressor and is characterized by a rapid response by the body's appropriate mechanisms to stop and reverse all adverse effects the stressor is causing. During this initial stage, the individual is able to perceive the cause-and-effect relationship between the stressor and its adverse effects on the body.

The second level of adaptation also has two substages. The first is known as *adapted*, or *masked*. "Here, appropriate mechanisms automatically upregulate to deal with a stressor and prevent it from causing any adverse reactions," Dr. Oberg explains. "In this stage, the individual has no symptoms and does not perceive that the stressor is even burdening biological mechanisms; that is, the potentially harmful nature of the stressor is masked from the person's awareness." This stage continues as long as the exposure to the stressor is ongoing, and the mechanisms to neutralize it are not depleted of their required nutrient fuels. However, if the exposure is too great for the body to handle, or if the mechanisms' nutrient supplies become exhausted, the effectiveness of the body's mechanisms to prevent adverse reactions to stressors breaks down, and *maladaptation*, the second substage, occurs. This is the point at which nutrient fuels become depleted, and the individual begins to perceive pathological symptoms. Sufficient maladaptation will result in the occurrence of acute symptoms of illness, and this is considered by the patient to be the onset of the present disease condition. Symptoms are still reversible at this stage.

Stage three, known as the *nonadapted state of exhaustion*, is characterized by clinical symptoms based upon how much damage has been done to the various biological mechanisms affected by the total load of stressors. Nutrient fuels continue to be depleted, and irreversible end organ and system damage, and even death, may result.

When the body's response to a potential stressor is returned to the state of nonadapted alarm, where an acute reaction will occur to a challenge exposure to the stressor, this is known as *de-adaptation*. "De-adaptation is achieved by completely avoiding the stressor for at least several days before giving a diagnostic challenge of it," Dr. Oberg explains. "This must be done to accurately assess the state of susceptibility to a particular stressor, and is the reason behind elimination and challenge protocols which are used to assess true susceptibility. If a substance is challenged while the person is still adapted to it, no symptoms will occur, and the true potentially dangerous susceptibility to it will be missed."

Bipolarity of responses refers to the way a biological mechanism responds when challenged with exposure to a stressor. There are two forms of bipolarity. Phase I bipolarity occurs in all three stages of adaptation and is characterized by stimulation followed by withdrawal. Stimulation (upregulation or an increasing level of biological activity) occurs when the acute exposure to a stressor stimulates the body's appropriate biological mechanisms to neutralize the stressor's potentially harmful effects. Withdrawal (downregulation, or a decreasing level of biological activity) occurs when the removal of the stressor and its adverse effects allows the involved biological mechanisms to wind down.

Phase II bipolarity occurs only in the third stage of adaptation, which is characterized by end-stage organ damage. Clinical symptoms of phase II bipolarity are determined by the depletion of the biological mechanisms' nutrient fuels and the effects of end-stage organ damage. During this phase, stimulatory and withdrawal functions continue within the remaining capabilities of the involved biological mechanisms. "In phase II bipolarity, the timing of clinical symptoms is influenced more by the malfunctioning status of the compromised or damaged biological mechanisms and the effects of end-stage organ damage, than by the timing of the presence or absence of the stressors themselves," Dr. Oberg says. "This makes it more difficult to recognize that the stressors are what are actually causing the illness."

Spreading phenomenon manifests itself in two ways. The first type refers to the acute or chronic spreading of susceptibility over time to previously tolerated stressors; for example, over time, the list of stressors that makes a person ill may increase from just dust to include molds, foods, and chemicals. The second type of spreading phenomenon refers to the acute or chronic spreading of susceptibility over time to new target organs or body systems; for example, over time, a person's symptoms may go from just a runny nose to include asthma, fatigue, and irritable bowel. According to Dr. Oberg, both types of the spreading phenomenon generally occur while biological mechanisms are maladapting to a total load overload. "Appreciation for this biological principle allows one to understand the preventive power of such activities as maintaining a clean environment and a good diet," he notes. "As the saying goes, 'A stitch in time saves nine.'"

The switch phenomenon is the clinical pattern that occurs as the individual's symptoms switch back and forth over time from one target organ or body system to another. This phenomenon may occur acutely or more slowly over time and is further modified by the individual's total load and level of adaptation. The physician's chronological history, so critical to an appropriate environmental medicine workup, helps to identify a pattern of symptom switching over time. According to the model of environmental medicine, nine levels of clinical manifestations may present themselves over time:

Level +4: Manic (with or without convulsion)
Level +3: Hypomanic (toxic, anxious, egocentric)
Level +2: Hyperactive (irritable, agitated, hungry, thirsty)
Level +1: Stimulated, but relatively symptom-free
Level 0: "On an even keel"
Level −1: Localized reactions (rhinitis, asthma, colitis, etc.)
Level −2: Systemic reactions (fatigue, vasculitis, myalgia, etc.)
Level −3: Moderate depression, brain fog, aphasia
Level −4: Severe depression (with or without altered consciousness)

Practitioners of environmental medicine take all of the above principles into consideration in order to properly diagnose the underlying cause, or causes, of their patients' health complaints, as well as devising treatment plans that are tailor-made for each patient's specific needs. "The goal of treatment is to restore patients to a pre-illness level of functioning and to improve their tolerance to the stressors that previously caused adverse reactions," Dr. Oberg explains. "In addition, through education, patients learn to develop and adopt appropriate lifestyles to prevent the recurrence and development of new illnesses."

Dr. Oberg points out that several major requirements must be met by a patient's physician or other health care professional in order for patients to benefit consistently from environmental medicine. "The first requirement is that the physician must know how and when to supplement the current model of conventional medicine with the environmental medicine model, as dictated by the needs of each patient," he says. "This involves determining when the use of temporary symptomatic drugs alone may be appropriate, and when it is necessary to actively seek the actual nature of the disease in order to identify and correct its actual causes. In the case of acute and self-limiting diseases, it is often appropriate to employ drugs to minimize the patient's symptoms until the body's own homeodynamic functions recover from the acute illness and restore health again."

In cases of chronic or more complex illnesses, however, a different approach is usually necessary. "When treating illness that has become more chronic and not self-limiting, it is more useful to identify the specific biological dysfunctions that are present," Dr. Oberg says. "Rather than just masking symptoms, the goal is to repair whatever dysfunctions are discovered to be present in order to return the mechanisms to their proper homeodynamic state, so that health may be restored."

In order to properly diagnose the true nature of their patients' illnesses, environmental physicians are also trained to test for the complex range of potential external and internal stressors that can contribute to ETI, as well as to understand and assess the functional status of the body's many biological mechanisms, Dr. Oberg adds. "The physician must appreciate the true complexity of the relationships between biological mechanisms and the environment and diet as they interact to create either health or disease," he says.

Once the physician has made a diagnosis and a determination as to its underlying causes, the goal is to devise an effective treatment plan that addresses each patient's individual situation. "Treatment modalities should be those that are the most cost-effective, convenient, and useful for restoring the patient to good health and preventing further disease," Dr. Oberg says. "In addition, the physician must be able to educate patients about the dynamic natures of their illnesses in a clear and useful manner. This is necessary because there is no more powerful way for a patient to control his or her chronic disease than to understand its very nature, and to be able to manipulate its causes to reverse and prevent it."

Diagnostic Techniques

Environmental medicine physicians use a variety of diagnostic techniques to determine the underlying nature of their patients' illnesses. These include a comprehensive history, physical examination, diagnostic in vitro and in vivo laboratory tests, dietary testing, skin testing, and diagnostic medical imaging techniques.

Comprehensive history. Each diagnosis begins with a comprehensive patient history, which Dr. Oberg says is the most important part of the evaluation. To be effective, the history must be chronological, sufficiently detailed, and focused on the dietary and environmental factors that can play a role in ETI. During the history, patients will be asked to list chronologically all previous health problems they have had throughout their lives and any patterns in timing, location, or triggering substances, as well as questions about their diet and home and work environments and any physical, mental, or emotional stresses they may be exposed to. In addition, histories of family members are also included, to determine genetic predisposition to specific diseases, as well as the patient's individual susceptibility to ETI.

Physical examination. The physical exam helps to assess the patient's current degree of organ system dysfunction, with each organ system examined in light of the patient's comprehensive history. This allows physical clues to dysfunction and any fixed end-stage organ damage to be detected. According to Dr. Oberg, physical signs of dysfunction will depend on the organ system involved, the severity of involvement, the patient's total load, level of adaptation, type and virulence of the stressors involved, and the patient's nutrititional status at the time.

Diagnostic in vitro and in vivo laboratory techniques. Various diagnostic in vitro tests measure the current status of the various biological mechanisms of the body's organ systems, as well as the patient's nutritional status. For allergies, quantitative in vitro serum antigen-specific antibody assays (IgE, IgG) may also be employed, using a variety of techniques (MAST, RAST, ELISA, etc.) as well as live cell bioassays and environmental testing, in order to detect a variety of allergens, such as pollens, molds, dust, and foods. Functional in vivo laboratory tests are also used to assess the status of the biological mechanisms of the patient's various organ systems, as well as his or her nutrient status. Among the biological mechanisms that are evaluated using these tests are energy production, detoxification mechanisms, reproductive mechanisms, and the mechanisms of building, repair, and maintenance (anabolic, catabolic, anti-inflammatory, and pro-inflammatory).

Dietary testing. Undiagnosed food susceptibility is often implicated in ETI. For this reason, environmental physicians include a history of the patient's diet as part of the comprehensive history and may also ask their patients to keep a diet diary to record the foods they eat and any subsequent reactions. The most accurate way to assess a patient's susceptibility, according to Dr. Oberg, is the elimination/challenge diet, which involves having patients avoid eating all foods for which allergy or sensitivity is suspected for four days and then eating an oral challenge meal of each food one at a time, one per day. There are a variety of elimination dietary approaches, ranging from complete fasts to avoidance of only the most common food allergen groups (milk, dairy products, wheat, corn, citrus fruits, sugars, coffee, and alcohol, as well as food additives). Suspected foods are completely eliminated for three to seven days and then reintroduced one at a time, to see if their reintroduction provokes symptoms. This reintroduction process is known as a food challenge. As offending foods are identified, they are then avoided altogether or eaten on a rotation of one out of four days, depending on the severity of the reaction they provoke.

Skin testing. There are two categories of skin tests, nonquantitative and quantitative. Nonquantitative skin tests include the scratch test (generally not recommended), prick test, and the single strength intradermal test. The nonquantitative test forms have significant limitations to their usefulness. Quantitative skin tests are preferred, and include intradermal serial dilution end point titration (SDET); provocation/neutralization testing (P/N), which can be administered intradermally or sublingually; maximum tolerated intradermal dose testing (MTID); and enzyme potentiated desensitization (EPD). SDET skin testing is effective for determining sensitivity to inhalant allergens. P/N, MTID, and EPD help diagnose food sensitivity as well as inhalant sensitivity.

Diagnostic medical imaging techniques. Two types of medical imaging techniques can be used: static and functional. Static tests include sinus x-rays, sinus CAT scans, and magnetic resonance imaging (MRI), while functional tests include PET or SPECT scans of the brain, and computerized EEGs. In rare circumstances, diagnostic surgical techniques may also be used.

Types of Therapies

"The practice of environmental medicine is both strategic and comprehensive, rather than a limited treatment modality," Dr. Oberg says. "In addition to being customized to the specific needs of each patient, the therapies employed by practitioners of environmental medicine are also proactive, and emphasize early assessment and proper intervention to maintain each patient's optimal physical, mental/emotional, and spiritual well-being."

The goals of environmental medical treatment include:

ongoing optimal nutritional and metabolic functioning
adoption of lifestyles intended to minimize as much as possible exposure
    to all identified stressors
improvement of the biological mechanisms of all organ systems

significant reduction or elimination of acute and chronic symptoms in all
  involved mechanisms and organ systems
improved tolerance to all stressors that previously caused symptoms; sustained optimal physical, neuro/cognitive, psychological, social, and
  spiritual well-being
improvement in the patient's ability to carry out the tasks of daily living
  (employment, school attendance, etc.)
adoption of a lifestyle designed to prevent the development of new illnesses

"The best outcomes will be achieved by a cooperative partnership
consisting of a well-educated and motivated patient working with a
physician and staff well trained in the principles and practices of environmental medicine," Dr. Oberg advises.

To achieve these goals practitioners of environmental medicine
might use some of the following treatment therapies.

Patient education refers to the attention practitioners of environmental medicine give to educating their patients about the various factors
that may be causing their illnesses, as well as their treatment options, and
any dietary and lifestyle changes they can make to help regain their
health. "The most important thing that physicians in our field have to
offer patients is the knowledge of what is going on with them, and the
multiple levels of opportunities they have for dealing with their conditions," Dr. Oberg says. "This is the heart of what being a doctor involves,
since the word itself is derived from the Latin verb 'docere,' meaning 'to
teach.' There is no more powerful way for patients to control chronic
disease than to understand its very nature and to be empowered to know
how to manipulate its causes to reverse and prevent it. And the best way
to achieve that is for the patient to have an ongoing and dynamic partnership with a physician who is well trained and experienced in the practice of environmental medicine."

Therapeutic customized diets are tailored to each patient's specific
health care needs and designed to provide optimal nutrition, reverse
nutritional deficiencies, and address diet-related problems such as food
allergies and sensitivities and food-borne toxins. In addition to a whole
foods diet, the physician might prescribe nutritional supplements, as well
as a rotation diet, in which the patient eats specific foods four or more
days apart to reduce triggering susceptibility. Foods that patients are
found to be reacting to are rotated if tolerated this way or avoided altogether for at least three to six months.

Detoxification therapies are employed when the patient is found to have an overload of toxins stored in various tissues. Toxins can include pesticides, volatile organic hydrocarbons, heavy metals, and various other chemical compounds. When the body is overburdened by toxins, its biological functions become impaired, diminishing its ability to heal itself. Detoxification therapies can be taken orally, as when nutritional supplements, herbal remedies, or homeopathic formulas are employed, or be administered intravenously, intramuscularly, or injected beneath the skin. Exercise, massage, sauna, and hyperthermia (the application of heat) can also help to stimulate the removal of toxins from body tissues and organs.

Nutritional therapy involves the judicious balanced use of various nutrients, such as vitamins, minerals, amino acids, and fatty acids, tailored to each patient's unique biochemistry, nutritional status, and current overall health status. "The goal of nutritional therapy is to correct or enhance specific biological functions, including the detoxification, antioxidation, and anti-inflammatory pathways," Dr. Oberg explains.

Immunotherapy involves the use of customized vaccines composed of specific inhalants, foods, chemical, or other compounds, in order to build up patient tolerance to such substances. Immunotherapy is especially useful for helping patients deal with dietary and environmental stressors that they cannot easily avoid. By taking customized treatment doses determined by quantitative testing techniques, adverse reactions can be decreased or eliminated fairly quickly as patient tolerance is increased. Typically, the immunotherapy vaccines are administered as subcutaneous (under the skin) injections, or taken sublingually (under the tongue as drops).

Psychotherapy or counseling can be prescribed in cases where patients are suffering from an illness-related emotional overload, in order to enhance their neurocognitive, psychological, social, and spiritual well-being, according to Dr. Oberg.

Environmental controls refer to the various protocols designed by environmental medicine physicians in partnership with their patients in order to achieve clean air, water, and food. The goal of such controls is to decrease or eliminate the "fuel supply" of stressors that patients come in contact with in both their work and home environments, in order to increase the likelihood of a full return to health.

Pharmaceutical drugs are another treatment option regularly used by environmental medicine physicians, especially in cases of illness that are acute or self-limiting. "The purpose of pharmaceuticals from the model of environmental medicine is to relieve patient symptoms while the underlying causes of their illnesses are being found and corrected," Dr. Oberg says. "However, the potential for adverse reactions when using drugs must always be remembered, as well as the fact that they tend to be far less useful for treating complex and chronic illness."

The above therapies are used to achieve the therapeutic goals of environmental medicine, which focus on detoxifying the body, improving biological function, and eliminating or minimizing the effects of environmental and dietary stressors. The therapies themselves range in complexity, with some of them being as safe and simple to employ as self-care approaches, while others should be administered only under the care of a physician well-trained in their use. How any particular therapy should be employed is best decided after a full examination and consultation with an experienced practitioner of environmental medicine. Since it is rare for the health problems of patients suffering from ETI to be due to a single environmental or dietary stressor, treatment is most effective when patients are willing to participate in treatment protocols that address all contributing causes, including making any necessary changes in their lifestyles, diets, and home and work environments.

CONDITIONS THAT BENEFIT FROM ENVIRONMENTAL MEDICINE

Because of modern society's ongoing exposure to more and more chemical compounds, as well as the increasing proliferation of devitalized foods and commercial farming methods that rely on pesticides, preservatives, and other chemical agents, potentially any health condition can fall under the category of environmentally triggered illnesses. "While diseases are not always the result of ETI, physicians should be alert to this possibility, especially when patient histories suggest the likelihood that environmental or dietary stressors are involved in their conditions," Dr. Oberg advises. "When an illness is determined to be due to one or more components of ETI, the primary goal of treatment should be correcting the underlying causes, with symptom care being used adjunctively as appropriate."

According to Dr. Oberg, the primary categories of illness that can result from environmental stressors are cancer; cardiovascular disease (angina, arrhythmia, edema, fluid retention, hypertension, migraine headache, myocardial infarctions, thrombophlebitis, vasculitis); endocrine disorders (fibrocystic breast disease, premenstrual syndrome, thyroid dysfunction); eye, ear, and throat disorders (blurred vision, conjunctivitis, eczema of the eyelids, frequent colds, hearing loss, laryngeal edema, Ménière's disease, otitis media, photophobia, pressure in the ear, rhinitis, sinusitis, tinnitus, vertigo); gastrointestinal disorders (chronic gastritis, Crohn's disease, eosinophilic gastroenteritis, gastric and duodenal ulcers, gut flora dysbiosis, ileitis, infantile enterocolitis, irritable bowel syndrome, malabsorption syndromes, mouth ulcers, ulcerative colitis); genitourinary conditions (chronic cystitis, dysmenorrhea, enuresis, glomerulonephritis, infertility, nephrotic syndrome, recurrent vaginitis, vulvodynia); hematologic disorders (certain anemias, thrombocytopenia); neurobehavioral and psychiatric disorders (anxiety, attention deficit disorder, bipolar disorder, eating disorders, irritability, panic disorders, schizophrenia, sexual dysfunction, somatoform disorders, spaciness); neurological conditions (Alzheimer's disease, cognitive and memory disorders, fatigue, multiple sclerosis, Parkinson's disease, seizure disorders, sleep disorders); pulmonary conditions (asthma, chronic bronchitis, certain pneumonias); rheumatologic disorders (arthralgia, fibromyalgia, lupus erythematosus, myalgia, rheumatoid and other forms of arthritis); skin conditions (angioedema, dermatitis, eczema, scleroderma, urticaria); and systemic disease (alcoholism, nicotine addiction, chronic fatigue syndrome, obesity). "All of the diseases that fall into these categories have been documented in peer-reviewed, published medical studies to be potentially due to ETI," Dr. Oberg says.

In addition, Dr. Oberg further ranks the following disease conditions according to how responsive they are to environmental medicine.

Primary level: Asthma, gut flora dysbiosis, irritable bowel syndrome, Ménière's disease, rhinitis, and somatoform disorders (a group of disorders for which symptoms of disease are present, but for which there is no evidence of a physical disorder to explain them) are all conditions for which environmental medicine is ideally suited as a primary form of evaluation and treatment. Environmental medicine is also well suited as an adjunctive treatment for cancer, due to the various environmental and dietary factors that often contribute to its manifestation.

Secondary level: Research indicates that environmental medicine also serves as a valuable therapy for treating attention deficit disorder, chronic bronchitis, chronic fatigue syndrome, dermatitis, dysmenorrhea, eczema, enuresis, fatigue, fibrocystic breast disease, fibromyalgia, infantile enterocolitis, laryngeal edema, migraine, muscle spasm headache, myalgia and arthralgia, premenstrual syndrome, recurrent otitis media, regional ileitis, ulcerative colitis, irritable bowel syndrome, rheumatoid arthritis, sinusitis, and urticaria (hives).

Adjunctive level: According to Dr. Oberg, environmental medicine can serve as a beneficial adjunctive therapy for numerous other disease conditions in which environmental and dietary stressors are involved. These include alcoholism, Alzheimer's disease, angina, angioedema, arrhythmia, bipolar disorder (manic depression), certain forms of anemia, chronic cystitis, chronic gastritis, conjunctivitis, eating disorders, eczema of the eyelids, edema and fluid retention syndromes, eosinophilic gastroenteritis, frequent colds, gastric and duodenal ulcers, glomerulonephritis, hearing loss, hypertension, infertility, irritability, lupus erythematosus, malabsorption syndrome, multiple sclerosis, myocardial infarction, nephrotic syndrome, obesity, panic disorders, Parkinson's disease, pneumonia, pressure in the ear, recurrent vaginitis, schizophrenia, scleroderma, sexual dysfunction, spaciness, thrombophlebitis, thyroid dysfunction, tinnitus, vasculitis, vertigo, vulvodynia, and various cognitive and memory disorders, as well as certain other forms of arthritis.

HEALING CHRONIC FATIGUE: ❧ A CASE HISTORY ❧

The following case history, involving one of Dr. Oberg's patients, a thirty-eight-year-old woman, clearly illustrates the comprehensive nature of environmental medicine.

As Dr. Oberg explains, the woman's major complaint was her long history of severe chronic fatigue. She also had many other ongoing and evolving complaints involving many other body systems. Despite multiple medical evaluations and treatments, over time, all of these symptoms were increasingly compromising the quality of her life.

"My evaluation of her began with an initial comprehensive chronological listing of her complaints. As a child, she began having recurrent eye, ear, nose, and sinus allergies, along with frequent ear, throat, and sinus infections, all of which still persisted when she came to see me. As a teenager, she developed asthma, which cleared after several years. After puberty, she began having chronic gastrointestinal complaints, including alternating diarrhea and constipation, bloating, gassiness, cramps, and occasional mucus. In her twenties, she had three pregnancies, and her GI complaints increased after each one. After her second pregnancy, she developed recurring fatigue, irritability, depression, and anxiety which, over time, evolved into several specific patterns. She also developed recurring diffuse muscle aches and joint aches, weakness, cold intolerance, and various rashes that came and went. Many of these symptoms increased in the second half of her menstrual cycle."

Prior to coming to Dr. Oberg, the woman had consulted with several other physicians of different specialties. An allergist diagnosed her eyes, ear, nose, and throat (EENT) symptoms as allergic rhinitis with recurrent secondary upper respiratory infections. These were treated with antihistamines, decongestants, steroids taken orally or as nasal sprays, and antibiotics as needed. Her gastrointestinal complaints were diagnosed by a gastroenterologist as irritable bowel syndrome, and treated with anticramping agents and increased fiber in her diet. Her muscle and joint aches were diagnosed by a rheumatologist as fibromyalgia and treated with SSRI medications and various anti-inflammatory medications. A neurologist diagnosed her central nervous system complaints as chronic fatigue syndrome, and treated this with Ritalin. "The various medications for her many symptoms helped to varying degrees, temporarily, or actually made her worse over time, so she discontinued them," Dr. Oberg says. "By the time she arrived in my office, she was most distraught with her lack of success in correcting her problems and was at her wit's end with all of this."

Dr. Oberg began his treatment with a further evaluation of each of her complaints, beginning with an environment- and diet-oriented history based on the model of environmental medicine, as he looked for specific patterns to identify her potential stressors. He was able to identify multiple patterns, implicating many types of stressors. He then performed a physical examination. Pertinent physical findings included puffy dark eye circles, lavender-colored and hypertrophied nasal turbinates with clear rhinorrhea, tenderness over and below the eyes, cool dry skin with diffuse rough red patches on her cheeks, chin, and upper chest, a blood pressure of 95/65 with a pulse of 48/minute, a soft abdomen with bloating and increased bowel sounds, and normal joints. She was also distraught and restless.

"Based upon the above assessment, my initial impression of her current situation was that she was suffering from allergic rhinitis and sinusitis; gastrointestinal dysfunction caused by fungal-type dysbiosis; multiple endocrine dysfunctions of her thyroid, adrenal, ovarian, and pancreatic glands; multiple inhalant sensitivies; and chronic fatigue due to all of the above," Dr. Oberg says.

The woman's testing and treatment evolved as follows: First, a comprehensive stool analysis was obtained, which showed a high concentration of *Candida albicans* (level +4). This was treated with the drugs Diflucan and Nystatin, along with a processed carbohydrate-free diet, and a probiotic (live bacteria) supplement. "This resulted in a significant decrease in her GI complaints, elimination of her recurrent rashes, and partial decrease in her fatigue, but she still had alternating irritability with fatigue and depression," Dr. Oberg says.

An endocrine evaluation revealed an elevated TSH (thyroid-stimulating hormone), and low levels of the thyroid hormones free T-4 and free T-3 as determined by a blood test. Additional testing using the saliva adrenal stress index, saliva female hormone panel, and a five-hour glucose/insulin tolerance test revealed the woman was also suffering from adrenal exhaustion, progesterone deficiency with estrogen dominance, and reactive hypoglycemia. "She was treated over the next couple of months by giving her physiologic doses of cortisol, followed by adding Armour Thyroid, a hypoglycemic control diet, and progesterone in oil capsules in the second half of her menstrual cycle," Dr. Oberg explains. "This resulted in elimination of more of her fatigue and other central nervous system symptoms, and her muscle and joint aches."

Finally, the woman's susceptibility to inhalants was tested with Maximum Tolerated Intradermal Dose skin testing and she was begun on vaccines for dusts, danders, and various pollens, as shots at home. "This controlled her EENT symptoms and the rest of her fatigue," Dr. Oberg reports. "Within several months, she was functioning better than she had in years, and cried with gratitude during her follow-up visits with my staff." 〽

YOUR FIRST SESSION

Unlike initial consultations with conventional physicians, which can be as short as five minutes in length, your first session with an environmental medicine physician will last from thirty to ninety minutes, and begin with a comprehensive patient history. "A sufficiently detailed, chronological history that focuses on the patient's diet, environment, and symptom history is the most important and revealing part of an evaluation," Dr. Oberg says. "Environmental medicine physicians move forward through their patients' life history, asking questions that are oriented to discovering patterns for symptoms and causes, and when the history is completed it's usually quite clear why patients have arrived where they are, and what needs to be done to correct their problems." In order to complete your medical history, your physician will want to know everything that you can remember about when, where, and under what circumstances your symptoms occurred, the order in which they evolved, and how they have been evaluated and treated up to now. The history can be assembled through an interview between you and your physician or a trained assistant, or by filling out a comprehensive questionnaire.

Once the history is complete, it will be followed by a physical examination. Laboratory testing to assess the functional status of your biological systems may also be performed during your first visit or scheduled soon thereafter. Testing methods can include blood, saliva, and hormone profiles; hair analysis, urinalysis, and stool specimens, as well as medical imaging techniques, and other diagnostic techniques helpful to the practice of environmental medicine.

After your physician has compiled a complete picture about the total nature of your health complaints, he or she will create a comprehensive treatment plan specific to your problems. The length of treatment will vary according to the severity and uniqueness of your condition and your own health goals. The costs of patient visits are on par with those of conventional physicians and are covered by most health insurance plans if your practitioner is an M.D. or D.O.

SELECTING A PRACTITIONER

Although a variety of holistic and conventional health practitioners have received training in environmental medicine through the American Academy of Environmental Medicine, at this time only physicians (M.D.'s and D.O.'s) may be certified by the American Board of Environmental Medicine. For referrals to such physicians in your area, contact either of these organizations (see the "Resources" section at the end of this chapter). To better understand how environmental medicine is intended to be practiced, you may also wish to review *Practice Guidelines for the Field of Environmental Medicine*, published by the AAEM. When selecting an environmental medicine practitioner, ask if he or she follows these guidelines and is certified or has received training from the AAEM and ABEM.

THE FUTURE OF ENVIRONMENTAL MEDICINE

"Our goal at the AAEM is to get the entire medical profession to shift from its current symptom-oriented paradigm of fixed diagnoses and fixed treatments to a cause-oriented paradigm that is patient-centered and provides customized, individualized forms of diagnoses and treatments, because that's the only method of treating complex, chronic illnesses that really works," says Dr. Oberg, speaking about the future of environmental medicine. "Physicians need to be trained to look at all the different pieces of their patients' etiology, and to understand how they interact with each other. By doing so, they will be better able to effectively improve their patients' functioning, so that patients can go from being a helpless victim of some unknown disease process and at the mercy of their physicians' drugs and surgical therapies, to becoming captains of their own ships and able to understand the multiple options they have to regain whatever level of health they wish to attain. Only when this shift in paradigms occurs will patients be afforded the opportunity for a consistently good-quality diagnosis and treatment regimen that will not just treat their symptoms but will help them to heal their whole system. The sooner conventional physicians are willing to deal with this, the more effective health care will be, and costs will drop significantly."

Dr. Oberg readily admits, however, that achieving the paradigm shift he envisions will be difficult, in large part because of how medicine is currently taught. "Medical education is heavily influenced by the pharmaceutical industry, the hospital industry, and the medical appliance industry," he points out. "As a result, medical students learn how to make a diagnosis and to use the products of these industries, but at present, as far as I know, few of the principles of environmental medicine are taught in any medical school."

Dr. Oberg believes that it will be the patients themselves, along with the continued efforts of organizations like the AAEM and the

ABEM, who will ultimately be responsible for wider physician acceptance of environmental medicine. "As the incidence of chronic illnesses continues to multiply, increasing numbers of patients are becoming dissatisfied with the current medical paradigm and demanding more effective treatments for their problems," he says. "As a result, more and more physicians are now searching for better health care approaches, and becoming more receptive to the programs that the AAEM is making available."

Currently, the AAEM has several hundred members, and hundreds of other physicians have also received training by the organization. Both numbers are expected to grow in the years ahead. In addition, the AAEM continues to expand its programs. "The amount of material that is required to practice environmental medicine is growing by leaps and bounds, so we are expanding our courses and training to accommodate this new knowledge," Dr. Oberg reports. All of the AAEM's programs are fully accredited for M.D.'s and D.O.'s by the Accreditation Council for Continuing Medical Education, and plans are underway to seek accreditation for the many non–M.D./D.O. practitioners who are also seeking training from the AAEM.

RESOURCES

To learn about environmental medicine, and for referrals to environmental medicine physicians, contact:

The American Academy of Environmental Medicine (AAEM)
American Financial Center, Suite 625
7701 East Kellogg Avenue
Wichita, Kansas 67207
Phone: (316) 684-5500
Fax: (316) 684-5709
E-mail: aaem@swbell.net
Web site: *www.aaem.com*

The American and International Boards of Environmental Medicine
    (ABEM/IBEM)
65 Wehrle Drive
Buffalo, New York 14255
Phone: (716) 837-1380
Fax: (716) 833-2244

For referrals to support groups that assist people suffering from environmentally triggered illness, contact:

Human Ecology Action League (HEAL)
P.O. Box 49126
Atlanta, Georgia 30359
Phone: (404) 248-1898

Also of interest is

Immuno Labs
1620 West Oakland Park Blvd. Suite 300
Fort Lauderdale, Florida 33311
Phone (800) 321-9197

A lab specializing in allergy testing, that also provides referrals to environmental medicine physicians worldwide.

RECOMMENDED READING

Crook, William G. *Detecting Your Hidden Allergies.* Professional
    Books/Future Health, 1988.
Randolph, Theron. *An Alternative Approach to Allergies.* Bantam Books,
    1987.
Randolph, Theron. *Human Ecology and Susceptibility to the Chemical Environment.* Charles C. Thomas Publishing, 1962.

CHAPTER 5

Mind-Body Medicine

The link between the mind and the body in relation to overall health has been a central tenet for a variety of holistic approaches to health care, including homeopathy, Ayurveda and traditional Chinese medicine (see Chapters 11, 12, and 13). Only in recent decades, however, have Western scientists and physicians started to give credence to the importance of this mind-body connection to overall well-being. Among the most exciting developments in the field of medicine in the past few decades is the scientific validation that our physical health is directly influenced by our thoughts, emotions, attitudes, and beliefs.

Today, a growing number of scientists recognize that *body* and *mind* are not separate aspects of ourselves, but interrelated expressions of who and what we are. In addition, many researchers now believe that our physiology also has a direct influence on the ways we habitually think and feel. Such views are based on findings in the field of psychoneuroimmunology (PNI) and the discovery, in the 1970s, of "messenger molecules" known as *neuropeptides*. Neuropeptides are biochemicals composed of amino acids that are capable of causing alterations in mood, pain, pleasure, and immune and hormone function at the cellular level in direct response to our thoughts, emotions, attitudes, and beliefs. "In practical terms, this means that all of us are capable of both weakening and strengthening our immune system by virtue of how we think and feel," explains Robert S. Ivker, D.O., a past president of the American Holistic Medical Association, who incorporates mind-body medicine in his clinical practice. "Moreover, scientists have also proven that these chemical messages can originate not only in the brain, but in every cell in the body. As a result, many scientists now believe that the immune system actually functions as a type of circulating nervous system that is actively and acutely attuned to our every thought and emotion."

Based on the growing body of research within the field of PNI, practitioners of holistic medicine incorporate a variety of mind-body medicine techniques to help their patients become more aware of how their thoughts and emotions are affecting their health, and to empower them to think and feel more efficiently and effectively. The first step in this process, according to Dr. Ivker, lies in making patients aware of what it actually means to be mentally and emotionally healthy. "From the perspective of holistic medicine, being mentally healthy means that you recognize the ways in which your thoughts, feelings, beliefs, and attitudes affect your well-being and limit or expand your ability to enjoy your life," he says. "It also means knowing that you always have choices, and that you are aware of your priorities, values, and goals." According to Dr. Ivker, patients who are treated with various mind-body techniques increasingly come to recognize how their habitual limited and inappropriate thoughts and emotions can cause or contribute to their illnesses, while at the same time learning how to create a mind-set conducive to experiencing optimal health and more effectively achieving their personal and professional goals. "Once patients accept the fact that there is an ongoing, instant, and intimate communication occurring between their minds and bodies via the mechanisms of neuropeptides, they can also see that they, themselves, are the ones who are best qualified to direct that communication. Learning how to do so effectively enables them to become their own twenty-four-hour-a-day healers as they become more conscious of their thoughts and emotions and how to manage them better to improve all areas of their health."

🌿 FAST FACTS 🌿

Research in the field of mind-body medicine deals with the influence that psychosomatic factors (thoughts and emotions) can have on physical health. Disease conditions now known to be affected by thoughts and emotions include addiction, asthma, back pain, cancer, cardiovascular disease, gastrointestinal conditions, immunological conditions, and obesity.

Additional research in the field of psychoneuroimmunology has shown that:

Feelings of sorrow, loss, depression, and self-rejection can significantly lower immune function and contribute to a number of chronic disease conditions, including heart attack.

Chronic stress has a broad suppressive effect on immune function and can diminish natural killer cell function, thereby exacerbating chronic conditions, including cancer. Stress and anxiety also lead to increased adrenal corticosteroid production, thereby compromising immune function and inhibiting the ability of cells to repair themselves.

Repressed anger has been shown to be a contributing factor in a variety of diseases, including bronchitis, candidiasis, headache, heart attack, hypertension, and sinusitis.

Feelings of grief, depression, hopelessness, and loneliness can also greatly increase the risk of heart attack, cancer, and gastrointestinal disorders.

Saliva levels of the protective antibody immunoglobulin A have been shown to increase in response to laughter, humor, compassion, and caring; and to decrease in response to anger.

A thirty-year study conducted by the Mayo Clinic in Rochester, Minnesota, found that people who are prone to pessimism die earlier than expected, based on normal survival rates for their age and gender, while people who are generally optimistic live longer.

Acknowledging and expressing one's emotions strengthens immune response.

Feelings of joy and exhilaration produce a measurable increase of a neuropeptide analogous to the powerful anticancer drug interleuken-2. The same emotions improve tissue repair and enhance circulation.

Feelings of peace and calm produce a biochemical in the body with tranquilizing effects similar to those of the drug Valium.

A variety of disease conditions are now known to potentially be due, at least in part, to inhibited or inappropriately expressed emotions. These include asthma, back pain, bronchitis, cancer, colitis, constipation, diabetes, eczema, endocrine disorders, fatigue, headache, heart disease, hypertension, migraine, obesity and overeating, peptic ulcer, psoriasis, rheumatoid arthritis, and spastic colon. 🔥

HISTORY OF MIND-BODY MEDICINE

The concepts forming the basis of mind-body medicine are a central part of most holistic healing traditions, especially the idea that health and disease are both reflections of the whole person—body, mind, and spirit. In the East, such concepts originated in the spiritual traditions of Vedanta (the underlying philosophy of Hinduism), Buddhism, and Taoism, and are reflected in Eastern healing practices such as Ayurveda, traditional Chinese medicine, yoga (see Chapter 14), and meditation. In the West, the link between body, mind, and spirit was emphasized by Hippocrates 2,500 years ago and was also a central tenet in the teachings of the noted Greek healer Galen (A.D. 130–200) and the Swiss alchemist and physician Paracelsus (1493–1541), both of whom influenced the Western practice of medicine until the seventeenth century. It was primarily due to the influence of the French philosopher René Descartes (1596–1650) that the schism between mind and body first occurred. In Descartes' view, mind and body were separate and different from each other, with little or no influence over each other. Ever since this Cartesian model grew to dominance in the West, modern conventional medicine until recently has accepted this artificial division between mind and body as one of its basic tenets. As a result, allopathic medicine has witnessed an increasing trend toward specialization, with an emphasis on treating specific organ systems and body parts rather than "whole person" therapy, and focusing on symptom care rather than addressing the underlying causes of disease.

Not all healers and physicians abided by this separation, however. Samuel Hahnemann (1755–1843), the founder of homeopathy, for instance, made note of patients' mental and emotional predispositions when determining their homeopathic remedies. Friedrich Anton Mesmer (1734–1815), one of Hahnemann's contemporaries, was also able to demonstrate the influence the mind has over the body through the use of his "mesmerizing" techniques, which he used to effect patient cures by harnessing their mental energy. Although Mesmer's results varied widely, in 1841 they led Scottish physician James Braid (1795–1860) to develop his own series of trance-inducing techniques. Braid coined the word *hypnosis* to describe the trance state itself, as well as the terms *hypnotist* and *suggestion*, as used in that context. Soon thereafter, hypnosis was used as an aid to a variety of medical procedures, especially anesthesia during surgery, most notably by Braid's friend and fellow physician James Esdaile (1818–1859), whose use of hypnotic anesthesia during his tenure with the British East India Company in India lowered the surgical mortality rate to less than 5 percent. Sigmund Freud (1856–1939) also initially employed hypnosis techniques in order to access the unconscious, but he ultimately rejected it in favor of psychoanalysis, due in part to the fact that he was unskilled as a hypnotist. As a result, the popularity of hypnosis waned until the 1950s, when it was approved as a useful technique by the American Medical Association.

Another pioneer in the field of mind-body medicine was the French pharmacist Emile Coué (1857–1926), whose work with the imagination and "conscious auto-suggestion" was a central aspect of the free health clinic he operated between 1910 and the mid-1920s. In addition to standard hypnosis techniques of the time, Coué encouraged patients to notice their thoughts and emotions and to deal with melancholy or woeful thoughts by placing their attention on something happier or more positive. He also instructed patients to repeat out loud his famous affirmation "Every day in every way I am getting better and better," twenty times a day upon awaking. Coué firmly believed that all physical illness, as well as all other external events in a person's life, was the direct result of how he or she thinks. According to Coué, listening to repeated suggestions of illness is enough to cause the actual illness to manifest, while feeding the unconscious with positive suggestions can lead to healing. As a result, he created a series of positive suggestions for specific disease conditions, instructing his patients to repeat them daily with confidence but no force of will; he was convinced that doing so enabled the unconscious to accept the suggestions as fact, and would lead to a resolution of symptoms. Coué treated a variety of chronic disease conditions in this manner, including constipation, asthma, tuberculosis, varicose ulcers, and fibrous tumors.

Chicago physician Edmond Jacobson was another early-twentieth-century innovator in the field of mind-body medicine, and the developer of progressive relaxation, which he first wrote about in 1929. According to Jacobson, the simple act of relaxation itself is enough to maintain health and heal disease. By teaching his patients how to achieve simple, yet deep, muscle relaxation, Jacobson was able to successfully treat a variety of illnesses, including anxiety, cardiac neurosis, colitis, depression, fatigue, hyperthyroidism (Graves' disease), phobia, and stuttering. In addition, after learning how to relax, his patients typically demonstrated clinically significant improvement in functions controlled by the autonomic nervous system. Overall, Jacobson found that 80 percent of his patients responded favorably to daily practice of thirty minutes of deep relaxation regardless of what type of illness they suffered from.

Around the same time as Jacobson's work, German neurologist Johannes H. Schultz developed autogenic training after researching previous German studies on both sleep and hypnosis. Schultz, who was later assisted by Wolfgang Luthe, spent the 1930s refining the techniques of autogenic training in order to allow patients to mentally manipulate and voluntarily control normally involuntary physiological functions.

Further research into how the mind can influence health continued throughout the next three decades, but it was not until the 1970s that the mind-body connection began to be truly understood and accepted by mainstream researchers and physicians. The beginning of this paradigm shift first occurred in the 1960s with the seminal experiments of Elmer Green, Ph.D., a psychologist and physicist then working at the Menninger Foundation in Topeka, Kansas, and Alyce Green, his wife. While monitoring the skin temperature of a woman they were guiding through a series of relaxation exercises, they notice an abrupt increase in the temperature of the woman's hand at the same moment that she reported that the headache she'd been experiencing had vanished. Intrigued, the Greens went on to develop a biofeedback temperature device, which they employed as an aid in teaching their patients how to ease migraine pain by the simple act of raising their hand temperature. Elements of autogenic training were also included in the Greens' experiments, and approximately 80 percent of all patients who were taught the technique were able to use it successfully to decrease both the severity and frequency of migraine attacks. Based on the Greens' work, the applications for biofeedback training have since been extended to a wide range of disease conditions.

Later in the same decade, the Greens used EEG biofeedback to test the well-known yoga master Swami Rama. During a series of experiments, they observed, and were able to record, that Swami Rama was able to voluntarily alter and regulate a variety of normally involuntary physiological functions. Among the effects that Swami Rama demonstrated were significant changes in heart pulse rate, and an 11-degree difference in the temperatures of his right and left hands. As a result of the Greens' clinical studies, the possibility that the mind could influence physical behavior became more widely accepted by other Western researchers and physicians, and additional research into a variety of mind-body approaches soon followed.

The 1970s was another important decade in the development of mind-body medicine, especially with regard to the field of psycho-neuroimmunology. Among those in the vanguard of PNI research is Candace Pert, Ph.D., research professor at Georgetown University Medical Center's Department of Physiology and Biophysics, and formerly a chief researcher at the National Institute of Mental Health. In 1972 Dr. Pert discovered, and was able to quantify, the existence of the opiate receptor, a molecule occurring on the surfaces of cells in the brain and throughout the body. Dr. Pert's discovery was crucial to subsequent neuropeptide research, which showed that neuropeptides are capable of altering mood, pleasure, and pain. More important, research by Dr. Pert and her colleagues resulted in the discovery that endorphin and other neuropeptides, which were previously thought to be present only in the brain, are actually found throughout the body, including the immune and endocrine systems. This discovery revealed that emotions, which until then were considered solely psychological in nature, were in actuality linked to precise biochemical reactions that occur throughout the body. Moreover, neuropeptides, which Dr. Pert describes as "the biochemical correlates of emotions," are affected by our emotional states, with emotions such as calm, compassion, happiness, and joy enhancing the chemicals' ability to positively impact a variety of biological functions, including improving immunity. Repressed, or so-called negative, emotions, by contrast, which are now known to decrease immune function and increase the risk of disease, are capable of diminishing the amount of neuropeptides present in cellular receptor sites, opening the way for viruses that share the same sites to more easily invade the cells themselves.

Other recent pioneers in the mind-body field include O. Carl Simonton, M.D., who in 1971 first began to demonstrate the ability of patients to stabilize, reverse, and in some cases completely recover from cancer by harnessing the power of their imaginations to visualize themselves becoming healed; Herbert Benson, M.D., associate professor of medicine at Harvard Medical School and founder of the Mind/Body Institute of Deaconess Hospital, whose research into the "relaxation response" and the power of belief has empowered thousands of patients to gain better control of their health using various mind-body techniques; Patricia Norris, Ph.D., and Steven Fahrion, Ph.D., founding members of the Life

Sciences Institute of Mind-Body Health in Topeka, Kansas, whose use of advanced biofeedback techniques is proving remarkably effective in the treatment of alcoholism and addiction; and noted physician, author, and researcher Larry Dossey, M.D., whose writings continue to document the power that faith and spiritual practices such as prayer and meditation can have on health and healing.

Today, the principles of mind-body medicine are incorporated into the programs and curricula of many major hospitals and universities across the United States and abroad, and further research continues to substantiate the role that mind-body techniques can play in reversing disease and enhancing optimal health.

THE THERAPIES OF MIND-BODY MEDICINE

The underlying goal of all of the therapies that comprise the field of mind-body medicine is to teach patients about the influences, both positive and negative, that the mind and body have upon each other and to empower patients to more effectively manage their thoughts, emotions, attitudes, and beliefs in order to create and maintain optimal health. The therapies themselves are many, and vary extensively in their therapeutic approaches. A number of them, once learned, easily lend themselves to self-care techniques that can be used safely on a daily basis, while others require the supervision of a skilled practitioner trained in their use. The most common forms of mind-body medicine include autogenic training, biofeedback training, breathwork, Eye Movement Desensitization and Reprocessing (EMDR), flower essences, guided imagery and visualization, hypnotherapy, journaling, meditation, progressive relaxation, psychotherapy and counseling, somatic psychology, and Thought Field Therapy.

AFFIRMATIONS:
❧ REPROGRAMMING THE MIND ❧

Affirmations serve as a means of identifying habitual limiting or unhealthy beliefs, while reprogramming the mind with positive thoughts, ideas, and images intended to produce a specific outcome. One of the most famous affirmations is the one developed by Emile Coué and cited above. More recently, the use of affirmations has been popularized through the writings of Louise Hay, author of the book *You Can Heal Your Life*. According to Hay and other practitioners who encourage their use, affirmations create images that directly affect the unconscious and stimulate the body-mind's innate healing energies. According to Dr. Robert Ivker, when affirmations are practiced regularly, they have the power to create optimal health by generating the life energy of hope, which, in turn, triggers the activity of neuropeptides in the cells and stimulates the immune system. Besides illness, affirmations can be used to address virtually all aspects of one's life, such as enhancing self-esteem, improving the quality of relationships, or launching a more rewarding career.

"Because of the simple nature of affirmations, the greatest challenge in beginning to work with them is to suspend judgment long enough to allow them to produce the results you desire," Dr. Ivker says. "Keep in mind that the way your life is today is the direct result of the thoughts and beliefs you have held for most, if not all, of your life. Replacing these old thought patterns can take time, although it is quite possible that you will begin to experience the results you want much sooner than you might expect." ❧

Autogenic Training

Autogenic training was primarily developed by German neurologist Johannes Schultz in the early 1930s after he reviewed earlier research related to sleep and hypnosis conducted by physiologist Oskar Vogt. During the course of his research, Vogt discovered that many people were able to induce states of autosuggestion during hypnosis and prior to falling asleep. While conducting his own studies as a follow-up to Vogt's work, Schultz found that his patients invariably experienced heaviness in their extremities, accompanied by increased sensations of warmth. With further experimentation, Schultz discovered that these same physiological perceptions could be triggered by autosuggestion. Moreover, as his patients entered into the reverie, or autogenic, state that accompanied these physical sensations, they usually also experienced renewed energy levels and reduced bodily tension. By regularly experiencing the autogenic state, Schultz maintained, the patient was able to regulate the normally involuntary processes of the autonomic nervous system, while counteracting the effects of stress.

Over time, Schultz found that there were six basic suggestions necessary for invoking these health benefits, each of which was directed to a specific part of the body, and that they are best practiced regularly during times of quiet, while sitting or lying comfortably, with eyes closed. In this relaxed state, practitioners silently tell themselves: My arms and legs are heavy. My arms and legs are warm. My heartbeat is calm and regular. It (the heartbeat) breathes me. My abdomen is warm. My forehead is cool. Initially, the exercises are intended to be practiced for five to fifteen minutes, two to three times a day, usually under the supervision of a teacher trained in the method. With regular practice, however, most practitioners become able to quickly and easily induce the effects each phrase is meant to induce simply by saying them. As they become more proficient, many practitioners are able to induce and maintain a calm state of relaxation even when they are physically active.

Most people are able to experience the full benefits of autogenic training with six months or less of regular practice. In addition to the basic six exercises Schultz developed, more advanced applications of autogenic training are also available for dealing with specific disease conditions and to elicit heightened states of awareness.

Caution: While autogenic training is extremely safe, some people may initially experience feelings of dizziness or muscle strain due to the exercises' ability to spontaneously release stress in the body. For this reason, it is recommended that new practitioners work with someone trained in the method to ensure proper training.

Biofeedback Training

Biofeedback training refers to the use of various devices to help people become more aware of, and gain greater control over, their various physiological processes. By monitoring and "feeding back" changes in body temperature, muscle tension, heart and respiration rates, skin conductivity, and brain waves, biofeedback devices enable users to become more conscious of such activity, and to learn how to adjust it in order to achieve greater degrees of relaxation and reduce stress.

There are a number of biofeedback approaches, including electroencephalogram (EEG), to monitor brain wave activity; electrocardiogram (EKG), to monitor changes in heart rate; electromyogram (EMG), which tracks changes in muscular tension; galvanic skin response (GSR); and monitoring of skin temperature (ST). During the course of biofeedback training, patients learn to recognize the physiological activity that is indicative of normal, healthy readings, such as a slow, relaxed heart rate;

deep, even breathing; warm skin; and low rates of perspiration. Then, through the use of techniques such as progressive relaxation, autogenic training, meditation, or guided imagery, they learn how to create for themselves the same levels of relaxation without the aid of the device they are using.

Currently, biofeedback training is used to treat or manage over one hundred disease conditions, particularly those that are stress- or anxiety-related. EMG biofeedback training has been approved by the American Medical Association as a treatment for tension headaches. Depending on each person's nature and particular need or disease condition, training time can range from a few sessions to more extensive training lasting a few months or longer.

A more advanced form of biofeedback training, known as brain-wave, or neurofeedback, therapy has been shown to be effective as a treatment for alcoholism and addiction. An outgrowth of pioneering biofeedback studies conducted by former University of Chicago research psychologist Joseph Kamiya in the 1950s, and Elmer and Alyce Green at the Menninger Foundation during the 1960s and '70s, brain-wave therapy works by normalizing alpha and theta brain-wave states, while simultaneously rebalancing brain chemistry. According to Drs. Patricia Norris and Steven Fahrion, individuals struggling with alcohol or drug addiction typically have low levels of alpha and theta activity, making it difficult for them to experience satisfaction from everyday life events that normal people take for granted. As a result, they live in a state of depression that is only alleviated by alcohol or drug use. Through the use of brain-wave therapy, however, addicts, even those whose addictions have been long-term, are taught how to normalize their alpha and theta activity levels, resulting in a much higher incidence of successful, long-term recovery than those normally achieved by conventional means. Brain-wave therapy has also been shown to benefit people suffering from anxiety, depression, attention deficit disorder, closed head injury, and stroke, among other conditions.

Breathwork

Breathwork refers to various breathing approaches that enable practitioners to learn how to breathe more consciously and freely in order to improve health, increase vitality, and deal more effectively with emotional pain. All forms of breathwork focus on the breath itself and its ability to move energy through the body. Most breathwork therapies also use the technique of connected breathing, in which there is no pause between each inhalation and exhalation. The pattern of respiration employed by breathwork therapists varies according to method. Sometimes it is rapid; other times it is deep, slow, and full. In addition, some approaches recommend breathing in and out through the mouth, instead of the nose, and both abdominal and chest breathing can be used. A more complete overview of the various approaches to breathwork therapy is provided in Chapter 9.

Caution: Because of the emotional release that often results from performing breathwork techniques, it is recommended that they initially be learned and performed under the direction of a skilled breathwork therapist. Certain forms are also not recommended for people with a history of mental illness, pregnant women, people with cardiovascular conditions, or people prone to epileptic seizure.

Eye Movement Desensitization and Reprocessing (EMDR)

Developed in the late 1980s by Francine Shapiro, Ph.D., senior research fellow at the Mental Research Institute in Palo Alto, California, EMDR has been hailed as a breakthrough therapy for relieving a variety of psychological conditions, particularly anxiety, depression, phobias, recurrent nightmares, and post-traumatic stress disorders (PTSDs). When such conditions are initially triggered and experienced, the emotional distress that accompanies them often remains unresolved, making it extremely difficult for people who suffer from trauma to integrate their experiences and move beyond them in a healthy fashion. EMDR works by having clients focus on the images, thoughts, and physical sensations they associate with their emotional or mental problems while the EMDR therapist moves his or her hand from side to side before their faces. Clients are instructed to follow these hand movements with their eyes while maintaining their attention on the experiences that disturb them. By doing so, a reprocessing occurs relating to how they perceive and respond to the triggering events. In addition to these directed eye movements, EMDR therapists will sometimes use other methods of side-to-side lateralization, such as tapping on alternate sides of their clients' bodies or employing sound tones that shift from ear to ear. Once the reprocessing occurs, therapists then proceed to replacing negative thoughts associated with their patient's trauma with thoughts of a more positive nature that are more congruent with the present.

Although how and why EMDR works is yet to be fully explained, numerous studies have verified its ability to achieve permanent resolution of deep-seated emotional issues related to trauma and stress, often in as few as one to three sessions. Numerous victims of rape and abuse, war veterans afflicted with PTSDs, and survivors of both man-made and natural disasters have all experienced documented long-lasting relief from the traumas associated with such experiences, even when other therapies failed to produce results. Because of its success with these and other conditions, EMDR is one of the fastest-growing therapies in the entire field of mind-body medicine, with over twenty thousand EMDR therapists in the United States alone.

Caution: Dr. Shapiro cautions that directed eye movements comprise only one aspect of EMDR, and that reprocessing can occur without them when other elements of EMDR are used. In addition, a number of reports indicate that pyschological harm can result when eye movements are used alone, without following the procedures and protocols of the entire EMDR method. People interested in experiencing EMDR are advised to work only with EMDR therapists trained and licensed by the EMDR Institute or the EMDR International Association (see the "Resources" section at the end of this chapter).

Flower Essences

Flower essences refers to a system of medicine originally developed by the English physician Edward Bach (1886–1936), who believed that "our fears, our cares, our anxieties and such like open the path to the invasion of illness." In his book *Heal Thyself*, Bach wrote, "Disease will never be cured or eradicated by present materialistic methods, for the simple reason that disease in its origin is not material." Convinced that physical illness could be healed once stress and emotional disorders were resolved, Bach abandoned his successful medical practice in 1930 to retire to the countryside, where he spent the remaining years of his life researching the healing properties of flowers. Ultimately he identified thirty-eight flowers that had therapeutic benefits, which today are known as the *Bach Flower Remedies*.

Using his knowledge as an accomplished practitioner of homeopathy (see Chapter 11), Bach conducted a series of experiments that led to his discovery that the morning dew on flowers, when warmed by the sun, became imprinted with each flower's specific healing properties. Eventually, he classified the flowers according to their ability to relieve seven specific types of emotional imbalances, which he determined to be fear, loneliness, despondency or despair, uncertainty, insufficient interest in present circumstances, oversensitivity, and "over-care for welfare of others." He also created "Rescue Remedy," a general formula consisting of five flower essences that can be used during times of crisis or acute stress. Today, flower essences are created by picking flowers in the early morning when they are in full bloom. The flower blossoms are then soaked in unfiltered spring water and exposed to the sun for three hours, after which the blossoms are removed and the water is poured into sterile bottles and mixed with equal amounts of brandy. Following the potentization process of homeopathy, the liquid is then repeatedly diluted until only minute amounts of the original "mother essence" remain in the final preparation. The remedies can be taken sublingually (beneath the tongue) or placed in water and sipped throughout the day.

At the time of his death, Bach felt certain that his original thirty-eight remedies, along with his Rescue Remedy, were all that were necessary for treating all conditions, based on his belief that physical illnesses were the result of one or more of the seven categories of emotion he'd identified. Since his death, however, a number of other flower essence systems have been developed, some of which also focus on treating specific diseases. Overall, flower essences are easy to learn how to use, extremely safe, and effective as a self-care approach for enhancing mental and emotional well-being. Although little clinical research currently exists to satisfy mainstream scientists about the efficacy of flower essences to treat disease, a wide body of anecdotal evidence involving both human and animal subjects has been collected since Bach's time in support of his claims, and today flower essences are used by a variety of health care professionals as part of their overall practice.

Guided Imagery and Visualization

"Guided imagery and visualization work to improve and maintain health because of their ability to directly affect our bodies at a cellular level, particularly with regard to stimulating neuropeptides," Dr. Ivker says. "In addition, the use of imagery can often provide greater insight about causes and treatment for chronic conditions, guiding us towards the most personalized and effective solutions for our particular health problem."

Since the 1970s, researchers, physicians, and other health care professionals have been examining how guided imagery and visualization techniques can be used to consciously create improved states of well-being. Since 1971, radiation oncologist O. Carl Simonton, M.D., for instance, has been a pioneer in developing imagery as a self-care tool cancer patients could use to bolster their response rate to traditional cancer treatments, with remarkable success. The first patient he taught his techniques to was a sixty-one-year-old man who had been diagnosed with a "hopeless" case of throat cancer. In conjunction with his radiation treatments, the man spent five to fifteen minutes three times a day imagining himself healthy. Within two months, he was completely cancer-free. Numerous studies also confirm the health benefits of imagery and visualization. In addition, the regular practice of imagery and visualization techniques has been shown to engender greater feelings of peace and relaxation, enhanced creativity, greater fulfillment in relationships, improved professional success, and improved ability to reshape negative habit patterns.

There are two types of guided imagery and visualization: preconceived or preselected images employed by you or your health care professional in order to address a specific problem and achieve a specific outcome, and imagery that occurs spontaneously as you sit comfortably, eyes closed and breathing freely. Both forms have been shown to have value for treating a variety of disease conditions.

Hypnotherapy

Hypnotherapy is the use of hypnosis to deal with a variety of conditions, both physical and psychological. It is also one of the most paradoxical therapies within the field of mind-body medicine, in that its effectiveness has been scientifically verified, yet it remains misunderstood, due to public perception influenced by movies and television shows, as well as by stage hypnotists. Perhaps the most common misconception about hypnotherapy is that the hypnotist can use it to gain control over his or her subjects and command them to perform acts that they would otherwise object to. In actuality, hypnotherapy is entirely safe, with subjects being entirely aware of the process and of any suggestions that are made as they occur, and they are able to end the experience at any time should they so choose.

While the exact mechanism of hypnotherapy has yet to be fully explained, there is no longer any question that hypnotherapy can be an effective therapy for treating a variety of illnesses, and is also useful for creating beneficial changes in subjects' beliefs, attitudes, thought processes, and behavior patterns. At the heart of hypnotherapy is what is known as the "hypnotic trance," a naturally occurring state of consciousness similar to the experience of daydreaming and the twilight reverie that often precedes the moments before sleep. There are numerous ways in which hypnotherapists can induce this state in their clients, and with training self-hypnosis is also easy to achieve. Contrary to popular belief, the trance does not have to be deep, in order to be effective. Once the trance state has been achieved, subjects usually experience a detached state of calm, accompanied by a heightened sense of awareness in which it is possible to retrieve unconscious memories, reframe limiting beliefs, alleviate both physical and emotional pain, and accept positive suggestions intended to facilitate the subject's specific intentions. In addition to helping people achieve their goals and gain better control over their moods and emotions, hypnotherapy has been shown to be an effective aid for a diverse range of disease conditions, including anxiety, addiction (alcohol, nicotine, drugs, food cravings, etc.), headache, migraine, dermatitis, impotence, gastrointestinal disorders, immune dysfunctions, stress, pain, and obesity. Because of its proven effectiveness for treating such conditions, hypnotherapy has been recognized as a valid medical treatment option by the British Medical Association since 1955, and by the American Medical Association since 1958. Today it is taught in many conventional medical schools across the United States and abroad and is used by an increasing number of physicians, dentists, psychologists, and other health practitioners, in addition to the growing body of clinical hypnotherapists themselves.

Note: Although hypnotherapy is an entirely safe process, it is not advisable for people suffering from psychotic conditions, or those under the influence of drugs or alcohol. It is also not effective for most children under the age of five. In addition, people considering hypnotherapy should be sure that they work with a qualified practitioner certified in its use. For referrals to such practitioners, see the "Resources" section below.

Journaling

Journaling is a simple but very effective way to become more conscious of your mental and emotional life, and to help you better express your feelings. The practice of journaling entails keeping a written record of your thoughts, emotions, and any other daily experiences that you would like to better understand. When done on a regular basis, journaling can result in increased self-knowledge, often with insights that are both enlightening and enlivening. "Many people who begin the practice of journaling are amazed to discover how the simple act of writing about one's daily experiences can lead to sudden or deeper insights into what they are feeling," Dr. Ivker says.

Journaling can also help people become better aware of their beliefs, enabling them to better recognize and change those that may be limiting them. Studies of people who journal regularly indicate that they exhibit greater control over their thoughts and emotions, become less reactive to life experiences over which they have no control, and more creative in their approaches to dealing with them. A number of researchers, including James W. Pennebaker, Ph.D., author of the book *Opening Up*, have also documented the physical health benefits that journaling can provide by writing about upsetting or traumatic experiences.

Meditation

There are a variety of meditation techniques, each of which can serve as a useful tool for enhancing health. Meditation's many benefits include increased oxygen intake, greater relaxation, improved focus on the present instead of regrets and worries for the past and future, enhanced creativity, heightened spiritual awareness, and an improved ability to be aware of, and manage, your emotions. Other benefits include reduction in blood pressure, heart rate, adrenaline, cortisone, cholesterol, muscle tension, blood sugar, triglycerides, free radicals, and improvement in immunity, reaction time, auditory perception, and pain tolerance. Meditation also aids in the treatment of heart disease, migraine, allergies, headache, seizures, and many other physical ailments.

The regular practice of meditation can provide many psychological benefits, as well. These include increased feelings of calm and peace, improved mental functioning and enhanced powers of concentration, more frequent feelings of joy and happiness, and a heightened sense of awareness and compassion for others.

❧ PRAYER AND HEALING ❧

In addition to being the most common form of spiritual exercise engaged in by most Americans, prayer has in recent years been the subject of a great deal of scientific study focused on its bene-

ficial health effects. Among the pioneers in the study of the physiological effects of prayer is Herbert Benson, M.D., a Harvard
cardiologist. Since 1988, Dr. Benson and psychologist Jared Klass
have conducted a series of programs at the Mind/Body Medical
Institute at New England Deaconess Hospital investigating the
spiritual and health implications of prayer. Their studies reveal
that people high in spirituality, which Dr. Benson defines as a
feeling that "there is more than just you" and as not necessarily
religious, scored higher in psychological health. They also were
less likely to get sick, and better able to cope if they did; had fewer
stress-related symptoms; showed the greatest rise on a life-purpose
index; and exhibited the sharpest drop in pain. Dr. Benson's
research has also shown that praying regularly can reduce stress,
lower metabolic rates, slow heart rate, reduce blood pressure levels, and result in slower, calmer rates of respiration, and that these
and other psychophysiological benefits of prayer increase according to the degree of faith on the part of the person praying. ❦

Progressive Relaxation

While relaxation techniques have existed for thousands of years, modern-
day progressive relaxation therapies are an outgrowth of the research
conducted by Chicago physician Edmond Jacobson in the early twentieth century. The goal of relaxation methods is to induce what Dr. Herbert Benson terms the "relaxation response," a psychophysiological state
of bodily calm that is the opposite of the stress-induced "fight or flight
response." During relaxation, a number of health benefits accrue, including reduced blood pressure, and a normalization of heart, respiration,
and metabolic rates.

Despite the obvious benefits, researchers in the field of mind-body
medicine have found that many people are incapable of releasing mental
and physical stress without some form of help or training. Moreover,
many people are also unaware of their stress levels, often believing
themselves to be relaxed when in fact their bodies are exhibiting chronic
tension patterns. Progressive relaxation techniques help people become
more aware of when and how they are holding stress in their bodies, and
they provide people with the means to release it. One of the most common relaxation techniques is based on Dr. Jacobson's method of teaching his patients how to relax by first recognizing how stress caused their

muscles to contract. He accomplished this by having them lie down or sit comfortably while tensing various muscles groups, initially focusing on only one group each day, for a period of five to fifteen minutes. Over time, they became adept at quickly contracting and then relaxing each muscle group in turn, until a state of total relaxation was achieved. Today, this exercise is usually performed in its entirety, with patients lying down with their eyes closed as they first tense, then relax, their toes and feet, and then progressively move upward, tensing and relaxing each muscle group until they end with the muscles of the face and skull.

All progressive relaxation techniques are safe to perform and can be effective for relieving a host of health complaints, including pain, respiratory conditions, irregular blood pressure patterns, anxiety, depression, and other physical and mental/emotional conditions related to stress. Once learned, progressive relaxation techniques are also well suited as self-care techniques.

Psychotherapy and Counseling

The field of psychotherapy, an outgrowth of the theories and discoveries of Sigmund Freud, continues to evolve more than a hundred years since its inception. In addition to the mental and emotional benefits commonly attributed to psychotherapy, a growing body of research has documented that physical benefits can also occur. Today the most popular forms of psychotherapy are Classical or Freudian, Jungian, cognitive/behavioral therapy, brief/solution-focused therapy, humanistic/existential therapy, and family therapy.

Classical, or Freudian, psychotherapy is based on the principles Freud developed to investigate and improve mental functioning through the understanding of past emotional traumas contained in the unconscious. Freud believed that the purpose of psychotherapy "was to elucidate the darkest recesses of the mind and soul and to enable the individual to integrate the emotional and intellectual sides of his nature." Classical psychotherapy is similar to conventional medicine in that its treatment approach to mental and emotional disorders is disease-oriented, meaning that patients engage in the process in order to be "fixed" and be made "normal." How this is accomplished, however, can substantially differ. Although there are a variety of therapeutic methods, many psychiatrists and psychoanalysts currently rely heavily on drug therapy.

Jungian therapy is based on the work of Carl Gustav Jung, one of Freud's earliest and closest disciples, who broke ranks with Freud in order to develop a psychotherapeutic approach that, while still involving the unconscious, was more spiritual in orientation. It was Jung who coined the term *collective unconscious* to explain what he believed were archetypal patterns common to all human beings at a threshold below our normal conscious minds. Jungian psychotherapists emphasize working with these archetypes (also referred to as personality types), along with an exploration of the patient's *animus* and *anima*, which relate to the masculine and feminine aspects of the individual's psyche. Dreamwork also plays an important role in Jungian therapy.

Cognitive/behavioral therapy holds the view that our beliefs significantly determine our emotions and behavior. Developed by Albert Ellis, Ph.D., cognitive therapy emphasizes the role that cognition (one's beliefs, ideas, assumptions, interpretations, and thinking processes) plays in both the creation and treatment of mental and emotional problems. While there are various types of cognitive therapeutic approaches, all of them teach patients how to critically evaluate their thought processes and to trust in their own unique reasoning abilities instead of following the standards of others. Unlike other psychotherapeutic approaches, cognitive therapy focuses on the present, not the past, and is based on the view that if you can change what you think, you'll change how you feel.

Brief/solution-focused therapy has become increasingly popular in recent years, especially in managed care settings. Its objective is to break down larger life issues into smaller, more manageable parts in order to resolve each part in turn. Solution-focused therapy is short-term in nature, usually occurring in one to eight sessions. It is also focused on the present and geared toward goal achievement.

Humanistic/existential therapy recognizes each person's innate ability to resolve problems through the choices he or she makes. The goal of this therapy is to help patients develop an awareness of their uniqueness, with an emphasis on discovering and using their individual strengths, talents, and other positive attributes.

Family therapy is based on systemic thinking that views the family as an interconnected structure. A patient's mental and emotional problems are not due to individual flaws but, rather, result chiefly from the way his or her family is structured and how the family members relate to one another.

Other types of psychotherapy include *client-centered therapy*, developed by Carl Rogers and emphasizing reflective listening on the part of the therapist; *transactional analysis*, developed by Eric Berne, M.D., and emphasizing interactions of three ego states—parent, adult, child—in leading clients to greater functionality; and *psychosynthesis*, developed by

Roberto Assagioli, M.D., an early colleague of Freud who broke ranks with him to emphasize the higher unconscious and the "Higher Self" or Soul. (Psychosynthesis is the only form of psychotherapy to deal openly with the Higher Self and has become known as "Psychotherapy with a Soul.") In all of these therapies, counselors usually go far beyond merely listening to their clients. Using a variety of proactive approaches, they help their clients to resolve past issues, validate themselves, and take charge of their decisions as they learn the skills necessary for creating meaningful change in their lives.

Note: Psychotherapy, by its very nature, is not a self-care protocol, but can be extremely valuable for individuals struggling with deep-rooted mental and emotional problems. If you feel that you might benefit from psychotherapy, use the overviews of the therapies outlined above to choose the approach best suited to your needs. In addition, be aware that the work of psychotherapy is increasingly being conducted by nonpsychiatrists, such as psychologists, social workers, and pastoral counselors. One of the reasons for this, perhaps, lies in the fact that the majority of today's patients seeing psychiatrists are given a psychiatric diagnosis (manic-depressive, obsessive-compulsive, etc.) and then treated with drugs, such as the antidepressant Prozac. While psychotherapeutic drugs can be effective at times, especially short-term, each of the drugs commonly prescribed by psychiatrists has the potential to cause unpleasant, and even dangerous, side effects. Equally important, according to Dr. Ivker, is the fact that by focusing on treating psychological symptoms with drugs, many psychiatrists are depriving their patients of the opportunity to change their attitudes and behavior and to learn how to understand and grow from their emotional pain.

Whichever type of psychotherapist you choose, make sure that he or she is someone with whom you are comfortable. Psychotherapy can be effective only in a situation of trust, so you may wish to interview a number of therapists before making your choice.

Somatic Psychology

Somatic psychology refers to various bodywork methods that, like other therapies in the field of mind-body medicine, acknowledge the interrelationship between the body (soma) and the mind (psyche), as well as how each influences the other to affect overall health. According to Christine

Caldwell, Ph.D., founder of the Naropa Institute's Somatic Psychology Program, somatic psychology "draws upon philosophy, medicine, physics, existing psychologies, and countless thousands of hours of human observation and clinical experience to unify human beings into an organic and inseparable whole for the purpose of healing, growth, and transformation." A more complete overview of somatic therapies and their health benefits is provided in Chapter 9.

Thought Field Therapy

A fairly recent development in the field of mind-body medicine, Thought Field Therapy (TFT) is also one of the most potentially exciting approaches for treating stress- and phobia-related conditions of both a physical and mental/emotional nature. Originally developed by psychologist Roger Callahan, Ph.D., beginning in the 1970s, Thought Field Therapy addresses the fundamental causes underlying such conditions, while balancing the body's bioenergy system. Research has shown that TFT techniques can eliminate most negative emotions within minutes and stimulate the body's innate healing mechanisms.

TFT combines elements of cognitive therapy with muscle-testing techniques similar to those common to applied kinesiology (AK) and behavioral kinesiology, developed by George Goodheart, D.C., and John Diamond, M.D., respectively (see Chapter 9), along with acupressure along specific points within the body's meridian system (see Chapter 13). Based on research conducted by Dr. Goodheart and other AK practitioners, it is now known that muscle testing is a useful tool for diagnosing and correcting structural imbalances and weakness in the body. Additional research by Dr. Diamond using muscle testing has also determined that various meridian points are associated with specific emotions. Building upon such discoveries, Dr. Callahan discovered that muscle testing can also reveal unconscious, or hidden, limiting thoughts and beliefs, which he terms "psychological reversals." In addition, Dr. Callahan found that the negative effects of such self-sabotaging patterns, which serve to block or otherwise thwart one's conscious intentions, can be eliminated when certain meridian points are activated (usually by tapping on them) while subjects focus on specific thoughts or affirmation-like statements.

Although his discoveries were initially resisted by the American Psychological Association and other health organizations, today Dr. Callahan's methods, known as Callahan Techniques Thought Field Therapy, are increasingly being utilized by psychologists and other health counselors to rapidly eliminate phobias, addictions, and other mental/emotional conditions, as well as enhancing performance and social skills, including eliminating the fear of public speaking. Today, a number of other TFT methodologies are also available, such as Emotional Freedom Techniques, Emotional Self-Management, Energy Diagnostics, and Thought Energy Synchronization Therapy. In addition to being effective for treating most mental/emotional conditions, TFT has also been found to be useful for treating other conditions such as jet lag, nasal congestion and premenstrual syndrome. Many of the techniques also lend themselves to effective self-care approaches.

In addition to the above therapies, other mind-body approaches to health and healing include *art therapy*, which combines art with psychotherapeutic techniques and can enhance self-awareness, heal unresolved emotions, and promote greater emotional expression; *dance therapy*, which has been shown to be effective in helping people deal with cognitive and emotional issues, enhance self-esteem, and increase energy levels; *dream therapy*, which can provide clues to the underlying nature of disease and guidance on how to treat it; *humor therapy*, which can neutralize stress, increase circulation, improve respiration, enhance heart and muscle tone, and stimulate the immune response; and *music therapy*, which has been shown to ease pain and anxiety, increase learning and memory skills, enhance immunity, promote feelings of peacefulness and joy, reduce insomnia and depression, and aid in the treatment of conditions such as autism, Alzheimer's disease, childhood cerebral palsy, and schizophrenia.

SOCIAL AND SPIRITUAL COMPONENTS ❦ OF MENTAL HEALTH ❦

Practitioners in the field of mind-body medicine emphasize that optimal health, in addition to physical well-being and emotional and mental stability, involves strong positive connections to one's spouse or intimate partner, friends, family members, and members of one's community. The importance of social relationships with respect to health has also been well documented by a variety of scientific studies. Research, for example, shows a high incidence of illness and death after the loss of a loved one. Other studies point to a lack of healthy social relationships as a common denominator among patients with heart disease, particularly when accompanied by feelings of hostility and a sense of isolation. Conversely, the longevity of terminal cancer patients with long-term survival rates has been attributed to a relatively high degree of social involvement.

One of the most convincing studies highlighting the importance of being socially connected found that Hispanic people, despite poverty, lack of health insurance, and poor access to medical care, are surprisingly less likely than whites to die of major chronic diseases, including all forms of cancer, heart disease, and respiratory ailments. Moreover, with the exception of diabetes, liver disease, and homicide, their overall health outlook is significantly better than for whites. Some health experts, including former Surgeon General Coello Novello, the first Latina to serve in that post, postulate that the reason for this stems from Hispanic culture, which promotes strong family values and frowns on health risks such as drinking and smoking. Lending credence to Dr. Novello's hypothesis is a growing body of evidence indicating that people with the fewest social connections are more prone to illness and less likely to recover once illness strikes. One long-term study also found that people with the fewest number of meaningful social relationships had a 200 to 300 percent greater overall risk of death, compared to people with the greatest amount of significant social connections. A growing number of other relationship studies have led researchers to conclude that social isolation is statistically just as dangerous as smoking, high blood pressure, high cholesterol, obesity, or lack of exercise.

Recent research shows that spiritual and religious observances, practices, and beliefs can provide significant health benefits, as well. In addition to engendering a greater sense of peace and acceptance of life events, spiritual and religious practices can result in increased self-confidence and a greater sense of purpose. Spiritual and religious traditions also reduce health risks by discouraging harmful activities such as unsafe sexual practices, and the use of alcohol, drugs, cigarettes, and other toxic substances. Studies show that spirituality and religion can also contribute to a deeper sense of connectedness to life, making it easier to deal with life challenges while reducing feelings of anxiety, depression, fear, and loneliness, all of which have been shown to suppress immune function. But perhaps the most important health benefit of a committed spiritual or religious practice, according to Dr. Ivker, lies in its ability to connect us to the underlying life force energy to which all spiritual and religious traditions refer. "In holistic medicine, this energy is referred to as unconditional or divine love," Dr. Ivker explains. "By allowing yourself to become more open to receiving and expressing unconditional love, you will begin to experience a profound reduction in your feelings of fear, a greater acceptance of yourself and others, and a heightened awareness of your purpose and unique talents. This process of spiritual growth will enable you to more fully experience the power of the present moment." ❧

CONDITIONS THAT BENEFIT FROM MIND-BODY MEDICINE

Mind-body medicine is a valuable treatment for all diseases of a poten-tially psychosomatic nature. This is particularly true of conditions caused or exacerbated by stress, which is estimated to be a co-factor in at least 85 percent of all disease conditions. By learning how to better manage and control their thoughts and emotions, patients are more empowered to more actively participate in, and influence the outcome of, the healing process, including bolstering immune function and reducing the impact of mental and emotional stressors. What follows is an overview of some of the benefits of the various mind-body therapies discussed above.

Autogenic Training

Over six hundred published clinical studies on the benefits of autogenic training were conducted prior to 1959, when its developer, Johannes Schultz, along with his colleague Wolfgang Luthe, published the first English translation of their original work *Das Autogene Training*. Among the conditions for which autogenic training has been shown to be clinically effective are alcoholism, bronchial asthma, angina pec-toris, cardiovascular conditions, impaired circulation, endocrine disor-ders, epilepsy, hypertension, insomnia and other sleep disorders, skin conditions, stuttering, vision problems, and conditions of the urogeni-tal tract. In addition, autogenic training can alleviate problems associ-ated with pregnancy. According to C. Norman Shealy, founding president of the American Holistic Medical Association, autogenic training has also been shown to help patients cope with associated disorders (fatigue, muscle cramping, tremor, and lack of emotional control) related to diseases of the central nervous system, such as Parkinson's disease, multiple sclerosis, and Huntington's chorea. Dr. Shealy reports that autogenic training has also shown benefit for people suffering from anxiety, depression, melancholia, and phobia, as well as schizophrenia when used in conjunction with conventional psychiatric procedures. People suffering from drug and nicotine addiction have also been shown to benefit from regular practice of standard autogenic training exercises.

The conditions for which autogenic training has been shown to be most effective are those that are psychophysiological or psychosomatic in nature, including constipation, colitis, gastritis, hemorrhoids, and other gastrointestinal conditions; nausea; loss of appetite; vomiting; and gallbladder dysfunction. It also relieves anxieties associated with being overweight or obese, resulting in more effective weight loss. According to Dr. Shealy, autogenic training,when practiced daily for six to ten weeks, provides an 80 percent success rate among patients suffering from headache, respiratory conditions, muscle tension and spasm, insomnia, cardiac conditions, and sexual dysfunction. Moreover, it is capable of triggering a "relaxation response" similar to that achieved by the regular practice of meditation or biofeedback.

Biofeedback Training

Literally thousands of scientific studies show that biofeedback training can be effective for a variety of health conditions, including many that often fail to respond to conventional medicine.

Brain-wave, or neurofeedback, therapy, a form of biofeedback that helps normalize and regulate the normal alpha and theta wave activity in the brain, has been shown to be very effective in treating alcohol and drug addiction when used in conjunction with traditional counseling. This was demonstrated by a three-year study conducted by leading neurofeedback researchers Patricia Norris, Ph.D., and Steven Fahrion, Ph.D., at Ellsworth Correctional Facility in Kansas during the late 1990s. The study involved prison inmates diagnosed with alcohol or drug problems, almost all of whom had previously and unsuccessfully undergone a variety of other treatment programs. Training was provided prior to the prisoners' release back into society, after which time they were closely monitored by parole officers and submitted to frequent urinalysis. After two years of follow-up, 63 percent of the study's participants remained drug- and alcohol-free. Just as significantly, recidivism for new crimes was only 4 percent. Based on the success of the study, Kansas's Depart of Corrections has tripled the number of Ellsworth inmates who are receiving neurofeedback therapy,with similar programs being planned at other prisons throughout the state.

By training patients to relax sphincter muscles, biofeedback can also help alleviate severe cases of constipation. In one study involving twenty-six children, those who received biofeedback training had noticeably less constipation and fewer incidences of painful bowel movements after sixteen months, compared to those receiving conventional treatments, including laxatives, enema, and changes in diet.

Additional research has shown that biofeedback is effective for treating headache and migraine, due to its ability to teach patients how to increase hand temperature and regulate stress levels. Studies show that biofeedback is capable of achieving success rates of between 44 to 100 percent for headaches caused by tension related to muscle contraction, and that 84 percent of migraine sufferers who were taught biofeedback techniques achieve long-term (five years or more) improvement, as well. Similar decreases in patient pain and need for medication have also been documented.

Hypertension is another condition that responds well to biofeedback training, particularly when it is used with other forms of relaxation training. In one study involving nineteen patients suffering from high blood pressure, patients who received biofeedback training and were taught muscle relaxation techniques were able to significantly decrease their blood pressure levels, compared to those who used the relaxation techniques alone. For most patients, biofeedback is most useful for learning how to control systolic, rather than diastolic, pressure. Still, other studies have shown that biofeedback used in conjunction with relaxation can result in significant reduction in diastolic pressure for up to a year or more. Overall, biofeedback is most effective for cases of mild hypertension, while conventional drugs are usually more effective for cases that are moderate to severe.

Other conditions benefited by biofeedback include circulatory problems related to diabetes, gastrointestinal disorders, hypertension, insomnia, respiratory conditions, sexual dysfunction, stroke, temporal-mandibular joint syndrome (TMJ), and urinary and bowel incontinence.

Note: While biofeedback can be useful as a self-care technique, for it to be most effective, regular practice under the guidance of a certified biofeedback therapist is usually required.

Breathwork

Although not a health care therapy per se, breathwork therapies result in improved respiration patterns that can result in numerous physical and psychological benefits. Researchers in the field of breathwork point out that in infancy nearly all children breathe diaphragmatically, which allows for deeper, more relaxed respiration. By adulthood, however, most people, due to a lifetime of reacting to stress and trauma, breathe shallowly and inefficiently through the chest. Such unconscious breathing patterns tend to increase the likelihood of tension and fatigue. Learning how to breathe consciously and properly, by contrast, can result in improved energy levels, a greater ability to manage stress, and enhanced mental functioning. Fuller respiration patterns also result in greater oxygen delivery to the cells and can trigger the "relaxation response," resulting in overall improvement in how the body functions. Research also indicates that proper breathing can be helpful to people suffering from anxiety and depression, improve mood, and help resolve mental and emotional pain.

Eye Movement Desensitization and Reprocessing (EMDR)

EMDR is best known for its ability to rapidly and, in most cases, permanently heal anxiety, stress, and trauma. In 1987, EMDR's developer, Dr. Francine Shapiro, conducted the first controlled study involving EMDR. The study involved twenty-two randomly selected subjects, ranging in age from eleven to fifty-three, all of whom were suffering from post-traumatic stress disorder (PTSD). Study participants first received traditional "therapy," in which they would focus on the traumatic event responsible for triggering their PTSD, while talking about it. Using a scale known as Subjective Units of Disturbance (SUD), developed by behavioral therapist Joseph Wolpe in the 1950s, Dr. Shapiro assessed "how disturbing the traumatic memory felt to the subject before, during, and immediately after" treatment. Talk therapy produced no long-term benefits for the test subjects, but when they received EMDR treatment, nearly all of them were able to resolve their trauma after only one session. Follow-up research showed that the results remained in place one and three months later. In addition, all of the subjects' self-images improved, with feelings such as denial, fear, guilt, shame, and anger being replaced with self-esteem, confidence, forgiveness, and acceptance. Since the publication of Dr. Shapiro's study in 1989 in both the *Journal of Traumatic Stress* and the *Journal of Behavior Therapy and Experimental Psychiatry*, hundreds of other studies have confirmed her original findings, resulting in the fast growth of EMDR as a therapeutic intervention for PTSD and other stress- and anxiety-related conditions. In addition, EMDR has also shown benefit as a treatment for attention deficit hyperactivity disorder (ADHD), alcoholism and drug addiction, bipolar disorder (manic depression), cognitive disorders, depression, grief, nightmare and night terrors, panic attacks, personality disorders, phobias, and sleep disorders. Based on such results, today the use of EMDR continues to increase among psychotherapists, and it has been used to successfully treat more than one million people worldwide.

Flower Essences

As originally developed by Dr. Bach, flower essences were not intended to treat specific disease conditions, but rather to alleviate and resolve the underlying mental and emotional factors that Bach believed were at the root of all illness. As Bach wrote in 1934, "The action of these remedies is to raise our vibrations and open up our channels for the reception of the Spiritual Self; to flood our natures with the particular virtue we need, and wash out from us the fault that is causing the harm.... They cure, not by attacking the disease, but by flooding our bodies with the beautiful vibrations of our Higher Nature, in the presence of which, disease melts away as snow in the sunshine."

Based on this perspective, health practitioners who use flower essences tend to focus less on patients' disease conditions and more on their predominant emotional states. As limiting emotions, thoughts, and beliefs are resolved through the use of the appropriate flower essence, however, improvement in a variety of illnesses has also been reported. These include psychological conditions, such as anxiety, depression, and nervous tension; headache and migraine; asthma and other respiratory conditions; chronic fatigue; and acute trauma associated with accidents, bruises, and other injuries. One of the most powerful examples of how flower essences can help to heal illness is a clinical study conducted in the 1980s by John Bolling, Ph.D., a specialist in behavioral disorders and drug abuse. While serving as chief resident in psychiatry at New York University's Bellevue Medical Center, Dr. Bolling found that 80 percent of patients treated with flower remedies experienced significant improvements in their conditions. Not only did the essences serve to increase the patients' receptivity to receiving other treatment modalities, they also resulted in "dramatic improvement" in resolving blocked emotions in 20 percent of the group, who previously had been thought to be resistant to any form of therapeutic intervention.

Note: While flower essences can serve as an excellent self-care therapy for alleviating unresolved or limiting emotions, in order to be effective they usually require a period of weeks or months of regular use.

Guided Imagery and Visualization

The use of the imagination to stimulate wellness has been a part of Western holistic healing processes since the time of Hippocrates, who taught that imagery could influence the various functions of the body and produce changes in overall health. Since ancient times, imagery has also been used in the Ayurvedic healing tradition to encourage the body's healing mechanisms, often through the use of specific images known as *yantras.* Imagery is integral to shamanistic healing traditions, as well, and has become more widely accepted by modern scientists and physicians since Carl Simonton's early experiments using guided imagery and visualization with cancer patients in the 1970s.

Today, researchers recognize that imagery, in addition to helping stimulate the immune system, can relieve stress, ease pain symptoms, increase cell tissue oxygen levels, and positively affect brain, cardiovascular, and gastrointestinal function. As a result, guided imagery and visualization techniques are increasingly used in a variety of conventional and holistic modalities, including autogenic and biofeedback training, hypnotherapy, meditation, and psychotherapy. Imagery and visualization are also increasingly being used prior to surgical procedures, in order to help patients be better prepared and to reduce anxiety. Research shows that many patients who employ imagery techniques prior to, and during, their hospital stays, experience a reduction in pain, require less medication, and are able to return home sooner than usual. In addition, the use of guided imagery and visualization techniques can also help patients reach a better understanding of the nature of their illness, including, in some cases, how to more effectively treat it.

One of the most dramatic examples of how effective imagery can be to health involves Garrett Porter. When he was nine years old, Garrett was diagnosed with an inoperable, terminal brain tumor. Working with Dr. Patricia Norris, Garrett used biofeedback techniques in conjunction with guided imagery based on *Star Trek*, his favorite TV show. With Dr. Norris's help, within a year Garrett was able to achieve a complete remission of his condition, which was confirmed by brain scans showing his tumor's disappearance.

Numerous studies now confirm the health benefits of guided imagery and visualization. One study of volunteer college students, for example, found that those who practiced imagery twice daily over a six-week period experienced a marked increase in salivary immunoglobulin A (IgA), an indicator of increased immune activity, compared to the control group. Another study found that students who daily used imagery techniques prior to their final exams had far less of a decline in their helper T-immune cells than is normally experienced by students during such examination periods. Other clinical studies have shown that guided imagery and visualization techniques work to improve and maintain health due to their ability to directly affect the health of the cells, particularly with regard to neuropeptides. Among the conditions for which research shows imagery and visualization techniques have benefit are anxiety, autoimmune conditions, cancer, depression, diabetes, headache and migraine, heart disease, pain, and stress-related disorders. Imagery has also been shown to be helpful as an aid to quitting smoking, and as a means of enhancing performance and motor skills, including athletic performance.

Hypnotherapy

Hypnotherapy's proven efficacy for treating both physical and psychological problems is well established. Today, it is used by a variety of health care practitioners to treat a wide range of conditions, including addiction, anorexia, anxiety, asthma, arthritis (both rheumatoid and osteo), bedwetting, chronic pain, depression, gastrointestinal disorders, headache and migraine, hypertension, impotence, immune dysfunctions, nausea, phobias, skin conditions, and stress. It is also used by many dentists to help patients better cope with the anxiety and pain related to dental procedures, and has been shown to be effective as an aid during pregnancy and childbirth, and for enhancing creativity, relaxation, and performance skills. Hypnotherapy has also been shown to be beneficial for managing pain related to breast cancer, bone marrow biopsies, and oral pain as a side effect of chemotherapy.

One of hypnotherapy's most remarkable applications is as a substitute for anesthesia. First used in this regard by British physician James Esdaile and French physician Jules Cloquet in the early 1800s, hypnoanesthesia is now used by a growing number of physicians to help ease pain during and after surgery, as well as for treating the pain of serious burns. In 1960, the late Maurice Tinterow, M.D., Ph.D., published a dramatic case of hypnoanesthesia in the journal *The American Surgeon*. The case involved one of Dr. Tinterow's patients, a fifteen-year-old girl in need of open heart surgery who was allergic to all anesthetic chemicals. Due to the potentially fatal consequences of using the anesthetics on her, Dr. Tinterow opted to use hypnotherapy instead. For eight weeks prior to her surgery, he used hypnosis to help the girl enter a state of deep relaxation. He then hypnotized her before her surgery began, and she remained conscious and pain-free throughout the procedure, which lasted for four hours. While her heart was being repaired, Dr. Tinterow instructed her to picture herself waterskiing, an activity she very much enjoyed. To ensure that her mind was functioning properly, he also had her perform various arithmetic exercises. The operation was a complete success, and afterwards Dr. Tinterow reported that the girl required no medication of any kind, including aspirin to deal with postsurgical pain. Besides this event, Dr. Tinterow also successfully employed hypnotherapy to control pain during a number of other surgical procedures, including breast biopsies, cesarian section childbirths, hemorrhoidectomies, hernias, and hysterectomies, as well as for the treatment of second- and third-degree burns.

Two other areas for which hypnotherapy is popular are smoking cessation and weight loss. While certain hypnotherapists offer workshops purporting to help smokers quit their habit in one session, a review of seventeen studies involving smokers who had used hypnosis found that after six months the range of those who were still not smoking ranged from 4 to 88 percent. For smokers who receive several hours of hypnotherapy and follow-up treatment, however, research indicates that long-term success rates average 50 percent or higher.

Hypnotherapy's effectiveness for weight loss has also been clinically verified. In one study involving obese patients, for instance, those who received hypnotherapy alone, or in conjunction with listening to audiotape suggestions, lost an average of seventeen pounds over six months, compared to the control group, which actually gained weight.

Note: Hypnotherapy is most effective for people who are most susceptible to hypnotic suggestion. According to the World Health Organization, 90 percent of the population are capable of being hypnotized, but only 20 to 30 percent have high susceptibility.

Journaling

The practice of keeping a journal has been shown to help patients better cope with disease, more effectively communicate their thoughts and emotions, and bolster immunity. One of the original investigators of journaling's health benefits is research psychologist Dr. James Pennebaker. In one of his studies, Dr. Pennebaker instructed test subjects to spend fifteen to twenty minutes for four consecutive days writing about their emotional challenges. After they had done so, all of the subjects were found to have improved immune function, which lasted for an additional six weeks without the need for any further writing. Additional follow-up revealed that months later all of the subjects were reporting less need for doctor-assisted medical treatments for their illnesses than they had previously required.

Another study by Dr. Pennebaker compared the effects on journaling on forty-six college students, all of whom had previously visited the college health care clinic with similar frequency. The students were divided into two groups, with the first group instructed to record their thoughts and feelings about traumatic events they had experienced, and the second group told to simply write about everyday trivial occurrences. At the end of the study, the students who had written about their trauma had a 50 percent reduction in clinic visits, compared to the other group.

Until recently, most of the research conducted on journaling involved subjects who were already healthy. In 1999, however, a study involving sixty-one asthma patients and fifty-one patients suffering from rheumatoid arthritis revealed that journaling is effective for relieving disease symptoms, as well. In the study, patients were divided into two groups, with each group being asked to write either about the most stressful event of their lives or about emotionally neutral events. Both groups wrote for twenty minutes for three consecutive days. Four months later, those patients who had written about their trauma showed a 19 percent improvement of asthma symptoms, and a 28 percent reduction of arthritis pain, compared to patients in the other group. Additional research into the positive effects of journaling has shown that writing about traumatic events can enhance immune function by increasing lymphocyte levels in the bloodstream, and can also be beneficial for reducing hypertension.

Meditation

The health benefits of meditation have been scientifically verified since the 1960s, when researchers found that meditation masters from India could regulate and voluntarily control functions of the autonomic nervous system while in a meditative state. Since then, well over a thousand clinical studies have been conducted on the effects of meditation on a wide range of physiological processes.

In addition to the health benefits of meditation discussed above, research shows that:

Regular practice of meditation lowers resting heart rates, and can help lower blood pressure levels in cases of moderate hypertension, and that both benefits diminish or cease entirely when meditation is discontinued. Research by Dean Ornish, M.D., also shows that meditation when practiced as part of a comprehensive change in lifestyle, can stabilize, and in many cases reverse, heart disease.

Meditation produces marked changes in both alpha and theta activity, brain-wave states associated with heightened relaxation, creativity, concentration, mental functioning, and positive emotions such as pleasure, happiness, and joy.

Meditation results in metabolic and respiratory changes, suggesting a decreased need by the body for energy and oxygen in order to function.

Meditation reduces muscle tension and blood lactate levels linked to stress and anxiety and increases galvanic skin responses, another indication of lessened stress.

Meditation alleviates chronic pain. One study conducted by Jon Kabat-Zinn, Ph.D., founding director of the Stress Reduction Clinic at the University of Massachusetts Medical Center, found that after eight weeks of meditation, ninety patients suffering from chronic pain achieved pain reductions of 33 to 50 percent, along with significant reductions in accompanying anxiety and depression levels, compared to patients receiving conventional pain care.

In addition, meditation has also been shown to be an effective aid in the treatment of alcohol and drug addiction, and capable of creating deeper levels of relaxation than those normally achieved by ordinary rest. Meditation also has been shown to improve memory and intelligence skills, enhance reaction time, and increase motor skills, as well as promoting greater levels of emotional equanimity, detachment, and peace of mind.

Progressive Relaxation

The original research related to progressive relaxation was conducted by Edmund Jacobson, the physician who developed it. Included in Jacobson's research were the findings that progressive relaxation is capable of reducing anxiety, chronic muscle tension, hypertension, nervous irritability and excitement, and chronic stress. In addition, Jacobson achieved significant clinical results using progressive relaxation techniques to treat numerous other disease conditions, including cardiac neurosis, colitis, compulsive tic, depression, fatigue, hyperthyroidism (Graves' disease), mild cases of phobia, and generalized spastic paresis. More recent research reveals that progressive relaxation is also effective in reducing the effects of trauma, stimulating immune function, enhancing mood, and alleviating chronic pain.

In one study involving sixty-four patients suffering from orthopedic trauma due to incidents that included gunshot wounds and crushed ankles, patients who received relaxation training, either alone or with biofeedback training, exhibited significantly less anxiety and pain and had lower blood pressure levels compared to control groups. Another study involving forty-five elderly participants in nursing homes found that progressive relaxation can enhance immunity. In the study, the participants were divided into three groups. The first group was led through progressive relaxation exercises three times a week for a month. The second group received visitors three times a week for the same period, and the third group received no training or social contact. At the end of the month, those who received progressive relaxation reported greater levels of relaxation and had improved natural killer cell activity, compared to the other two groups, both of which exhibited no change in immune status or relaxation levels.

Progressive relaxation exercises can also be used to improve mood, as was demonstrated by a study involving 154 patients receiving radiation treatments for breast cancer. The patients were divided into three groups, with the first group taught progressive relaxation and deep breathing exercises, the second group receiving progressive relaxation and guided imagery, and the third group, which served as the control, instructed to discuss their situations among themselves. Prior to the study, all participants self-assessed their mood, with all of them sharing similar scores. Six weeks later, the first two groups reported significantly higher mood scores than those in the control group.

Studies show that progressive relaxation provides more effective relief for chronic low back pain than either biofeedback training or placebo, while additionally reducing associated muscle tension. Progressive relaxation is useful for relieving pain following surgery, as well. One study of one hundred patients who underwent surgery of the spine found that patients who received one hour of progressive relaxation training the night before their surgeries required less pain medication after the procedures and were able to leave the hospital sooner than those who did not. Another controlled study involving forty-two patients scheduled to receive elective surgery produced similar results, with patients who were taught progressive relaxation also requiring less pain medication, as well as exhibiting more rhythmical patterns compared to the control group.

Somatic Psychology

The various therapies that comprise the field of somatic psychology have been shown to be effective in treating a wide range of disease conditions of both a psychological and physiological nature. An overview of the research in this area is provided in Chapter 9.

Thought Field Therapy (TFT)

Since its development by Roger Callahan, Ph.D., more than twenty years ago, thought field therapy has demonstrated a remarkable track record for providing rapid, effective treatment of most problems of a psychological nature. Among the mental/emotional conditions TFT can benefit are anxiety, depression, alcohol and drug addiction, chronic anger, eating disorders, general stress, irrational guilt, panic attacks, phobias, post-traumatic stress disorder, and psychologically related sexual dysfunctions, as well as being able to reverse limiting or self-sabotaging belief and thought patterns. TFT is highly effective for resolving emotional pain and trauma due to child abuse and rape, and for alleviating fears related to such issues as acrophobia (fear of heights), public speaking, flying, or visits to doctors and dentists. It can also be used successfully to reverse negative habits, such as smoking.

More recent research has demonstrated that the Callahan Techniques can benefit various physical conditions, including food and environmental allergies, attention deficit disorder, hypertension, fibromyalgia, seasonal affective disorder (SAD), sinus conditions, and chronic pain. Through the use of a medical device that measures heart rate variability (HRV) and the health status of the autonomic nervous system (ANS), Fuller Royal, M.D., of Las Vegas, Nevada, has found that the Callahan Techniques help to dramatically improve his patients' symptoms, as shown by pre- and post-treatment measurements of HRV and ANS rates. One of the advantages of the HRV equipment Dr. Royal uses is that it is not influenced by suggestion or the placebo effect, meaning that its readings are based solely on the physiological status of each patient's heart rate and ANS, and therefore able to accurately detect any imbalances that may be present. Thus, when patients report an improvement or cessation of symptoms, the device is able to verify whether such improvement has in fact occurred.

Based on the growing acceptance of TFT by a variety of psychologists, physicians, and health counselors, as well as continued research regarding its benefits, its use is likely to become more commonly available in the near future.

YOUR FIRST SESSION

As with bodywork (see Chapter 9), your experience with mind-body medicine will vary according to the type of mind-body therapy you choose to explore. Some mind-body approaches, such as journaling, meditation, or working with affirmations, can easily be adapted as regular self-care routines, with positive benefits usually noticeable within a few weeks of daily practice. If you feel you require assistance in resolving mental or emotional issues, however, you will most likely receive greater benefit exploring the professional care therapies outlined above, some of which, such as autogenic training, biofeedback training, hypnotherapy, and progressive relaxation, can also be adapted as self-care approaches once you have received proper training in their use.

Session time and length of treatment will also vary according to the therapy you select, with sessions usually ranging from forty-five to ninety minutes. Some forms of therapy, such as biofeedback training, psychotherapy, and somatic psychology, can require a time commitment ranging from weeks to months, before full results are achieved, while other therapies can often yield results more quickly. In all cases, however, treatment results depend to a large degree on the nature of each person's problem and psychological makeup, as well as individual goals.

During the course of your therapy, deep-seated unexpressed or painful emotions may surface, as well as traumatic events from your past that may have been forgotten or suppressed. Such occurrences are normal, and rather than being cause for alarm, they offer you the opportunity to resolve or positively reframe them, while at the same time learning the lessons they carry. Due to the painful nature of such experiences, however, many patients find themselves resisting them. A skillful therapist can guide you past this resistance in a manner that is both safe and ultimately rewarding.

SELECTING A PRACTITIONER

Before selecting a practitioner, it is helpful to have a clear idea of what your goals are. The following guidelines apply for all practitioners, however, regardless of which form of mind-body medicine you choose.

Choose a practitioner who is properly trained and certified. While many of the therapies within the field of mind-body medicine are not required to be licensed, most competent practitioners are affiliated with at least one of the professional organizations or associations listed in the "Resources" section below. If you have any doubts about a practitioner's qualification, be sure to ask for information about his or her background. Also seek out recommendations from people you know and trust regarding practitioners they are satisfied with. In addition, because of the sometimes vulnerable nature of mind-body medicine, let your practitioner know when you are feeling uncomfortable, and don't hesitate to stop treatment if you feel he or she is not respectful of you or is ignoring the boundaries within which you are comfortable.

Before beginning treatment, also inquire about fees, which can vary widely, and determine whether your insurance policy will cover them. Depending on the therapy and practitioner you choose, costs can range from $50 to $150 per session, and even more, and insurance coverage is largely dependent on the type of treatment best suited to your needs.

THE FUTURE OF MIND-BODY MEDICINE

The continued acceptance and availability of mind-body medicine in the United States and around the world, on the part of laypeople and conventional and holistic practitioners alike, appears certain to accelerate throughout the twenty-first century, due to the increasing number of exciting studies that are demonstrating the inextricable link between our thoughts, emotions, beliefs, and physical health. Already throughout the United States, major hospitals and university medical centers are incorporating aspects of mind-body medicine as a means of offering more effective, "patient-centered" care. The many self-care elements of mind-body medicine are also likely to be increasingly promoted by physicians to their patients, due to the proven health benefits they provide. As this trend continues, it seems increasingly probable that before long all disease, regardless of type, will be treated according to the principles of holistic medicine that mind-body medicine exemplifies, with patients' specific mental, emotional, and spiritual needs receiving attention equal to that given their bodily and environmental requirements.

RESOURCES

Further information about mind-body medicine and the specific therapies discussed in this chapter can be obtained by contacting the following organizations and associations.

General

Center for Mind-Body Medicine
5225 Connecticut Avenue N.W., Suite 414
Washington, D.C. 20015
Phone: (202) 966-7338
Web site: *www.cmbm.org*

Mind/Body Medical Institute
110 Francis Street
Boston, Massachusetts 02215
Phone: (617) 632-9525
Web site: *mindbody.harvard.edu*

Biofeedback/Neurofeedback Training

Association for Applied Psychotherapy and Biofeedback
10200 W. 44th Avenue, Suite 304
Wheat Ridge, Colorado 80033
Phone: (800) 477-8892
Web site: *www.aapb.org*

Life Sciences Institute of Mind-Body Health
2955 S.W. Wanamaker Drive, Suite B
Topeka, Kansas, 66614
Phone: (785) 271-8686
Web site: *www.cjnetworks.com/~lifesci/*

Breathwork

Rebirth International
P.O. Box 118
Walton, New York 13856
Phone: (607) 865-8254

EMDR

EMDR Institute
P.O. Box 51010
Pacific Grove, California 93950
Phone: (408) 372-3900
Web site: *www.emdr.com*

Flower Essences

Nelson Bach USA Ltd
100 Research Drive
Wilmington, Massachusetts 01887
Phone: (800) 319-9151
Web site: *www.nelsonbach.com*

Guided Imagery and Visualization

Academy for Guided Imagery
P.O. Box 2070

Mill Valley, California 94942
Phone: (800) 726-2070
Web site: *www.interactiveimagery.com*

Hypnotherapy

American Psychotherapy and Medical Hypnosis Association
210 S. Sierra Street, Suite B-100
Reno, Nevada 89501
Web site: *APMHA.com*

American Society of Clinical Hypnosis
33 W. Grand Avenue, Suite 402
Chicago, Illinois 60610
Phone: (312) 645-9810

National Guild of Hypnotists
P.O. Box 308
Merrimack, New Hampshire 03054
Phone: (603) 429-9438
Web site: *www.ngh.net*

Journaling

Intensive Journal Program
Dialogue House
80 East 11th Street, Suite 305
New York, New York 10003
Phone: (800) 221-5844
Web site: *www.intensivejournal.org*

Center for Journal Therapy
12477 West Cedar Drive, Suite 102
Lakewood, Colorado 80228
Phone: (888) 421-2298
Web site: *www.journaltherapy.com*

Meditation

Insight Meditation Society
1230 Pleasant Street

Barre, Massachusetts 01500
Phone: (978) 355-4378
Web site: *www.dharma.org*

Washington Center for Meditation Studies
1834 Swann Street, N.W.
Washington, D.C. 20009
Phone: (202) 234-2866

Somatic Psychology

The Naropa Institute
Somatic Psychology Department
2130 Arapahoe Avenue
Boulder, Colorado 80302
Phone: (303) 444-0202

Thought Field Therapy

Callahan Techniques, Ltd.
78-816 Via Carmel
La Quinta, California 92253
Phone: (760) 564-1008
Web site: *www.tftrx.com*

RECOMMENDED READING

General

Benson, Herbert, with Marg Stark. *Timeless Healing: The Power and Biology of Belief.* Scribners, 1996.
Dossey, Larry. *Healing Words.* HarperSanFrancisco, 1993.
Gordon, James. *Manifesto for a New Medicine.* Perseus Books, 1996.
Pert, Candace. *Molecules of Emotion.* Scribners, 1997.
Shealy, C. Norman. *Sacred Healing.* Element, 1999

Biofeedback

Norris, Patricia, and Garrett Porter. *Why Me? Harnessing the Healing Power of the Human Spirit.* Stillpoint Publishing, 1985.

Breathwork

Orr, Leonard. *Breaking the Death Habit: The Science of Everlasting Life.* North Atlantic Books, 1999.

EMDR

Shapiro, Francine, and Margot Silk Forrest. *EMDR: The Breakthrough "Eye Movement" Therapy for Overcoming Anxiety, Stress, and Trauma.* Basic Books, 1997.

Flower Essences

Bach, Edward, and F. J. Wheeler. *The Bach Flower Remedies.* Keats, 1979.

Guided Imagery and Visualization

Gawain, Shakti. *Creative Visualization.* Bantam Books, 1983.
Simonton, O. Carl, Stephanie Matthews and James L. Creighton. *Getting Well Again.* Bantam Books, 1992.

Hypnotherapy

Elman, David. *Hypnotherapy.* Westwood Publishing Company, 1984.

Journaling

Progoff, Ira. *At a Journal Workshop.* Tarcher/Putnam, 1992.

Meditation

Goleman, Daniel. *The Meditative Mind.* Tarcher/Putnam, 1988.
Kabat-Zinn, Jon. *Wherever You Go, There You Are.* Hyperion, 1994.

Somatic Psychology

Caldwell, Christine, ed. *Getting in Touch: The New Guide to Body-Centered Therapies.* Quest Books, 1997.

Thought Field Therapy

Callahan, Roger. *Five Minute Phobia Cure*. Enterprise Publishing, 1985.

Callahan, Roger and Joanne. *Thought Field Therapy and Trauma*. TFT Training Center, 1996.

Lambrou, Peter, and George Pratt. *Instant Emotional Healing*. Broadway Books, 2000.

CHAPTER 6

Osteopathic Medicine

Osteopathic medicine, sometimes referred to as *osteopathy*, is a complete system of primary health care that is both an integral part of mainstream medicine and firmly rooted in the principles of holistic medicine. It is also the most comprehensive holistic therapy to originate in the United States. Osteopathic medicine is most noted for its emphasis on the musculoskeletal system and the interrelationships of the body's nerves, muscles, bones, and organs, yet its overall scope is far more encompassing, says AHMA trustee Todd Alan Bezilla, D.O., a full-time faculty member in the Osteopathic Manipulative Medicine Department at the Philadelphia College of Osteopathic Medicine in Philadelphia and a certified specialist in a variety of osteopathic medical techniques.

"The primary goal of osteopathic medicine is to educate patients while working with them as active participants in their journey to optimal health in body, mind, and spirit," Dr. Bezilla says. "To achieve this goal, osteopathic physicians take a multifaceted approach towards disease prevention and treatment, and seek to learn as much about their patients as possible." Osteopathic physicians (D.O.'s), along with M.D.'s, are also the only qualified physicians licensed to prescribe medications and perform major surgery. In addition, like many M.D.'s, many D.O.'s specialize in specific health fields, such as cardiology, ophthalmology, rheumatology, pediatrics, psychology, and surgery. They also generally receive more training in preventive medicine than do conventional allopathic M.D.'s, and are more oriented to treating the whole person. In recent years, osteopathic medicine has emerged as one of the fastest-growing medical professions in the United States, with many D.O. candidates choosing to become osteopathic physicians because of its original holistic philosophy.

❧ FAST FACTS ❧

Osteopathic medicine's basic philosophy and scientific principles were first set forth by physician Andrew Taylor Still in 1874. Dr. Still went on to found the first school of osteopathic medicine in 1892.

All fifty states and the District of Columbia license osteopathic physicians for the unlimited practice of medicine and surgery.

Currently, there are approximately 44,000 osteopathic physicians (D.O.'s) practicing in the United States, and nineteen fully accredited U.S. colleges of osteopathic medicine. In the college year 1998–1999, these colleges had a combined enrollment of approximately 9,630 students, attesting to osteopathic medicine's growing popularity.

All D.O.'s must complete four years of osteopathic medical training, followed by an additional three years of postgraduate osteopathic medical education in the form of a residency, undergoing an extensive training program parallel to that of conventional M.D.'s. Like M.D.'s, D.O.'s who choose to pursue a specialty discipline must often complete additional postgraduate training that typically extends their training another two to six years, depending upon the specialty.

Approximately 64 percent of all D.O.'s practice in primary care areas such as family practice, internal medicine, obstetrics/gynecology, and pediatrics.

Each year in the United States, over 100 million office visits are made to D.O.'s, many of them from referrals by conventional M.D.'s ❧

HISTORY OF OSTEOPATHIC MEDICINE

The founder of osteopathic medicine was Dr. Andrew Still (1828–1917), a conventionally trained physician who served as a soldier and surgeon for the North during the Civil War and was also an abolitionist and early supporter of woman's suffrage. Still developed the philosophy and techniques of osteopathic manipulation after becoming disillusioned with the medical approaches of his time, which failed to prevent the deaths of his first wife and six of his seven children, three of whom died in the same year during a meningitis epidemic. In 1864, saddened by the limitations of his chosen profession and rejecting its reliance on harmful drugs and practices to treat disease, Still sought alternate approaches to medicine that worked with the body's natural healing abilities. For the next ten years, he actively studied and experimented with the structures and functions of human anatomy, after observing that problems in the musculoskeletal system were always present in patients, regardless of their presenting disease condition. Still theorized that musculoskeletal imbalances, as well as the impaired functioning of the circulatory and nervous systems that accompanied them, significantly contributed to illness. To counteract these conditions, he manually manipulated the body to restore proper nerve function and circulation. Based on the success he achieved, Still came to regard the musculoskeletal system as a key component to overall health, leading him to formulate the principles of a system of health care he called osteopathy, which he derived from the Greek root words *osteo* (bone) and *patheia* (suffering).

At the core of Still's philosophy was his belief that "structure governs function," a tenet that remains one of the primary principles of osteopathic medicine today. His research also led him to the realization that true health entailed not only physical well-being but also harmony in mind and spirit. Presaging the philosophy of health espoused by holistic physicians today, he wrote, "Man is triune when complete. First, the material body; second, the spiritual being; third, a being of mind which is far superior to all vital motions and material forms.... Thus to obtain good results, we must blend ourselves with, and travel in harmony with, nature's truths." Compared to most American physicians of the nineteenth century, Still was a visionary in a number of other ways, as well. In addition to emphasizing preventive medicine and teaching that physicians should treat *patients*, not *symptoms*, he was one of the first American healers to identify the human immune system and develop natural methods for enhancing its function. He also pointed out that women were far too often subjected to needless, and even harmful, surgeries, and warned that allopathic medicine's overreliance on addictive prescriptive drugs would result in an increase in alcoholism and drug addiction that would escalate throughout the twentieth century.

In 1874, Still officially introduced osteopathic medicine to the world, declaring, "To find health should be the object of the doctor. Anyone can find disease." Almost immediately, however, he was branded a quack due to the fierce opposition his teachings faced from the medical establishment of his time. Undaunted, he spent the next eighteen years crisscrossing the United States in order to demonstrate his techniques to whoever would listen. Finally, in 1892, he gained enough supporters to found the American School of Osteopathy in Kirksville, Missouri, which became the first institution to grant Doctor of Osteopathy (D.O.) degrees. Once again he demonstrated his visionary instincts, by seeing to it that the college welcomed both women and minorities as students, making it the first U.S. medical school to do so. In keeping with the principles Still formulated, students at the college were taught a curriculum that emphasized the body's self-healing capacities and disease prevention, including proper diet and exercise. They also received instruction in palpation, osteopathic manipulation techniques, and noninvasive diagnosis and treatment methods that Still developed. Following the college's inception, and based largely on word-of-mouth recommendations from satisfied patients, osteopathic medicine grew in popularity. In 1896, Vermont became the first state to license D.O.'s, and in 1896 the American Association for the Advancement of Osteopathy was founded. In 1901 the association renamed itself the American Osteopathic Association, which remains the leading organization in the United States devoted to promoting and overseeing osteopathic medicine.

Throughout the first half of the twentieth century, the American Medical Association (AMA) remained staunchly opposed to osteopathic medicine, despite research conducted as early as 1898 that validated its effectiveness. In addition to continuing to classify D.O.'s as quacks, the AMA threatened to prevent its members from practicing in the military during World War I if D.O.'s were also allowed to practice. This tactic was repeated during World War II, as well, although ironically it led to an increase in the popularity of D.O.'s among patients who were led to try it because of the number of M.D.'s called away from home to tend to American troops. By the time of Still's death in 1917, there were more than five thousand licensed D.O.'s practicing in the United States, and the first osteopathic college had been established in England.

Another early pioneer in the osteopathic medical field was Dr. William Garner Sutherland (1873–1954), who enrolled in the American School of Osteopathy in 1895. Like Still, Sutherland was regarded as a medical heretic, because of his research devoted to the body's self-healing mechanisms and his theories about what he termed "the Primary Respiratory Mechanism." Sutherland postulated that the body's central nervous system maintained a constant rhythmic motion that was essential to health and comprised of five components. Sutherland identified these components as motion at the cranial sutures, or joints, that link the skull's twenty-six bones; motion (expansion and contraction) of the brain's left and right hemispheres; motion of the membranes enfolding the brain and spinal cord; motion within the cerebrospinal fluid bathing the brain and spinal cord; and involuntary motion of the sacrum, or tailbone. By correcting impediments to these five elements of Primary Respiration using cranial osteopathic manipulation, Sutherland was able to successfully treat numerous patients suffering from a broad range of disease conditions. Despite this, his theories were soundly rejected by the medical establishment, even after he published a book to explain them in 1939. By the mid-1940s, however, Sutherland's views began to take hold, leading to the establishment in 1946 of the Osteopathic Cranial Association, now known as the Cranial Academy. Following advances in technology in the late twentieth century, Sutherland's theories were eventually validated using computerized diagnostic devices.

The second half of the twentieth century witnessed the acknowledgment of osteopathic medicine by the conventional medical establishment, spurred in large part by growing public acceptance and, beginning in 1936, the inspection and approval of osteopathic hospitals for the training of interns. During 1936–1937, 18 hospitals received such approval, and 81 physicians served internships within them. By 1996, there were 144 accredited osteopathic health care facilities in the United States, with 1,456 internships and 4,511 residencies being served. In 1952, osteopathic medicine was further validated when the U.S. Office of Education, Department of Health, Education and Welfare (now known as the Department of Health and Human Services) officially recognized the American Osteopathic Association as the accrediting body for osteopathic education in the United States. Today, osteopathic physicians practice in all branches of medicine and surgery, many of them working side by side with conventional M.D.'s in hospitals and health clinics nationwide. In 1993, osteopathic medicine became the first holistic therapy to acquire legal statutory recognition in Europe with the signing of the Osteopaths Bill by England's Queen Elizabeth.

HOW OSTEOPATHIC MEDICINE WORKS

Inherent in osteopathic medicine's approach to treating disease and restoring health are the principles formulated by Dr. Still, beginning with the recognition of each patient as a "complete entity" of body, mind, and spirit. According to Dr. Bezilla, the following principles also underlie osteopathic medicine:

Each person has inherent homeostatic, self-regulatory mechanisms that have the capacity to repair and heal following injury or other nociceptive (pain- or injury-related) challenges. When nociceptive challenges occur, the body will palpably express observable changes that allow for early detection of such disturbances. Unless they are appropriately diagnosed and treated, these changes, via the central and autonomic nervous system, and intra- and intercellular communication, can contribute to the continuation of the imbalances caused by the original nociceptive challenge.

The unrestricted flow of air, nerve impulses, and body fluids (blood, lymph, cerebrospinal, and excretory) is essential to the maintenance of optimal health.

Structure (form) and function are reciprocally interrelated, and influences on one also influence the other.

All living beings are greater than the sum of their collective parts and animated by an unseen, vital energy (spirit) that needs to flow freely and without obstruction throughout each organism for health to be realized.

Air, sunshine, water, plants, and animals help to sustain, maintain, and promote health and vitality, and should regularly be experienced, consumed, and enjoyed in their pure, unaltered forms, as free of pollution, chemical toxins, and other artificial substances as possible.

A healthy diet, proper nutrition, appropriate regular physical activity, a positive mental attitude, and the ability to properly manage stress are all essential for good health.

While genetics can be a major factor in predisposition to disease, modification or removal of other contributing disease factors can often significantly compensate for genetic susceptibility.

Prevention of disease is far superior to its treatment.

Guided by these principles, osteopathic physicians focus on detecting the underlying causes of their patients' illness, rather than simply treating their symptoms. In addition to evaluating their patients' physical conditions, they consider mental and emotional factors, including home and work environments and relationships, as well as any other stress factors that may be present. They also take the time to educate patients about good health and preventive measures to safeguard against disease.

In addition to using many of the same diagnostic tools (blood and urine tests, X-rays, etc.) and treatment approaches used by M.D.'s, D.O.'s employ hands-on diagnosis and treatment techniques specific to their profession and place particular emphasis on the musculoskeletal system. "During the initial evaluation, a patient's entire body is examined to assess any areas of asymmetry, alterations in range of motion, and tissue texture changes," Dr. Bezilla explains. "Osteopathic physicians are interested in determining what is causing such changes to occur and how they are influencing the patient's health. They then explore how to best correct these imbalances from the standpoint of manipulative medicine."

Once nonmechanical causes for illness or injury have been ruled out, the D.O. will create a comprehensive treatment plan suited to each patient's individual needs. Treatment will usually include osteopathic manipulative treatment (OMT) in order to correct musculoskeletal imbalances and enhance the circulation of blood and other body fluids. The rationale behind using OMT lies in osteopathy's recognition that musculoskeletal problems can affect health in a variety of ways. Conversely, disease conditions can also affect the musculoskeletal system, which comprises approximately two-thirds of the body's mass. Once such imbalances are corrected and circulation improves, the body's self-healing and self-regulatory mechanisms are able to operate more efficiently. Osteopathic manipulation also increases respiration, which in turn delivers more oxygen into the bloodstream, improving energy levels and such body processes as digestion.

There are a variety of OMT techniques that D.O.'s can employ to correct musculoskeletal imbalances, depending on each patient's presenting condition. Among the most common are joint mobilization, soft-tissue technique, muscle energy technique, myofascial release, strain/counter-strain technique, thrust technique, and cranial manipulation.

Joint mobilization involves slowly and gently moving joints through their range of motion, with the motion being gradually increased. This technique helps to restore full range of motion and to free joints from restrictions. It is usually employed when restricted movements are found following an evaluation of all body parts using motion testing (bending, stretching, rotation, etc.).

Soft-tissue technique helps to relax and release restrictions in the body's soft tissue (ligaments and fascia), particularly the muscles surrounding the spine and the joints of the body. Soft-tissue work can involve traction, rhythmic stretching, or the application of deep pressure to tense or restricted muscles, helping to relax them while improving the circulation of body fluids.

Muscle energy technique is used to relax specific muscles or muscle groups and to improve their range of motion. When this method is employed, patients may be instructed to hold specific muscles in position while their D.O. gently tenses and releases each muscle in turn. Counterforce can also be used, with the D.O. gently resisting or pushing against the direction of movement by the patient.

Myofascial release involves releasing tension in the fascia to restore balance to the musculoskeletal system, and therefore the entire body. In this method, D.O.'s use long, gentle strokes to stretch the musculature in order to release tension and relieve muscle pain. Muscle function is also improved by myofascial release, as is range of motion. (Myofascial release is covered in more detail in Chapter 9.)

Strain/counterstrain technique is employed when abnormal patterns of joint movement create tenderness in the surrounding musculature. When such tenderness is present, the D.O. will move the corresponding limb, and sometimes the entire body, into a specific position that allows muscles to relax and release any tension or spasms that are causing the pain. In addition to relieving pain, the strain/counterstrain technique also restores proper movement to joints to help prevent the pain's recurrence.

Thrust technique can be used by D.O.'s when range of motion is severely limited. In such cases, high-velocity, low-amplitude thrusts similar to those sometimes used in chiropractic (see Chapter 7) are employed to restore joint motion. Neural reflexes can also be reset or improved by thrust technique.

Cranial manipulation uses various cranial manipulation techniques developed by William Sutherland to diagnose and release tensions in the head, spine, and temporomandibular joints of the jaw. Such techniques are extremely gentle and subtle and help enhance the flow of cerebrospinal fluids surrounding the brain and nervous system. Cranial manipulation is also effective for relieving a variety of conditions, including dizziness, headache, hyperactivity, mood disorders, spinal problems, and temporomandibular joint syndrome (TMJ).

In addition to OMT, many D.O.'s use massage techniques, and prescribe specific exercises to enhance musculoskeletal function. They may also prescribe dietary changes, as well as nutritional supplementation, to ensure that the body has the nutrients it needs to properly function. Some osteopathic physicians use botanical remedies and homeopathic formulas when warranted (see Chapters 8, 10, and 11). When necessary, appropriate drugs may also be prescribed, as well as surgery. "The primary goal of osteopathic physicians is to assess and treat all of the causative factors related to each patient's disease," Dr. Bezilla says. "This includes patient anatomy, biochemistry, diet, level and type of physical activity, lifestyle habits, psychosocial stressors, and personal and family history. Once these factors have been identified, osteopathic treatment helps patients heal from within by restoring balance to the body systems and altering whatever external factors are contributing to their disease process. Pharmaceutical agents and surgical procedures which act by doing for the body what the body should be able to do on its own are used only when absolutely necessary for the immediate survival of the patient."

The final aspect of osteopathic treatment involves educating patients about steps they can take on their own to maintain the benefits they derive from their D.O.'s care. Patients are taught how to use their bodies more efficiently in order to improve body function and minimize musculoskeletal tension. Postural correction techniques enable patients to change habitual patterns of mis- and overuse that can damage joints and soft tissues, limit motion, and reduce energy levels.

Relaxation techniques can help patients cope better with stress. Such techniques, when used in conjunction with physical exercises and stretches, aid in restoring and maintaining structural function and motor coordination while reducing joint stress.

Breathing exercises may also be recommended when a patient exhibits dysfunctional breathing patterns that can cause the musculoskeletal system, particularly areas of the back, neck, and shoulders, to become unduly stressed. By learning how to breathe fully and smoothly through the diaphragm, patients also experience improved lung capacity and a lessening of joint restrictions caused by improper breathing habits.

Where appropriate, D.O.'s may offer nutritional guidance as well, especially with regard to specific nutrients that are known to play a role in the overall health of the musculoskeletal system and various body tissues.

Each of these measures can greatly enhance the effectiveness of osteopathic treatment and help patients maintain the health benefits that osteopathic medicine can provide. Depending on the complexity or severity of patients' conditions, follow-up treatments may also be advised.

CONDITIONS THAT BENEFIT FROM OSTEOPATHIC MEDICINE

Because of the scope of their medical training, osteopathic physicians are qualified to treat the same types of disease conditions as those treated by M.D.'s, and can provide particular relief for conditions related to musculoskeletal dysfunction. Ongoing research on the clinical applications of osteopathic medicine continues to validate Dr. Still's belief that osteopathic manipulation, by restoring structural balance to the body, can be a valuable aid in treating nonstructural health problems. What follows are a few of the health conditions for which osteopathic manipulative treatment (OMT) has proven to be effective.

Back and Neck Pain

Osteopathic physicians have successfully treated back and neck problems since the days of Dr. Still, and studies continue to show that osteopathic medicine can relieve back and neck pain and help improve full range of motion in associated musculature. One recent study found that OMT is not only effective in treating chronic low back pain, but also more cost-effective than conventional low back pain treatment methods. In the study, which was conducted over a twelve-week period, low back pain patients were either treated with OMT or received standard treatment options such as analgesics and anti-inflammatory medication, physical therapy, Transcutaneous Electric Nerve Stimulation (TENS), and hot/cold packs. Although all of the treatment methods were found to be effective, OMT resulted in lower overall treatment costs and a need for less medication.

Another study found that OMT was able to provide more immediate relief of back pain symptoms compared to therapeutic massage treatments, and that the improvement continued to be more significant after treatment was completed.

Carpal Tunnel Syndrome

A number of studies have found that OMT, particularly myofascial release, is an effective alternative to drugs and surgery for treating carpal tunnel syndrome. In addition to relieving pain and other symptoms associated with the condition, OMT has also been found capable of improving nerve conductivity, while being able to widen the carpal tunnel itself, thereby significantly reducing the need for surgery in nonsevere cases.

Fibromyalgia Syndrome

Fibromyalgia syndrome (FMS) is characterized by chronic musculoskeletal pain. While little research into nonconventional treatments for FMS have been conducted so far, several studies have found that OMT and patient reeducation provided by osteopathic physicians can provide effective relief of FMS symptoms. One study, involving eighteen FMS patients who had suffered with the condition for one year or longer, found that OMT can be effective in reducing tender point pain specific to FMS, as well as reducing associated somatic dysfunctions and improving daily "quality of life" parameters. Such benefits were achieved after only nine treatment sessions spaced one to three weeks apart. In addition, thermographic analysis showed that the majority of test subjects also exhibited signs of improved musculoskeletal symmetry by the time of the study's completion.

A subsequent study of FMS patients divided test subjects into four groups. The first group received OMT alone, the second group received OMT and were taught reeducation techniques, the third group received moist heat applications, and the fourth group served as the control. Baseline data was collected from each group at weeks two, four, seven, eleven, nineteen, and twenty-three of the study, using a standard Pain Management Inventory, Depression Scale, and a portion of the McGill Pain Questionnaire. Both OMT groups had significantly lower levels of perceived pain than the other two groups, while results within the OMT group that also received patient reeducation indicated that such instruction can provide additional benefits, as well.

Hamstring Problems

A 1994 study of twenty-one subjects between the ages of sixteen and fifty-seven who suffered from tight hamstrings found that the OMT counterstrain technique was effective in both reducing hamstring and psoas (loin muscles) tension, and improving flexion and extension. Prior to treatment, each subject was evaluated using palpation, hip range-of-motion exercises, and electromyography (EMG). All twenty-one subjects experienced a reduction of hamstring tension following treatment, and nineteen also exhibited increased range of motion.

Immunity

In order to evaluate anecdotal evidence of improved immune function following OMT treatments, researchers conducted a pilot study of two groups of volunteers who were vaccinated with a recombinant hepatitis B vaccine. The vaccinations were administered at the onset of the study, one month later, and again six months later. The object of the study was to determine levels of antibody production in the group of twenty subjects who received the vaccine, plus OMT, compared to the control group of nineteen subjects who received only the vaccine.

The OMT group received three OMT treatments per week for two weeks after each vaccine was administered. Throughout the study, blood samples were drawn from both groups and analyzed for antibody production to measure immune system response. Six weeks after the first vaccine was administered, eight subjects from the OMT group, and six from the control group, showed a positive antibody response. Eight weeks after the second vaccine, eleven subjects in the OMT group had a positive antibody response, compared to eight in the control group. More significantly, however, the mean anti-hepatitis B antibody titers in the OMT group was 170, compared to only 18 for the control group, indicating that OMT can result in significant immunologic enhancement.

Neurological Development

Because of its ability to improve nerve function, OMT can be useful in treating conditions of impaired neurological development. This was demonstrated by a study involving children between the ages of eighteen months and three years, all of whom suffered from neurological impairments. All of the children in the study exhibited significant neurological improvement after receiving only six to twelve OMT treatments.

Otitis Media

A growing body of evidence suggests that otitis media (chronic middle ear infection) is due at least in part to structural problems that prevent the ear canal from properly draining. As a result, blockages can occur, becoming breeding grounds for bacteria and infection. A 1994 study supports the possibility of an underlying structural cause for otitis media.

The study involved eight children ranging in age from seven months to thirty-five months, all of whom had histories of recurrent otitis media. Following an osteopathic structural exam, each child received three OMT sessions spaced one week apart. During the following year, the children's parents and physicians were contacted to determine the number of episodes of otitis media each child had experienced after the last OMT session. Four children had no recurrences whatsoever, and two others experienced only one additional episode. Of the remaining two children, even though one had four additional episodes and the other required surgery, follow-up examination indicated that both children experienced a longer period of improvement prior to their subsequent episodes, compared to the period between recurrences before they received OMT treatment. The results of the study suggest that OMT can provide improvement in cases of otitis media even after medication fails to do so.

Parkinson's Disease

While there is no known cure for Parkinson's disease, recent research has shown that OMT can substantially improve the gait of patients with the disease and help manage its characteristic movement deficits, thereby improving quality of life. In one study, ten patients with Parkinson's disease were paired with eight normal control subjects of comparable age. The gaits of both groups were analyzed before and after a single OMT session. In addition, the gaits of ten other patients with Parkinson's disease were measured before and after they received a sham-control procedure. All patients were also asked to forgo their medication for twelve hours.

The OMT session was designed to reduce rigidity, improve spinal mobility, and increase flexibility and muscle length across the limbs. Each patient was treated with one standardized, thirty-minute session of OMT involving fourteen osteopathic techniques.

Testing before and after the OMT session used computerized gait analysis as each subject was filmed unawares while walking the length of a forty-foot pathway six consecutive times. Results indicated that patients who received OMT had "statistically significant increases in stride length, cadence, and the maximum velocities of the upper and lower limbs after treatment," while both the normal patients treated with OMT and the Parkinson's patients who received sham treatments showed no significant changes. As a result of the study, OMT is now being considered as part of a comprehensive treatment program for managing Parkinson's disease.

Reflex Sympathetic Dystrophy

Reflex sympathetic dystrophy, also known as "shoulder-hand syndrome," is a neurovascular condition characterized by severe shoulder pain and stiffness, swelling, and burning pain of the hands. A study conducted in 1993 examined children between the ages of seven and fourteen who suffered from chronic reflex sympathetic dystrophy of their upper left extremities. Prior to the study, all of the children had proved resistant to pharmacological and surgical attempts to treat their condition. Clinical examination of the children revealed that they suffered from similar symptoms related to their condition, including decreased range of motion in their elbow and wrist extension, audible stridor (harsh respiration), tender points beneath the scapula, and fascial restrictions of the left thoracic inlet and the left forearm and wrist. A number of the children also reported that they suffered from headache and had difficulty inhaling.

Each of the children received OMT treatments administered bimonthly over a six-month period. At the end of the study, researchers noted that all subjects had regained full range of motion in their wrists and elbows and had full resolution of their stridor. Their subscapular tender points also resolved, and their other fascial restrictions showed significant improvement, as well. As a result of the study, the researchers concluded that OMT is a beneficial adjunctive therapy for chronic reflex sympathetic dystrophy, and more effective than some costlier and more invasive conventional treatment approaches.

Shoulder Pain

Research shows that OMT can relieve shoulder pain and improve shoulder function and range of motion, as evidenced by a study involving twenty-nine volunteers with a median age of sixty-two. All of the volunteers suffered from chronic shoulder pain and diminished range of motion and shoulder function prior to the study's onset. Each of the volunteers received five randomized treatments of OMT or sham manipulation treatments over a five-week period. After each treatment, their affected shoulders were examined for pain, range of motion, and functional abilities by an assessor who was not informed as to which group the patients belonged to. By the study's end, patients who received OMT showed significant improvement in each of the three categories, indicating that OMT is an effective treatment for shoulder dysfunction.

Other conditions for which osteopathic medicine has been shown to be beneficial include asthma, arthritic joint pain, birth trauma, bronchitis, colic, gastrointestinal disorders, genitourinary conditions, headache, hiatal hernia, migraine, pneumonia, restless leg syndrome, sciatica, sinusitis, traumatic injury, and temporomandibular joint syndrome (TMJ).

HEALING CHRONIC PAIN AND
HEALING GASTROESOPHAGEAL REFLUX:
❧ CASE HISTORIES ❧

The following case histories involving two of Dr. Bezilla's patients illustrate the health benefits that osteopathic medicine can provide, as well as the range of treatment options that osteopathic physicians can employ.

The first case involved a twenty-one-year-old woman who came to Dr. Bezilla six months after being involved in a rear-end collision. As a result of her accident, she suffered from pain involving the cervical, thoracic, and lumbar vertebrae, was constantly fatigued, and experienced a tingling in her left hand. "She had been a restrained passenger in the car and experienced two extension impacts of her occiput on the headrest of the seat," Dr. Bezilla explains. "Following the accident, she was given a diagnosis of whiplash and strain/sprain of her cervical, thoracic, and lumbar regions by her primary physician. X-rays were also obtained at the time of the accident and interpreted as unremarkable. She participated in ten weeks of intensive physical therapy and received osteopathic manipulative treatment (OMT) by her primary physician following the accident. However, these measures were unsuccessful at alleviating the continuous discomfort of her neck and upper and lower back. Four months after the accident, she began to experience tingling sensations in her left and right hands after she increasingly used her hands and arms at work at a gym and fitness center, as well as increasing and constant fatigue which she had tried to ignore."

Dr. Bezilla conducted a thorough medical history and learned that the woman also suffered from a mitral valve prolapse and, during childhood, had undergone multiple surgical procedures for craniofacial abnormalities. During childhood, she had also dislocated her left olecranon (the bony prominence behind the elbow joint) and on separate occasions had fractured the distal radius of her left and right arms. At nineteen she also had surgery to realign her upper and lower jaws. In order to cope with her pain, she had been taking anti-inflammatory drugs, which provided only minimal relief.

After conducting an osteopathic structural exam, Dr. Bezilla confirmed the chronic strain/sprain to her cervical, thoracic, and lumbar regions, and also found that she suffered from congenital scoliosis, carpal tunnel syndrome in her left arm, and somatic dysfunctions in her cranial, cervical, thoracic, costal, lumbar, sacral, and hip regions, and in her lower and left upper extremities.

"After my initial evaluation, I discussed my findings and their possible implications with the patient, explaining to her that significant results should be obtained within three to five treatments if my findings were indeed accurate," Dr. Bezilla says. "We discussed the importance of her being an active participant in her treatment and recovery. She was very motivated and understood the treatment rationale and importance of the total treatment plan."

Dr. Bezilla's treatment plan included OMT using osteopathy in the cranial field, soft-tissue and myofascial release, muscle energy, and low-velocity high-amplitude maneuvers to increase motion and normalize her somatic dysfunctions. He also taught the patient specific carpal tunnel stretches and total body range-of-motion exercises, which he instructed her to perform several times a day. "I also taught her abdominal breathing exercises to facilitate relaxation, decrease thoracic accessory muscle activation, and promote balance of the autonomic nervous system," Dr. Bezilla reports. "Nutritional supplements were utilized as well. A high-dose regimen of B-complex vitamins, including methylcobalamin, a form of vitamin B_{12}, were recommended for improving nerve inflammation and repair, and Siberian ginseng was used to assist in stress tolerance and to alleviate fatigue. I then instructed her to return for evaluation and treatment in one week."

After only five treatments given over a span of ten weeks, the woman experienced a complete recovery from her injuries and symptoms. "The first two treatments following the initial evaluation and treatment were each spaced one week apart, the next treatment was spaced at two weeks, and the final treatment was six weeks later," Dr. Bezilla says. "After the first three treatments, she no longer had any symptoms of carpal tunnel syndrome, her cranial spheno-basilar compression had resolved, and she no longer experienced chronic pain or serious muscle spasm. After the fourth and fifth final treatments, other than some minor chronically recurrent somatic dysfunctions in her thoracic, cervical, and left upper extremity regions related to her scoliosis, she was fully recovered from her motor vehicle injuries, and I was able to discontinue her B-complex and ginseng supplementation. She reported she was back to her pre-injury exercise regimen, doing well in school, and looking forward to her summer sporting activities."

Dr. Bezilla attributes his success in this case to the accuracy of his diagnosis and subsequent treatment approach. "The most significant finding in my opinion was the patient's spheno-basilar compression, which I believed was induced when her head struck the car's headrest in the accident," he says. "I believe it was the cranial dysfunction that ultimately had thwarted the patient's healing process. The widespread effects of a severe compression due to its direct effects on the pituitary gland and alterations in the flow of cerebrospinal fluid and the subsequent changes in hormonal balance, neuronal nutrition and metabolism had significantly altered the patient's homeostatic state, resulting in fatigue, autonomic imbalance, mood changes, and heightened perception of pain and discomfort. Once the cranial dysfunction was removed, her recovery accelerated remarkably."

Another of Dr. Bezilla's cases provides an example of how structure and function are intricately related and how it is never too early to use osteopathic structural diagnosis and treatment when indicated. The case involved a baby boy who within his first month of life began to have difficulty with breast-feeding and soon thereafter developed symptoms of colic and vomiting, which occurred more frequently and with greater intensity. His parents brought him to their pediatrician, and at two months of age, the baby underwent an upper GI evaluation that confirmed that he had gastroesophageal reflux, a condition that can prevent adequate weight gain and development due to inadequate absorption of nutrients. "It also can cause inflammation and erosion of the esophagus, and if it occurs while the baby is sleeping, it can lead to aspiration and cause a chemical pneumonitis, which can lead to pneumonia," Dr. Bezilla explains.

The baby was placed on Zantac to decrease acid production, but his symptoms continued and began to worsen. He was then placed on Reglan, a medicine to quicken the transit of food out of the stomach, and a standard conventional medical approach for treating reflux.

"During this phase of the baby's care, one of his pediatricians brought him to my attention," Dr. Bezilla says. "He thought the baby might have a problem with his head that was causing his reflux. Although this pediatrician did not feel confident in his ability to adequately perform an osteopathic cranial evaluation, he nonetheless recognized that the child had a functional disorder, and since function and structure are directly related, he surmised that there must be a structural etiology. My subsequent evaluation showed that he was correct, and that the problem causing the reflux was in fact in the baby's head. Certain parts of the baby's occiput bone at the back of his head were compressed on both sides, affecting the various cranial nerves which control swallowing, esophageal, and stomach function."

Dr. Bezilla first treated the baby by adjusting his sacrum (the tailbone), since this is connected to the head via membranes known as the *dura mater.* "I then evaluated the baby's head using cranial osteopathic methods, and was able to partially decompress the left side on the first treatment," he says. "A week later, his parents brought him back for another treatment, reporting significant improvements. Where before the baby had been vomiting an average of four to five times per day, in the week following my first session with him he had only vomited five times. I reevaluated and treated him again, further releasing the sacrum and the left and right occipital compression. During follow-up treatment a week later, his parents noted still more improvement, and I was able to completely release the sacrum and occipital compression. At my final evaluation one month later, his parents informed me that they had been able to discontinue his medicines after my last treatment, and that other than an occasional burp after feeding, there were no more incidents of vomiting." 🌿

YOUR FIRST SESSION

An office visit with an osteopathic physician is in many ways similar to a consultation with an M.D., with the added element of a hands-on structural assessment of the musculoskeletal system, patient posture, body symmetry, and the condition of the joints, muscles, tendons, ligaments, and soft tissue. An initial consultation generally includes a detailed patient medical history, with attention also given to such factors as diet, lifestyle, stress factors, home and work environments, and any psychosocial issues that may be affecting the patient's health. A standard physical examination is normally also part of the consultation, and medical tests (blood tests, urinalysis, X-ray, etc.) may also be conducted to determine nutrient status, organ health, and other causative factors, and to rule out the presence of more serious, undetected illness.

During the consultation, most D.O.'s will also observe how a patient sits, stands, and walks in order to screen for structural problems and to evaluate posture and gait. Motion testing of the body's moving parts (limbs, joints, tendons, ligaments) will usually also be conducted to determine the health of the spine, overall flexibility, body symmetry, and possible restrictions. Palpation and soft-tissue inspection are generally also employed to detect pain, tenderness, hardened musculature, excessive fluid retention, reflex activity, and skin and temperature changes, all of which provide further clues about the patient's condition. By integrating the findings of the structural exam with the patient's medical history and a complete physical exam, D.O.'s are better able to develop a comprehensive treatment plan, which will usually include OMT, both to relieve pain associated with disease and to speed the healing process by improving circulation. When indicated, D.O.'s will also prescribe medication and can provide surgical intervention when it is required. Appropriate dietary and nutritional suggestions may also be made, as well as specific exercises and lifestyle changes designed to assist in the patient's full recovery.

On average, initial consultations last for one hour, with fees on a par with those charged by M.D.'s. Most health insurance policies provide coverage for osteopathic care, as does Medicaid.

SELECTING A PRACTITIONER

Although osteopathic medicine is truly holistic in nature and origin, a certain percentage of osteopathic physicians are not holistically oriented and practice medicine in much the same way as do conventional M.D.'s. In addition, not all D.O.'s are primary care physicians, choosing to specialize in a particular branch of medicine, such as cardiology or rheumatology. Therefore, it is important that patients inquire about their D.O.'s area of specialty, medical philosophy, and his or her approach to treating disease. For best results, patients should choose a D.O. who uses OMT as an integral part of his or her practice and who takes a holistic, comprehensive, "whole person" approach to providing health care. Recommendations from satisfied patients you know and trust provide another useful basis for making your selection.

THE FUTURE OF OSTEOPATHIC MEDICINE

Already accepted as an integral part of mainstream medicine, osteopathic medicine is certain to continue to grow in popularity in the years ahead. One reason for this is the steady increase in the number of osteopathic physicians nationwide, as well as the dramatic surge in enrollments in U.S. osteopathic colleges. Equally heartening is the fact that many new osteopathic students are turning to the profession because of its original holistic philosophy and treatment methods. In the meantime, osteopathic physicians continue to build a bridge between conventional and holistic medical paradigms through the example they provide as comprehensive primary care providers.

RESOURCES

To learn more about osteopathic medicine and to locate an osteopathic physician near you, contact the following organizations.

American Osteopathic Association
142 East Ontario Street
Chicago, Illinois 60611
Phone: (800) 621-1771
Fax: (312) 202-8200
Web site: *www.am-osteo-assn.org*

American Academy of Osteopathy
3500 DePauw Blvd., Suite 1080
Indianapolis, Indiana 46269-1136
Phone: (317) 879-1881
Fax: (317) 879-0563
Web site: *www.academyofosteopathy.org*

The Cranial Academy
8202 Clearvista Parkway, Suite 9-D
Indianapolis, Indiana 46256
Phone: (317) 594-0411

Fax: (317) 594-9299
E-mail: cranacad@aol.com

RECOMMENDED READING

Fulford, Robert C., with Gene Stone. *Dr. Fulford's Touch of Life*. Pocket Books, 1996.

Northrup, George W. *Osteopathic Medicine: An American Reformation*. 3d Edition. American Osteopathic Association, 1987.

Still, Charles, Jr. *The Frontier Doctor: Medical Pioneer*. The Thomas Jefferson University Press, 1991. (Andrew Still's biography, written by his grandson.)

CHAPTER 7

Chiropractic

Chiropractic (derived from Greek words *cheir* and *praktikos* and meaning "done by hand") is the most widespread natural system of health care in the United States and serves the health care needs of an estimated 20 to 30 million Americans each year. With over 50,000 chiropractors nationwide, chiropractic ranks behind only conventional physicians (M.D.'s) and dentists in terms of health professions requiring a doctorate in order to practice. In addition, chiropractors receive more patient visits per year than any other health care practitioners, and according to a recent Gallup Survey, 90 percent of people who receive chiropractic care say it is effective, making it the highest-rated system of health care in terms of patient satisfaction.

"The most common perception of chiropractic by the general public is that of forceful manipulation of the spine to address back and neck pain," explains chiropractic researcher and educator Michael Stern, D.C. "Indeed, some chiropractors themselves would agree with this view of chiropractic as a form of manual manipulation limited to mobilizing joints and helping to repair joint damage. The majority of the profession, however, along with most patients who use chiropractic as their primary form of health care, recognize that chiropractic adjustments also free up the nervous system by reducing nerve interference. In doing so, chiropractic helps the various body systems to work better and promotes greater health and healing, both on a symptomatic basis for various disease conditions, and for the general, overall health of the body and mind."

☙ FAST FACTS ☙

Chiropractic education focuses on health, instead of disease, making it a primary form of preventive care. In addition to helping to maintain the healthy function of the spine, most chiropractors also carefully evaluate a variety of factors related to overall health, including nutrition, exercise, and patient susceptibility to stress.

Between 80 to 90 percent of patient visits to chiropractors are for neuromusculoskeletal complaints and conditions. Within this category, 35–45 percent of all visits per year are specifically for back pain. Chiropractors annually perform 94 percent of all spinal manipulations and adjustments in the United States. Other conditions routinely treated by chiropractors include spine and joint dysfunction, joint sprains, postural abnormalities, osteoarthritis and degenerative joint disease, muscle strain, headache, peripheral neuritis and neuralgia, and tendinitis.

The first state law licensing chiropractic was passed in 1913. Today chiropractic is licensed and regulated in all fifty states, the District of Columbia, Puerto Rico, the U.S. Virgin Islands, and in over thirty foreign countries. Chiropractic is also officially recognized as a viable health care approach by the World Health Organization.

Currently, approximately 85 percent of insurance health care plans in the United States cover chiropractic treatments, and all fifty states plus the District of Columbia authorize chiropractic care as part of their workers' compensation programs. Chiropractic has also received federal authorization and recognition for Medicare, Medicaid, and vocational rehabilitation programs. In addition, the model bill for state health insurance programs adopted by the National Conference of Insurance Legislators stipulates that the term *physician* include "doctor of chiropractic (D.C.)."

Doctors of chiropractic receive an average of seven years of higher education, beginning with a minimum of two years of college education focused on the basic sciences. Once in chiropractic college, students complete four to five years of additional training, receiving a minimum of 4,200 hours of combined classroom, laboratory, and clinical experience. Areas of study include anatomy and embryology, physiology, nutrition, pathology, biochemistry, neurology, microbiology, orthopedics, first aid and emergency procedures, and diagnosis and diagnostic imaging, including X-ray.

In the United States, there is approximately one chiropractor for every five thousand people, with nearly three thousand additional chiropractors entering the health care profession each year. According to the U.S. Department of Labor, by the year 2005, "chiropractic will be the number one licensed profession among those with graduate degrees, in terms of level of education and training." Other surveys project that by the year 2020, the number of practicing chiropractors in the United States is likely to double, due to continued patient satisfaction and demand. ✺

HISTORY OF CHIROPRACTIC

Although chiropractic itself was not discovered until 1895, spinal and soft-tissue manipulation has been practiced since early recorded history, in most world cultures. The earliest known records of spinal manipulation can be found in cave paintings discovered in Point le Merd, France, dating back to 17,500 B.C. While obviously crude in terms of technique, these depictions nonetheless suggest that the importance of the spine in relation to good health was understood, at least rudimentarily, even then.

One of the earliest texts referencing soft-tissue manipulation originated in China around 2700 B.C. Known as the Kong Fou Document, it was introduced to the Western world by Christian missionaries thousands of years later and is a clear indication that manipulation was part of traditional Chinese medicine from its inception. Archaeological records reveal that the ancient Japanese, Egyptians, Babylonians, Syrians, Hindus, Tibetans, and Polynesians also practiced some form of soft-tissue manipulation. Manipulation was also part of the health practices employed by various native peoples throughout North, Central, and South America, especially "back walking," in which patients had their backs manipulated by the feet of tribal healers and others. Among the Amerindians who used back walking were the Lakota (Sioux), Winnebago, and Creek people in North America; and the Aztecs, Toltecs, Zoltecs, and Mayans, in Mexico and Central America. In South America, the Incas developed a sophisticated form of manipulation that was well documented in their written records.

Papyrus records dating from 1500 B.C. show that the Greeks were also familiar with the health benefits of manipulation, as they contain instructions for manipulating the legs and lower body to treat low back pain. Hippocrates, the father of Western medicine, also emphasized the importance of the spine in relation to health and disease. Convinced that the physician's primary role was to relieve the impediments that interfered with the body's natural ability to heal itself, in his books he instructed his students to "get knowledge of the spine, for this is the requisite for many diseases." To this end, he wrote two books on the subject, *Manipulation and Importance to Good Health* and *On Setting Joints by Leverage.*

The famed historian Herodotus, a contemporary of Hippocrates, was also well aware of the importance of the spine and its proper alignment. While best known today as the Father of History, in his time Herodotus was also famed for his ability to cure many disease conditions with exercises specifically designed to relieve spinal dysfunction. For those who were too ill to exercise, he would first manually adjust their spines, causing Aristotle to write of him, "He made old men young and thus prolonged their lives too greatly." Archaeological artifacts reveal that the Greeks also employed a form of back walking to correct spinal distortions, and that they invented a number of mechanical aids for this purpose, as well. In certain cases, patients were hung upside down in order to stretch their spines and release musculoskeletal tension.

Nearly four hundred years after Hippocrates died, Claudius Galen, another famed Greek healer, received the honorific Prince of Physicians after he healed Eudemus, an eminent Roman scholar, of paralysis of his right hand. After examining Eudemus, Galen adjusted the vertebrae of his neck, whereupon the scholar immediately regained full use of his hand. Like Hippocrates, Galen also exhorted his students to "look to the nervous system as the key to maximum health." Based on the teachings of both of these prominent Greek healers, the importance of the spine to health continued to be emphasized by physicians and other healers for the remainder of the Roman Empire's existence.

Following the empire's collapse in the fifth century A.D., however, this awareness was either lost or ignored by physicians, and spinal manipulation became the province of folk healers. Often known as "bonesetting" in later centuries, the technique was passed down from teacher to student, and parent to child, and was practiced in many regions of Europe throughout the Middle Ages and the Renaissance. In 1867, the practice was favorably written about in the *British Medical Journal* by noted English surgeon Sir James Paget.

But it was in the United States that chiropractic itself was invented by Canadian-born Daniel David Palmer in 1895. After several years as a successful magnetic healer, Palmer encountered Harvey Lillard, a janitor who had been deaf for seventeen years. Palmer learned that Lillard's deafness had occurred after he felt "something give way" in his back while he was working in a bent, cramped position. Upon examining him, Palmer discovered that one of Lillard's vertebrae was misaligned. He reasoned that Lillard's hearing might be restored if the vertebra was properly adjusted and persuaded Lillard to let him try. Shortly afterwards, Lillard's hearing returned. Palmer soon found himself using what he called "hand treatments" to treat other patients suffering from a variety of diseases, including sciatica, migraine, digestive disorders, heart conditions, epilepsy, and the flu. Palmer was able to alleviate their conditions without the use of medicines of any kind, and eventually one of his patients, a Christian minister, coined the term *chiropractic* to describe what he was doing.

Initially, however, Palmer was uncertain as to why his treatments worked, causing him to seek out a deeper understanding of the spine and its relationship to health. In the course of his studies, he realized that his adjustments were restoring proper nerve function by relieving misalignments in the spine, known as vertebral subluxations. Based on his research, Palmer reasoned that correcting subluxations enabled the body's own "Innate Intelligence" to restore itself to health. Although most members of the chiropractic profession today recognize other factors, such as exercise, lifestyle, and stress, that also have a bearing on health, Palmer's ideas about Innate Intelligence hold many parallels with the concepts of the body's "vital spirit" and "vitalism" espoused by Hippocrates and other ancient healers, which are still widely accepted today by most forms of holistic therapies.

Palmer passed on his discoveries through his published writings and lectures and by opening a school to train other chiropractors. Throughout most of his career, however, he was often branded a fraud, and in 1905 was even sentenced to 105 days in jail and a $350 fine after being indicted for practicing medicine without a license. Between 1906 and 1913, he published the original chiropractic texts, *The Science of Chiropractic* and *The Chiropractor's Adjustor*, both of which continue to be used in chiropractic colleges today.

After Palmer's death, in 1913, chiropractic was further developed by his son, Bartlett Joshua (B. J.) Palmer, who is credited with molding chiropractic into the licensed profession it is today. In the process, he purchased an amateur radio station that he renamed WOC radio (Wonders of Chiropractic), ultimately developing it into the nation's first 500-watt station. WOC eventually became part of the NBC radio network, and during his tenure as owner, B. J. employed future president Ronald Reagan as one of his radio announcers. Palmer went on to purchase other radio stations and is also credited with coining the word *broadcasting*. He was also a strong initial proponent of the X-ray machine, recognizing it as a useful diagnostic tool. A tireless spokesperson for chiropractic, B. J. was almost single-handedly responsible for chiropractic's acceptance as a viable healing method. His patients included presidents and international business leaders and celebrities, including Ronald Reagan, Herbert Hoover, Harry Truman, Jack Dempsey, and Harry Houdini.

Throughout its evolution in the twentieth century, chiropractors have continued to pioneer acceptance of holistic health care principles, including the importance of nutrition and numerous concepts that also inform the field of bodywork (see Chapter 9). "Chiropractors have also been at the forefront in promoting preventive wellness, natural health, and body-mind choices such as proper exercise, stress relief, internal cleansing, and Chinese and Ayurvedic medicine, often before these came into vogue," Dr. Stern points out.

The profession's growth has not been free of resistance, however, particularly from members of the American Medical Association (AMA). Both Palmers were strongly opposed by the controlling medical interests of their time, and B. J., who founded, and became president of, the International Chiropractors Association in 1926, publicly feuded with Morris Fishbein, editor of the *Journal of the American Medical Association*, in response to Fishbein's ongoing attempts to discredit chiropractic as quackery.

Two years after Palmer's death in 1961, the AMA's board of trustees established a Committee on Chiropractic, changing its name shortly afterwards to the Committee on Quackery. According to the committee's charter, its primary purpose was "first, the containment [and] ultimately, the elimination of chiropractic." In 1966, the AMA passed a resolution forbidding physicians to even associate with chiropractors, and its Judicial Council went so far as to charge that physicians would be acting unethically if they even gave a lecture on a medical subject before an audience of chiropractors. Physicians were also instructed to give up their membership in civic organizations whose members also included chiropractors if such organizations were to become involved, even indirectly, with health care issues. In addition, during the 1970s, hospital administrators were notified by the Joint Commission on the Accreditation of Hospitals that accreditation would be rescinded if hospitals granted privileges to chiropractors, even in cases where state law demanded that chiropractors be included on the hospital staff.

Spurred by such actions, in 1976, Chester Wilk, D.C., along with four other chiropractors, charged that the AMA, the American Hospital

Association, and six other medical associations were conspiring to eliminate chiropractic by means of a professional boycott. In 1987, the merit of Wilk's antitrust suit was established when the AMA and its codefendant parties were ruled guilty as charged. A permanent injunction preventing the AMA from restraining its members from associating with chiropractors was also issued. The AMA appealed the ruling, but in 1990 U.S. Court of Appeals Judge Susan Getzendanner rejected the appeal, upholding the previous court ruling that found the AMA and its codefendants guilty of engaging in a "lengthy, systematic, successful, and unlawful boycott" intended to eliminate chiropractic for primarily economic reasons. After a further appeal was rejected by the Supreme Court, the AMA relented, notifying its members that they were now free to associate with, and refer patients to and receive referrals from, chiropractors. Since then, a greater spirit of cooperation has existed between both professions, resulting in increased numbers of hospitals and other health care organizations that now offer chiropractic as a treatment option.

HOW CHIROPRACTIC WORKS

The primary aim of chiropractic care is to restore and maintain health by properly aligning the spine. "Central to the philosophy of chiropractic is the idea that the body's natural state is one of optimal health, no matter a person's age," Dr. Stern explains. "But in order for the body to function properly and heal itself, the nervous system needs to be free of interference, since it coordinates every function in the body and is the conduit through which life energy flows. While many chiropractors have moved away from the Palmers' concept of Innate Intelligence, due to its nonscientific connotation, there is no disputing that a healthy nervous system is essential for the experience of overall wellness."

The nervous system regulates all other body systems via the pathways of nerves that extend to every organ and cell. Health depends on the proper functioning of the nervous system's three interrelated subsystems: the central nervous system, comprised of the brain and spinal cord; the autonomic nervous system, which regulates automatic body functions such as heart rate and the digestive process; and the peripheral nervous system, which links the central nervous system to body tissues and voluntary muscles. The spinal column, in turn, is also integral to normal nerve function. Comprised of twenty-four vertebrae, it enfolds and protects the spinal cord, from which spinal nerves extend, reaching past each vertebra to connect with the body's muscles, bones, organs, and glands.

When subluxations of the spine occur, nerve interference is created by pressure placed on the nerves in the area of the vertebrae that are out of alignment. As a result, the nervous system's equilibrium can be disrupted and nerve function diminished. Over time, this can lead to pain, muscle weakness, impaired organ function, limited range of motion, or disease.

"A variety of factors can cause subluxations," Dr. Stern says. "The most obvious are those that are mechanical, or physical, such as physical trauma or injury. But psychological factors, such as stress or emotional pain, can also cause the vertebrae to become misaligned, as can illness, poor nutrition, exposure to excessive heat or cold, and environmental toxins. Since pain isn't always a presenting factor when vertebrae are subluxated, people are often unaware that their spines are out of alignment and therefore don't always recognize the ways in which their health is being affected. It's quite common, for instance, to see improved respiratory and digestive function after proper alignment has been restored, as well as improvement in a number of chronic illnesses that were being caused or exacerbated by impaired nerve function."

The lack of awareness people can have regarding subluxation and its effect on their health can be tied to the way spinal misalignment often affects brain function, according to Dr. Stern. "When your nervous system is unable to flow freely, which is what happens when subluxations are present, your ability to be in touch with yourself on all levels is diminished," he explains. "In my clinical experience, I've repeatedly noticed patients becoming more aware of themselves, not only physically, but also getting more in touch with their thoughts and feelings with greater clarity, once their subluxations are addressed and their nervous systems are restored to health. They also start making healthier life choices as a result."

❦ ARE YOU SUBLUXATED? ❦

According to Dr. Stern, it's not uncommon for people not to know their spines are subluxated or that their nervous systems are impaired, particularly those who have never experienced the benefits of a chiropractic adjustment. To help you determine whether you could benefit from chiropractic care, Dr. Stern suggests asking yourself the following questions:

Are your muscles tight, or do you feel persistent or chronic tension in your body?

Is your range of motion reduced?

Are your energy levels low?

Do you regularly experience feelings of being "uptight" or on edge?

Do you experience a lack of flexibility in your body?

Have you noticed that your ability to respond and adapt to the stresses of daily life has become more difficult?

If you answered yes to any of these questions, chiropractic care might make a noticeable improvement in your health and overall well-being. 🌿

The first step in chiropractic care usually lies in determining the cause and nature of each patient's specific problem or health complaint. This is accomplished by reviewing the patient's medical history, followed by a systematic physical examination. The examination usually encompasses the patient's vital signs, such as blood pressure and pulse rate; range of motion, and neurological and orthopedic status, as well as ruling out any pathologies that might be present and require other forms of medical attention. "Because their training enables them to differentially diagnose conditions, in many respects chiropractors serve as gatekeepers, or primary caregivers, providing preventive and maintenance care to reduce the need for more extreme or emergency treatments later," Dr. Stern says. "At the same time, when such treatments are needed, chiropractors can make that diagnosis and refer patients to the appropriate specialist."

As part of their diagnosis, chiropractors normally check a patient's posture and biomechanical status and perform a spinal analysis, using hands-on palpation procedures specific to their profession to assess any structural or functional problems that may be present. Many chiropractors also employ diagnostic techniques and instruments common to the medical profession at large, including X-ray, MRI, EMG, thermography, blood tests, and urinalysis, depending on their patients' needs and their own personal orientation. Following the diagnosis, treatment begins, with the goal of correcting the patient's particular subluxations and restoring the health of the nervous system and joint flexibility. When appropriate, lifestyle and nutritional counseling might also be provided, as well as stress management tips and general educational material designed to help patients participate more fully in their own healing process.

At the core of all chiropractic treatment is an adjustment of the misaligned spine in accordance with diagnostic findings. The adjustment involves precise contact along the appropriate areas of the spine and serves to increase the nerve supply to each area. Proper adjustment results in a greater range of motion and a free flow of life energy, as well as reduced tension in the musculature and connective tissue. Mobilization, which involves moving a joint as far as it will comfortably go, might also be employed when there is a need to improve the overall range of motion. Ice and heat applications are sometimes used, as well, as are ultrasound and other physiotherapy devices, in order to relax or stimulate muscles, break up scar tissue, and reduce swelling and pain.

There are approximately 150 different diagnostic and adjustment methods that chiropractors can employ, with "high velocity, low amplitude," or "short lever," adjustment techniques among the most common. "In general, the techniques can be categorized according to several different criteria and ideally are employed according to each patient's specific needs during each session," Dr. Stern explains. "Many people have the preconceived idea that the chiropractic adjustment is always forceful, and therefore won't risk going to a chiropractor for this reason. In actuality, the type of adjustment used can vary and really depends on the condition that is being treated and what approach will create the greatest benefit along with the greatest amount of ease. In many cases, soft-touch approaches can work best, particularly in the early stages of care."

In addition to the various techniques that chiropractors use, three different levels of chiropractic care are offered by many chiropractors, each of which varies in length according to the patient's specific needs. Acute care involves treating new injuries and other conditions. Usually the patient is experiencing some degree of discomfort during this phase of care, and the chiropractor's primary goal is to provide relief and bring the condition under control as quickly as possible. Acute care often entails chiropractic sessions ranging from daily to three times per week, depending on the severity of a patient's condition and the chiropractor's recommendations. It can last from one to two weeks to up to a few months or more. The second level of care, known as corrective care, occurs after a patient's acute care needs have been addressed, accompanied by a satisfactory reduction in nerve interference. During this phase, chiropractors work to stabilize and correct underlying structural imbalances and muscle weaknesses, as well as continuing to "reeducate" the nervous system as it begins to operate more efficiently and with greater ease. Corrective care usually requires fewer sessions per week than acute care and usually extends over a period of months. Maintenance, or wellness, care entails chiropractic treatments that vary in frequency, according to each patient's goals and needs. This level of care serves as a preventive measure, once a patient's more serious health concerns have been resolved and underlying imbalances corrected. "For people interested in achieving and maintaining optimal health, maintenance care is an excellent preventive measure for ensuring proper function of the spine and nervous system," Dr. Stern advises.

THE BRAIN
❦ REWARD CASCADE ❦

A new theory put forth by Jay M. Holder, M.D., D.C., director of the Holder Research Institute in Miami, Florida, may explain why people who receive chiropractic treatment often experience improved emotional well-being. Known as the "brain reward cascade," Dr. Holder's theory is based on over thirty years of research by Kenneth Blum, Ph.D., Candace Pert, Ph.D., and others, showing that positive emotions have a direct correlation to chemical messengers known as neurotransmitters, which must be released in the brain in a precise sequence in order for human beings to regularly experience pleasure, happiness, joy, and other positive emotions. Chief among these neurotransmitters is the chemical dopamine, which is essential for normal nerve activity in the brain. Working in concert with this process is the limbic system, which is biochemically associated with emotions, which Dr. Pert and her associates have shown resides along the length of spine, not just in the brain. According to Dr. Holder, misalignment anywhere along the length of the spine interferes with the proper function of the limbic system and therefore interrupts the flow of dopamine and other "brain reward" chemicals. By correcting spinal misalignment, he posits, chiropractic restores the proper flow of dopamine and rebalances the brain reward cascade. Dr. Holder's view seems to be borne out by the high level of success he and other chiropractors have achieved in treating addiction and alcoholism, both of which are characterized by chronic dopamine deficiency (see "Conditions That Benefit from Chiropractic," following page). ❦

CONDITIONS THAT BENEFIT FROM CHIROPRACTIC

Chiropractic's ability to improve the health of the nervous system makes it a valuable form of preventive care, and an effective primary care treatment for conditions related to the musculoskeletal system. Because unimpeded nerve function is also necessary for healing to occur, chiropractic can be useful as an adjunctive treatment for a wide range of other disease conditions as well. For this reason, holistic physicians may recommend chiropractic care to their patients as a complement to their own holistic treatment approaches in order to most fully address the underlying factors related to their patients' condition.

In addition, chiropractors are often able to resolve health complaints that are considered to be unrelated to the musculoskeletal system. "Because the nervous system and nerve function are central to optimal health, chiropractic can be of benefit, either primarily or adjunctively, for a broad range of disease conditions," Dr. Stern states. "I have seen chiropractic care help conditions ranging from organ related conditions like poor digestion and sexual dysfunction, to systemic problems like skin problems and high blood pressure."

Another benefit experienced by many people who receive regular chiropractic adjustments is an improvement in their overall quality of life. Not only does their physical health tend to improve and stabilize, but they also tend to experience diminished stress levels, more positive mental and emotional states, and greater resiliency in dealing with the challenges of their day-to-day routines. "This is because there is a direct relationship between the nervous system and one's mental and emotional states," Dr. Stern explains. "Chiropractic, through its ability to physically reduce tension within the structures of the nervous system, and therefore change neurochemical activity right down to the cellular level, can have many positive ramifications for a person's overall perceived quality of life, especially among patients who regularly benefit from chiropractic adjustments."

As a primary care treatment, chiropractic is best known for its effectiveness in treating back pain. Other conditions for which chiropractic has proven effective include headache and migraine, herniated discs, whiplash, addiction, and childhood colic, bed-wetting, and learning disabilities.

Back Pain

It is estimated that 80 percent of all Americans will suffer from some form of lower back pain at some point in their lives. Each year, some 20 percent of the population is affected with low back pain, with annual treatment and related costs estimated at $50 billion.

In 1994, the Agency for Health Care Policy and Research (AHCPR) of the U.S. Department of Health and Human Services, after conducting a comprehensive review of nearly 4,000 studies related to all current forms of treatment for low back problems, issued guidelines on the diagnosis and treatment of acute low back pain in adults. In their report, the AHCPR advised that adults suffering from low back pain choose the most conservative form of care first and recommended spinal manipulation as the only safe and effective form of drugless care for the condition. The AHCPR also wrote that spinal manipulation's ability to hasten recovery from low back problems was "statistically significant" in comparison to other forms of treatment and that "manipulation reduces pain and has positive short-term impact on daily functioning."

The AHCPR also advised against most other treatments for low back pain, including surgery and bed rest, both traditional mainstays of conventional medical care for back pain. The only other treatment that received high marks by the AHCPR for low back pain was the use of the over-the-counter medication acetaminophen, which is capable of masking pain symptoms but not hastening recovery time, and which can also cause serious side effects, including kidney failure. By contrast, the likelihood of spinal manipulation having serious complications has been shown to be one in one hundred million. Ninety-four percent of all spinal manipulations are performed by chiropractic physicians.

The AHCPR's findings closely reflect those of the Manga Report, funded by the Ontario Ministry of Health in 1993 to review all worldwide scientific literature related to back pain treatments. The authors of the Manga Report concluded "for the management of low back pain, chiropractic care is the most effective treatment, and it should be fully integrated into the government's health care system." The Manga Report also found that chiropractic treatment was more effective for low back pain than other forms of alternative treatment, and that adults diagnosed with low back pain returned to work "much sooner when treated by chiropractors."

In 1993, the *British Medical Journal* reported that the long-term benefits of chiropractic treatment of back pain were also significant, noting that "two and three years after patients with back pain were treated by chiropractors, they experienced far less pain than those who were treated by medical doctors." One of the most convincing studies of chiropractic's effectiveness for treating chronic back pain problems was conducted in the mid-1980s and involved 171 patients who had been completely disabled for an average of 7.8 years due to chronic low back pain. After receiving daily chiropractic adjustments for a period of two to three weeks, 87 percent of the group experienced a return to "full function, with no restrictions for work or other activities." Moreover, a reexamination one year later found that their success rate remained the same.

Not only is chiropractic care safer and more effective than other forms of back pain treatments, it is also significantly less expensive. In a 1995 study analyzing insurance claims and reported in *JNMS: Journal of the Neuromusculoskeletal System*, it was shown that mean outpatient costs for patients receiving conventional medical treatment for their low back pain problems was $1,027, while the mean cost for patients receiving chiropractic care was only $647. Work loss also varies significantly depending on which form of care patients select, with studies showing that chiropractic patients require an average of only 6.26 compensation days, compared to the average of 25.56 compensation days for medical patients. Finally, studies show that patients are more satisfied with chiropractic treatment for back problems than with any other form of care.

Headache and Migraine

Because nearly all pain conditions are due to diminished tissue function related to improper spinal function, chiropractic can be extremely useful in treating various types of headaches, as well as migraine. Research indicates that approximately 75 percent of patients suffering from recurring headaches or migraines are either cured or experience a noticeable reduction in symptoms following chiropractic treatments. In 1995 the *Journal of Manipulative and Physiological Therapeutics* reported that patients suffering from tension headaches still experienced "sustained therapeutic benefit in all major outcomes" four weeks after receiving chiropractic treatment, compared to patients whose initial symptoms returned after using conventional medications.

Herniated Discs

Commonly but inaccurately known as slipped discs, herniated discs can also respond well to chiropractic treatment. While chiropractic treatments do not affect the degree of disc protrusion, research has shown that disc protrusion in and of itself is not the cause of pain related to herniated discs. One study, for example, involving 98 people who were free of back pain found, through the use of magnetic resonance imaging (MRI), that 52 percent of them had at least one bulge along their vertebrae, despite being completely pain-free. In another study, 470 of 517 patients suffering from pain due to disc lesion experienced a decrease of symptoms following chiropractic treatment. Another study conducted in 1993 by researchers on staff at the Royal University Hospital in Saskatchewan, Canada, also found chiropractic treatments to be safe and effective for herniated discs in the lumbar region of the spine. Chiropractic has been found to be beneficial for cervical disc herniations, as well.

Whiplash

Whiplash affects more than three million Americans each year, and annual treatments for the condition run as high as $23 billion. Research indicates that chiropractic is the only therapy proven to be effective for treating chronic whiplash. When whiplash occurs, the affected areas of the body are the facet joint capsules and annuli (ring-like structures) of the discs, both of which are routinely treated by the very nature of the chiropractic adjustment. Recent studies have demonstrated that chiropractic can provide relief for both acute and chronic whiplash conditions, even in cases where conventional medical treatments have failed.

Addiction

Research conducted by Dr. Jay M. Holder indicates that chiropractic, as an adjunctive therapy, can substantially improve addiction treatments. An initial triple-blind study devised by Dr. Holder found that patients suffering from drug addiction were "ten times more likely" to complete drug treatment programs when chiropractic was included as part of their treatment, compared to patients who did not receive chiropractic care. In another randomized clinical trial overseen by Dr. Holder, patients who received chiropractic adjustments five times a week over a thirty-day period had a 100 percent completion rate for their overall drug treatment program, which also included amino acid therapy, auriculotherapy (ear acupuncture—see Chapter 13), and addiction counseling.

General statistics regarding addiction treatment show that patients who successfully complete three programs lasting three months or more have an 85 percent likelihood of being drug-free five years later. Dr. Holder's findings suggest that chiropractic's success in such programs is due to the fact that patients who receive regular chiropractic adjustments are far less prone to anxiety and depression and better able to respond to counseling than patients who do not receive chiropractic care. They also exhibit fewer symptoms of detoxification and withdrawal. According to Dr. Holder, the reason for this lies in chiropractic's ability to remove the interference of what he terms "the brain reward cascade" of brain chemicals necessary for the experience of pleasure and happiness. In 1991, Dr. Holder was awarded the Albert Schweitzer Prize in Medicine for his research on addiction.

Childhood Conditions

A number of childhood conditions have been shown to respond positively to chiropractic treatments, including colic, bed-wetting, and childhood learning disabilities. One study involving 316 infants with colic, most of whom had not responded to nutritional intervention or conventional medical care, found a 94 percent improvement of symptoms among the infants following chiropractic adjustment. After chiropractic treatments began, the infants also exhibited 75 percent fewer episodes of colic.

Incidents of bed-wetting can also improve following chiropractic care, as evidenced by a study of forty-six chronic bed-wetters, who were divided into two groups. The first group received chiropractic adjustments, while the other received sham treatments. Those receiving chiropractic care had fewer episodes of bed-wetting compared to the sham group.

Learning disabilities related to hyperactivity also respond favorably to chiropractic treatments. One study involving twenty-four students with learning disabilities found that those who received chiropractic care showed a 20 to 40 percent improvement in their learning abilities, compared to those who received medications such as Ritalin, the most commonly prescribed drug for children suffering from attention deficit hyperactivity disorder (ADHD). Moreover, chiropractic is free of adverse side effects, whereas the side effects of medication can be quite serious.

Other conditions for which chiropractic has been shown to be effective include pain in the neck, shoulders, or upper arms; sciatica; muscle strains; joint sprains; overall pain related to pressure on, or injury to, the musculoskeletal system; and menstrual problems, especially cramping.

Caution: Chiropractic is not an appropriate form of treatment for broken or fractured bones, or for bone diseases such as osteoporosis and bone cancer.

HEALING MULTIPLE SCLEROSIS: ❦ A CASE HISTORY ❦

The potentially dramatic benefits of chiropractic care are demonstrated by the following case history of one of Dr. Stern's patients, who came to him suffering from multiple sclerosis (MS). "She was in her mid-forties when she first came to me in 1998, and had been experiencing problems with her central nervous system since 1984," Dr. Stern says. "By 1987, her symptoms had exacerbated to the point where she was regularly experiencing numbness in her legs, and distorted vision, but it wasn't until 1995 that she was officially diagnosed with MS. By that point, she often had no feeling from her waist down, and her legs would give out on her when she was walking. Her vision also continued to deteriorate, and she was experiencing nausea, numbness and tingling in her hands, and periods of forgetfulness and poor concentration, as well as a lot of emotional stress due to the death of her mother to cancer and work-related pressures. By 1996, she was having serious problems with her equilibrium, memory, and strength, and suffering from chronic fatigue and depression. A nutritionist worked with her, placing her on a program of megavitams, essential fatty acids, and DHEA, but she wasn't having any results."

By the time Dr. Stern met her, the woman had no feeling in her legs, was barely able to walk, suffered from both short- and long-term memory loss, and would often spontaneously burst into tears. Determined to get well, she worked with both an acupuncturist and a homeopath, and upgraded her diet to include juicing, along with continued nutritional supplementation. She also explored counseling in the form of inner-child therapy. "At that point, acupuncture, which she received two to three times each week, was helping her the most," Dr. Stern says. "Eventually, it helped restore proper function to her hands. Due to my teaching and travel schedule at the time, I was able to treat her only occasionally that year. In addition to adjusting her, I showed her some breathing and mind-body exercises she could practice during times when she felt stressed or emotionally overwhelmed." Early in her treatment with Dr. Stern, the woman noticed that her numbness would temporarily disappear after each adjustment. She also began releasing stored feelings that she hadn't been fully aware of until they surfaced and were resolved. She began seeing Dr. Stern on a regular basis, during which time she continued to reconnect with and release the heavy emotional burdens she had unconsciously been carrying throughout her life. "Today, after approximately forty sessions with me, in addition to the other modalities she explored, she is completely free of symptoms, and leading an increasingly productive, energetic life," Dr. Stern reports, "and is continuing to receive wellness care to maintain the progress she's made." 🌿

YOUR FIRST SESSION

Normally, your initial consultation with a chiropractor will involve an assessment of your past medical history, as well as an opportunity to discuss what you hope to achieve by receiving chiropractic care. Any presenting symptoms or complaints that you are aware of will also be discussed, and an assessment might also be made of lifestyle, stress, and nutritional factors that may be contributing to your condition. Usually, this assessment will be followed by a complete physical exam that will enable your chiropractor to make an initial diagnosis of your condition. Depending on your practitioner, the exam may involve orthopedic and neurological testing, and analysis of your posture and range of motion, as well as chiropractic testing involving gentle palpating along your spine to determine where subluxations might be present. Most chiropractors also employ leg checks, which are performed with patients lying facedown while the chiropractor presses their heels together. Leg checks help your chiropractor to determine whether there are any imbalances along your spine, especially in the pelvis. Some chiropractors also use X-ray and other conventional diagnostic devices to rule out any damage to the spine itself, depending on each patient's specific condition and what is revealed by the rest of the examination.

Following your diagnosis, your chiropractor will discuss an appropriate treatment plan, giving you a general idea of your condition and the number of sessions you can expect before your health goals are achieved. Typically, you will then receive your first adjustment, although some chiropractors may suggest waiting until your next session for treatment to begin, especially if X-rays are involved.

A common concern among many first-time chiropractic patients is that the treatment will hurt or be uncomfortable. In reality, this is almost never the case, with most patients discovering that treatment not only relieves their pain, but also leaves them more relaxed, with feelings of greater ease in their body.

On average, initial consultations last from thirty to sixty minutes, with follow-up sessions usually ranging from fifteen to thirty minutes in length. The cost of initial visits can range from $70 to $150, with follow-up sessions generally averaging between $30 and $60. Chiropractic care is covered by an estimated 85 percent of all health insurance plans in the United States. A number of chiropractors also offer the option of monthly payment plans, allowing patients to receive multiple sessions for a set fee, which is particularly attractive to patients for whom frequent treatment sessions are advised.

SELECTING A PRACTITIONER

The same criteria that you would use for choosing any health professional apply for selecting a chiropractor. All chiropractors in the United States must be licensed in the state in which they practice. If in doubt, ask for proof of their credentials. Seek out recommendations from people you trust about chiropractors they have received benefit from. You can also find competent chiropractors in your area by contacting the organizations included in the "Resources" section at the end of this chapter. Don't be afraid to be selective. Although chiropractors in general abide by the standards set by their profession, their adjustment techniques and treatment approaches can vary. The better educated you are about what chiropractic is and what you can expect from it, the better able you will be to make an informed choice about your practitioner.

THE FUTURE OF CHIROPRACTIC

More than a hundred years after its inception, chiropractic continues to be the fastest-growing holistic health care profession in the United States, and is also experiencing rapid expansion worldwide. In addition, studies indicate that chiropractic has the highest patient satisfaction rate of any healing modality in the United States. These trends, along with ongoing research into the benefits of chiropractic, the widespread acceptance of chiropractic care by most medical plans, and greater receptivity to chiropractic on the part of the conventional medical establishment, suggest a bright future for the profession well into the twenty-first century. As Dr. Stern explains, "With increasing numbers of Americans seeking effective alternatives to drugs and surgery, as well as the greater emphasis today on preventive care and improved quality of life, chiropractors have never had a better opportunity to solidify chiropractic's position as the leading form of holistic primary health care."

RESOURCES

To learn more about chiropractic and to locate a chiropractor near you, contact the following organizations.

American Chiropractic Association
1701 Clarendon Blvd.
Arlington, Virginia 22209
Phone: (800) 986-4636
Web site: *www.amerchiro.org*

Foundation for Chiropractic Education and Research
704 East 4th Street
Des Moines, Iowa 50309
Phone: (515) 282-7118
Web site: *www.healthy.net/pan/pa/fcer/index.html*

International Chiropractors Association
1110 North Glebe Road, Suite 1000
Arlington, Virginia 22201
Phone: (703) 528-5000
Web site: *www.chiropractic.org*

World Chiropractic Alliance
2950 N. Dobson Road, Suite 1

Chandler, Arizona 85224
Phone: (800) 347-1011
Web site: *www.chiropage.com*

RECOMMENDED READING

Dintenfass, Julius. *Chiropractic: A Modern Way to Health*. Pyramid Books, 1975.
Rondberg, Terry. *Chiropractic First*. The Chiropractic Journal, 1998.

CHAPTER 8

Botanical Medicine

Botanical medicine in its broadest sense refers to all therapeutic approaches to healing that make use of plant-derived substances. In addition to the use of medicinal plants and herbs discussed in this chapter, other therapies that fall under the heading of botanical medicine include homeopathy (see Chapter 11), aromatherapy, and flower essence therapy (see Chapter 10), all of which can be used by practitioners of holistic medicine as part of a comprehensive treatment program.

More commonly known as herbal medicine, botanical medicine represents one of the oldest forms of healing and has been employed by nearly all world cultures since the beginning of recorded history. During the twentieth century, it evolved into a specialized form of medicine known as phytomedicine or phytotherapy (the study of medicinal plants). "Phytomedicine is the study of plants and their relationship to human health and wellness," explains AHMA member Steven Morris, N.D., a naturopathic physician and leading ethnobotanist. According to Morris, approximately 40 percent of all allopathic medicines (both prescription and over-the-counter) are plant-derived. "Such medicines were either originally derived from plants or they have been analogued to match plant substances," he says.

Today, botanical medicine is one of the largest and fastest-growing components of holistic medicine, largely due to increasing public interest in alternative self-care measures, coupled with consumer concern about drug-induced side effects. In 1991, approximately 3 percent of U.S. consumers purchased medicinal herbs; by 1998, that figure had leapt to 37 percent, accounting for nearly $4 billion in retail sales, with sales continuing to increase by an annualized rate of over 100 percent at the time of this writing. Despite their popularity, however, medicinal herbs should not be used injudiciously. Dr. Morris recommends that people on medication consult with their health care provider to ensure against possible interactions that are contraindicated. "Most herbs are very safe, but there are a handful that you need to be cautious with," Morris says. "Overall, though, the risks involved are very low, and with a bit of research you can actually alleviate what risk there is. Knowing the plants' properties and how to use them effectively is the key."

❦ FAST FACTS ❦

Some form of botanical medicine exists in nearly every culture throughout the world. The majority of these systems, such as those found within Ayurveda and traditional Chinese medicine (see Chapters 12 and 13), extend back thousands of years.

The word *drug* is derived from the old Dutch word *drogge*, meaning "to dry." Prior to the advent of modern medicine, physicians and other healers often dried plants before using them medicinally.

Throughout history, indigenous peoples have relied on herbs and other plants as a primary form of medicine. In most of these cultures, native healers known as shamans are responsible for exploring the benefits of herbs native to their lands, as well as properly preparing them for use. Shamanic training usually occurs within an apprenticeship structure, with the teacher passing on his or her knowledge to selected students in order to carry on the traditions. A number of shamanic traditions incorporate the use of intuition and sacred, psychotropic plants in order to perfect their understanding of how and when herbs should be used. In recent years, botanists from developed countries have worked directly with shamans from around the world to catalog an estimated ten thousand plant compounds each year.

Between 1983 and 1994, at least 40 percent of all new drugs were derived from plant products, including antibiotics. According to the World Health Organization, 74 percent of the most common pharmaceutical drugs derived from plants are used by doctors in ways that correlate exactly with how the plants themselves are used traditionally by native cultures.

One-third of all new cancer drugs are derived from plant sources.

The earth contains an estimated 250,000 plant species (double that number if subspecies are considered separately). Of these, fewer than 50,000 species have been studied extensively to determine their medicinal properties, suggesting that there is an abundance of potentially lifesaving plant substances awaiting discovery.

Common conventional medicines derived from plants include aspirin, digitalis, quinine, morphine, Taxol, AZT, and reserpine, as well as vinblastine and vincristine, the two primary drugs used to treat acute lymphocytic leukemia.

Herbs and herbal remedies are now available in nearly all retail outlets in the United States, accounting for nearly $4 billion in retail sales per year. Of all retail outlets, supermarkets account for the most rapid growth in the mainstream supplement market. Due to this growing demand, a number of pharmaceutical companies, including Smith-Kline Beecham; Bayer, Warner, Lambert; and American Home Products, have entered the herbal supplement market. A number of drugstore chains are also developing their own herbal product lines. 🌿

HISTORY OF BOTANICAL MEDICINE

The use of plants as medicine has been a part of nearly every world culture, beginning at least as far back as the Neolithic era of the Stone Age (8000 to 5000 B.C.), and well before the invention of written language. Initially, the use of medicinal plants was accompanied by magic rites and rituals and was to a large degree determined by religious superstitions and beliefs. Beginning around 3000 B.C., however, a number of world cultures began to codify the specific uses of herbs in medical texts. Some of the earliest writings occurred in ancient Mesopotamia and Egypt, a number of which are still preserved today, inscribed on clay tablets and papyrus. Babylonian priest-physicians often employed herbs in their healing practices, and written records dating as far back as 2600 B.C. indicate that they had developed prescription and compounding instructions for over two hundred herbs used to treat a number of illnesses. During that same period, Egyptian priests, physicians, and sorcerers also began to compile records of various herbs and their properties. The earliest known medical records originated around 1900 B.C. The Kahun Medical Papyrus, which deals with the use of herbs in relation to women's health and birthing practices, was written at that time, followed by the Edwin Smith Papyrus (1600 B.C.) and the Ebers Papyrus (1550 B.C.) Of these, the Ebers Papyrus is the most famous, and contains over 870 different prescriptions derived from approximately 700 drugs using vegetable, mineral, and animal sources.

During this same period, Chinese herbal medicine was developing as an essential component of traditional Chinese medicine (TCM). Around 2800 B.C., the emperor Sheng Nung, known to the Chinese as the Divine Plowman and father of Chinese agriculture, began the first systematic recording of the medicinal properties of plants. His efforts were preserved in *Sheng Nung's Herbal*, which described over 250 herbs according to their functions and health benefits and listed over 150 disease conditions that herbs could successfully treat. Sheng Nung's work was continued by Huang Ti, the Yellow Emperor, who came to power in 2687 B.C. and, along with his court physician, Qi Bo, established TCM as a complete system of medicine. Their work together resulted in the *Huang Ti Nei Ching* (The Yellow Emperor's Classic of Internal Medicine), which includes a listing of specific herbs and instructions in their use for treating a variety of illnesses. Both of these early medical texts laid the foundation for the rich and comprehensive system of Chinese herbology that remains an integral part of TCM today.

In India, the use of medicinal plants has also played an important role in relation to health care and the development of Ayurvedic medicine (Ayurveda). The *Charaka Samhita*, compiled by the physician-sage Charaka, who taught approximately three thousand years ago, lists over seven hundred plants and their medicinal properties. Nearly one thousand years after Charaka, another physician-sage, Sushruta, compiled the classic Ayurvedic text, the *Sushruta Samhita*, which built on Charaka's work and catalogued six hundred herbal combination formulas for treating disease. Both of these works continue to influence Ayurvedic physicians today, and much of the information they contain is now being scientifically validated. Interestingly, in both traditional Chinese medicine and Ayurveda, herbs are rarely used individually. Instead, carefully compounded herbal formulas are employed to restore balance in the body's organ and energy systems.

Herbs were prized for their medicinal value in early Greece, as well, due to the influence of the ancient Egyptians. Hippocrates (477 to 360 B.C.) emphasized preventive approaches to health that included proper diet, herbs, exercise, and hydrotherapy. Records of his works reveal that he employed over 250 medicinal plants in his herbal repertoire. Following him came Theophrastus (340 B.C.), a philosopher and natural scientist considered the "father of botany," due to his treatise *Inquiry into Plants*, in which he listed many types of plants, their medicinal values, and how they could be grown and harvested. Theophrastus is still recognized today for the accuracy of his observations and apt descriptions of the preparation and uses of drugs obtained from plants. Perhaps the most influential Greek herbalist was Dioscorides, a physician born in the first century A.D., who accompanied the armies of the Roman emperor Nero throughout Asia Minor, Greece, Italy, Spain, and Gaul, studying and recording plants and their uses according to the folklore of the lands he visited. Dioscorides' *De Materia Medica* was hailed by Galen, a Greek scientist of the second century A.D., as the supreme text of its kind and was repeatedly copied and recopied by physicians, herbalists, and scientists throughout Europe well into the sixteenth century.

Influenced by the Greeks, the Romans continued to explore and document the uses of medicinal plants and were responsible for spreading herbalism throughout much of Europe, where it was further influenced by various cultures. With the onset of the Middle Ages, however, much of the knowledge attained by the Greek and Roman civilizations was either destroyed or lost. During this time, herbal lore was often mixed with superstition, including the belief that plants possessed their own temperaments and were therefore best suited for treating individuals with similar personality traits. The use of herbs also increasingly became the province of women and of monks, who within their monasteries kept the knowledge of medicinal plants from disappearing altogether via Latin translations of older manuscripts from Greece, Rome, and other lands. Cultivating herb gardens also became a popular monastic practice, with the herbs being used to treat the sick and injured within the vicinity of the monasteries.

The knowledge and use of medicinal plants was taught and preserved by nuns in cloisters around Europe, as well, beginning in the seventh century. Within the Anglo-Saxon region, medical practitioners known as leeches also used herbs as a healing measure, although often in conjunction with rites and rituals that today are viewed as mere superstitions. The *Herbarium Apuleius*, which originated in A.D. 480 and continued to be added to until A.D. 1050, was one of the most widely copied and disseminated herbal manuscripts in the Anglo-Saxon world and contained instructions for the use of over one hundred herbs. Another work, the *Leechbook of Bald* (A.D. 925), also contained many therapeutic herbal formulas that are still valued by herbalists today, despite the myriad superstitious notions the book contains regarding application of the remedies. Both of these books are available in modern English translations.

Concurrent with these developments, herbalism was also being further developed by Arabic and Persian scientists and researchers, as part of an overall flowering of all the sciences that occurred within the Arabian world between A.D. 700 and 1300. Among the key figures who refined the practice of herbal medicine during this era are Ibn Sina, known to the Western world as Avicenna (A.D. 980–1037), and Jami Ibn-al-Baitar (A.D. 1197–1248). Considered one of the greatest minds of the Arabian School, Avicenna was an accomplished physician, botanist, poet, philosopher, and diplomat. Credited with refining and expanding the work of the renowned Greek physician Galen, Avicenna's writings held considerable influence in the Western world for over six hundred years, and he is still regarded as a healing authority in the Middle East and parts of Asia. Born in Spain, Jami Ibn-al-Baitar was another famed physician and botanist of the Arabian School, who compiled a sophisticated treatise on over two thousand medicinal plants and their usage. The influence of the Arabian School eventually entered Europe as a result of the Islamic invasion of Spain, and the work of physicians such as Constantine the African, who introduced the principles of Arabian medicine to the Salernum, a famous medical center in Salerno, Italy during the eleventh and twelfth centuries.

In 1498, the *Nuovo Receptario*, the first official Western pharmacopoeia (a guideline of standards for preparing and using herbal formulas), was published in Italy. Originally written in Italian, the information it contained was almost entirely derived from the Greek and Arabic approaches to herbology developed during the preceding centuries. In 1518, the work was translated into Latin and soon spread throughout the rest of Western Europe, eventually spawning the appearance of other pharmacopoeias in other European countries.

By the early seventeenth century, herbalism in Europe was further influenced by the interactions of European explorers with the Amerindian peoples of the New World, all of whom have employed herbal remedies as part of their healing traditions for thousands of years. The advent of settlers within the Americas led to an even greater exchange of information between European and Amerindian cultures, with many native American plants quickly finding their way into the herbal repertoire of Old World herbalists.

By the nineteenth century, a system of herbology combining elements of both Amerindian and European herbal lore was widely in use in

North America, while in Europe herbal practices fell increasingly under scientific scrutiny. These two trends set the stage for the emergence of phytotherapy as it is currently practiced. The modern-day father of phytomedicine, French physician Henri Leclerc (1870–1955), played a pivotal role in this development due to his research on the use of medicinal plants within the context of a clinical setting. He published numerous papers on this subject, and his textbook, *Précis de Phytothérapie*, remains a highly regarded reference to this day. During the twentieth century, the primary researcher who built on Leclerc's work was Rudolf Fritz Weiss (1898–1991), a German doctor whose efforts led to the organization of European scientists devoted to studying the benefits of herbal remedies. Weiss's textbook *Lehrbuch der Phytotherapie* (available in the United States as *Herbal Medicine*) is the leading reference on the medicinal use of herbs in the Western world.

Although interest in phytomedicine continues to grow in the United States today, its acceptance continues to lag behind Europe, Asia, and Central and South America. In France, for instance, all phytotherapists are also credentialed physicians, while in Germany 70 percent of all general practitioners prescribe herbal medicines to their patients. Germany is also home to the Commission E monographs on medicinal plants, which are reviewed by health care professionals from a variety of disciplines and describe the properties, applications, appropriate dosages, and contraindications of hundreds of herbal remedies. Many of these remedies are also covered by Germany's national health care insurance. The governments of both China and Japan also officially sanction and promote botanical medicine as part of their national health care systems. In India, herbal remedies also remain popular and are widely used within the system of Ayurvedic medicine. Given the growing consumer demand, as well as the entry of the pharmaceutical industry into the botanical medical field, it is likely that U.S. interest in medicinal plants will continue to flourish in coming years.

HOW BOTANICAL MEDICINE WORKS

Medicinal plants work in much the same way as drugs, in that both are absorbed orally and possess chemical compounds capable of triggering biological effects. Unlike pharmaceutical drugs, however, the actions of herbal remedies within the bloodstream and upon specific organs take an indirect route, meaning that their effects initially tend to be slower to occur and less dramatic than drugs that are administered directly. "Doctors and patients accustomed to the rapid, intense effects of synthetic medicines may become impatient with botanicals for this reason," explains leading holistic physician Andrew Weil, M.D. Yet, it is precisely because most herbs do act more slowly than pharmaceutical drugs that they are able to achieve results with far fewer side effects. Typically, too, once benefits are achieved, they tend to be longer-lasting. Not all herbs act slowly, however, and serious side effects can result if herbs are not properly prescribed or not of high quality in terms of preparation.

"One of the reasons phytomedicine can work so well," Dr. Morris says, "is because the whole of the plant is greater than the sum of its parts. Nature does things for a reason. In conventional medicine, the tendency is to isolate out the active compounds in plants that are considered to have medicinal value. This isolation process is sometimes called the 'silver bullet' approach and is in fact how drugs are produced. In the case of white willow bark, for instance, which was traditionally used by the Iroquois and many other first nation peoples to treat pain, the active compound salicylate was synthesized to make aspirin. Unfortunately, each year thousands of people in this country develop stomach bleeding as a result of using aspirin, something that does not happen when white willow bark is used in its entirety as a phytomedicine. When we start to isolate out these active compounds—and this is something that is starting to occur in the field of botanical medicine, as well, due to an emphasis on using standardized potencies—we tend to lose the art of healing, along with some of the other compounds that nature has put in plants to make them much more harmless and in many cases better absorbed."

❦ FORMS OF BOTANICAL MEDICINE ❦

Botanical medicines are available in a variety of forms, with various degrees of effectiveness. The most common commercial forms are whole herbs and powders, teas, capsules and tablets, tinctures, herbal extracts, essential oils, and balms and ointments.

Whole herbs and powders consist of all or part of herbs that have been cut and powdered. For the most part, herbs in this form undergo minimal processing and are often sold in bulk by herbal retailers and health food stores.

Herbal teas represent one of the most popular forms of herbal medicine and are now commercially available in mainstream drugstores and grocery chains, in addition to health food stores. Commercial teas are usually sold in the form of tea bags, but loose powders are also available. One of the simplest forms of herbal teas is known as an infusion, which is prepared by steeping dried or fresh herbs in boiling water. Infusions are an effective means of using herbs such as chamomile, rose hips, and herbs from the mint family. However, infusions are not an appropriate method for herbs containing active ingredients that are not water soluble.

Many herbalists also make use of medicinal teas known as decoctions, which are more concentrated and stronger than regular commercial teas and prepared by boiling bulk herbs in water. The mixture is then strained, and the liquid ingested. Decoctions are also commonly used by practitioners of Ayurveda and traditional Chinese medicine (see Chapters 12 and 13).

Capsules and tablets represent one of the fastest-growing sectors of the commercial botanical market due to their convenience. Both forms are prepared using dried herbal powders and are often standardized (see below) to ensure effective amounts of the herb's primary active ingredients. An additional benefit of capsules and tablets is that they often are free of the bitter taste common to many herbs when consumed in other forms.

Tinctures are also growing in popularity in the United States and are prepared by soaking herbs in a solvent for periods ranging from a few hours to a few weeks, depending on the herb in question. The most common solvents usually contain alcohol, due to its effectiveness as a carrier and for preserving shelf life. Water and glycerin can also be used. Typically tinctures contain one part herb (by weight) for every five to ten parts of solvent used. For the most part, tinctures are more quickly assimilated than herbs taken as capsules or tablets.

Herbal extracts can be either fluid or solid. *Fluid extracts* are also made from solvents, but usually in concentrations of one to one, making them much stronger than tinctures. *Solid extracts* are the most condensed types of herbal remedies and are prepared by steeping herbs in a solvent until all of the solvent evaporates. The remaining residue is usually sold as a powder in concentrations ranging from two to eight parts herb (by weight) to one part solvent. Increasingly, *standardized extracts*, both in liquid and solid form, have become the preferred methods of herbal preparation today. The standardization process focuses on extracting optimal dosages of an herb's primary active ingredients in relation to the overall weight of the extract. Since standardization is the most effective means of ensuring that the herb's active ingredients are contained in the remedy, it is the method most often recommended by health care practitioners who use botanical medicine as part of their treatment programs.

Essential oils have also grown in popularity in the United States in recent years, due to increasing interest in aromatherapy (see Chapter 15). Made from the distilled essences of various plant parts, most essential oils are applied externally and are usually diluted in water or a carrier oil, due to their high concentration. The oils may also be diffused throughout the room to promote feelings of relaxation and in certain cases can also be taken internally.

Balms and ointments made from plants have been used by world cultures for thousands of years to soothe muscle pain, treat wounds, and speed the healing process. Today, a variety of commercially prepared balm and ointment products are available for similar purposes. 🌿

The Medicinal Actions of Herbs

The medicinal actions of herbs correspond to the way the properties of specific herbs interact with the human body to enhance physiological performance, prevent illness, and aid in the treatment of disease. All medicinal plants directly affect physiological activity due to their various chemical components and primary active ingredients. Their actions vary, however, and many herbs also have more than one action for which they can be used. Knowing which herbs to use to perform an appropriate action is an essential component of botanical medicine.

The principal actions of medicinal plants fall into the following categories: adaptogens, antioxidants, anti-inflammatories, antimicrobials, anodynes, antispasmodics, astringents, carminatives, cholagogues, demulcents, digestive bitters, diuretics, emmenagogues, expectorants, immunomodulators, laxatives, nervines, stimulants, and tonics.

Adaptogens refer to a class of herbs that enhance the body's ability to resist and respond to stress. Adaptogenic herbs work by supporting the adrenal glands, while also balancing various other body systems, including the immune system, central nervous system, and metabolism. Adaptogens play an important role in both Ayurvedic medicine and traditional

Chinese medicine (see Chapters 12 and 13). Among the best-known adaptogens are ginseng, astragalus, and ashwagandha (an Ayurvedic herbal tonic).

Antioxidants are substances that protect cells from damage caused by free radicals, highly reactive atom clusters that have been linked to an assortment of chronic disease conditions, as well as premature aging. A variety of vitamins and minerals, such as vitamins C and E, carotenes, selenium, and zinc, are well known for their antioxidant properties, but a number of medicinal plants, especially those with high concentrations of bioflavonoids, also offer effective antioxidant support. These include green and black teas, ginkgo biloba, bilberry, and milk thistle.

Anti-inflammatory herbs work in a variety of ways to soothe or reduce inflammation of body tissues. Common herbs with anti-inflammatory properties include borage, chamomile, lobelia, mullein, slippery elm, wintergreen, and witch hazel.

Antimicrobials are herbs that aid the body in resisting or destroying disease-causing microorganisms (bacteria, viruses, and fungi). While certain antimicrobial plants contain chemicals that target the invading organisms themselves, in general this class of herbs work by stimulating the immune system. Echinacea is an increasingly popular herb with antimicrobial properties. Other herbs in this category include aloe vera, black walnut, burdock, cinnamon, garlic, Pau D'Arco, reishi and shiitake mushrooms, tea tree, and turmeric.

Anodynes refer to medicinal plants or plant compounds that relieve pain. Common herbal anodynes include black cohosh, ginger, kava kava, mullein, willow, and witch hazel (applied externally).

Antispasmodic medicinal plants are useful for relieving tension and cramping in the body's musculature. Psychological tension can also respond well to antispasmodic herbs, which include chamomile, feverfew, mugwort, mullein, kava kava, peppermint, and skullcap.

Astringent herbs cause cell tissue protein to coagulate, helping to tone tissue via a binding action that can also serve as a protective barrier against infection. Astringents are also helpful for reducing irritation in membrane and skin tissue, and for relieving inflammation. Such herbs improve blood circulation as well, and can be effective for alleviating edema, hemorrhoids, and varicose veins. American ginseng, angelica, black and green teas, black walnut, juniper berry, nettle, Pau D'Arco, rhubarb, sassafras, white willow, witch hazel, and yarrow are among the herbs containing astringent properties.

Carminatives refer to plants containing aromatic volatile oils that soothe and stimulate the digestive system. Carminative plants are also useful for reducing inflammation in the digestive organs and for relieving bloating and flatulence, as well as releasing trapped gas. Indigestion, heartburn, and irritable bowel syndrome are other conditions for which carminatives can provide relief. Chamomile and peppermint are two widely used carminative herbs recommended by herbalists and holistic physicians. Other herbs in this category include anise, cayenne, dandelion, fennel, ginger, juniper berry, spearmint, and thyme.

Cholagogues are herbs that aid the liver due to their ability to stimulate the production and proper flow of bile, thereby aiding in digestion and assimilation (particularly of fats), and reducing the likehood of gallstones. Among the most common cholagogues are milk thistle, dandelion root, turmeric, and artichoke.

Demulcents are herbs with a high mucilage content, a substance that helps soothe and protect irritated or inflamed mucus tissue. Demulcent herbs, which include aloe vera, borage, flax, licorice, mullein, and slippery elm, ease irritations in the bronchioles of the lungs and the gastrointestinal and urinary tracts and can provide effective relief from diarrhea, coughs, sore throats, and muscle spasms related to colic.

Digestive bitters aid the digestive process by triggering the release of saliva and stomach acids necessary to break down food. Digestive enzymes and bile flow can also be stimulated by digestive bitters. Barberry bark, centaury, dandelion root, and yellow dock are examples of bitters that can be effective in stimulating the production of stomach acid and aiding sluggish digestion.

Diuretics increase the production and elimination of urine, helping the body to eliminate wastes and diminishing unhealthy water retention. Examples of herbs that act as diuretics include angelica, arrowroot, bearberry, burdock, dandelion, fennel, feverfew, gotu kola, juniper berry, sassafras, and wintergreen.

Emmenagogues aid in menstruation and help regulate the overall health of the female reproductive system. Examples of emmenagogues include aloe vera, angelica, burdock, celery, chamomile, chasteberry, cohosh (both black and blue), feverfew, ginger, mugwort, parsley, passionflower, shave grass, willow, and wintergreen.

Expectorants promote the elimination of phlegm and mucus from the lungs. Expectorant herbs are of two kinds: irritants and relaxants. Irritant expectorants agitate the bronchioles, causing the expulsion of mucus and phlegm, while relaxants soothe bronchial distress, helping to loosen mucus secretions and easing dry coughs. Bloodroot, celery, chickweed, eucalyptus, fenugreek, licorice, myrrh, yam, and yerba santa all act as expectorant herbs.

Immunomodulators are a specific class of herbs that promote healthy immune function due to the polysaccharides they contain. Complex sugar molecules, polysaccharides act to improve immune cell function, especially lymphocyte cells, which act as the body's first line of defense against viral infections, including the HIV virus. Perhaps the most popular herbal immunomodulator is echinacea, which, according to Donald J. Brown, N.D., a noted phytotherapy expert, helps to improve immune function and speed recovery times from infectious disease. Dr. Brown cautions, however, that while for most people echinacea is well suited as a short-term immune system booster, it should be avoided by people whose immune systems are already overactive due to autoimmune conditions and progressively debilitating diseases such as multiple sclerosis. Other herbs that act as immunomodulators include Siberian and Korean ginseng, garlic, ginger, Pau D'Arco, and maitake, reishi, and shiitake mushrooms.

Laxatives refer to herbs that promote proper bowel movements. Herbal laxatives fall into two categories: bulking agents and stimulants. Bulking agents are laxatives that are rich in fiber and mucilage. As they come in contact with water, they expand and increase in volume in the bowel, causing the bowel walls to contract and empty. The most common laxative bulking agents are psyllium seed and guar gum.

Laxatives that act as stimulants directly trigger peristalsis, the wave-like contractions of the smooth muscles of the digestive tract. Examples of laxative stimulants include aloe vera, cascara bark, rhubarb, and senna leaves.

Caution: Stimulant laxatives, while often quite effective for short-term constipation, are not advised for long-term use without medical supervision, as they can cause dependency and lead to bodily dehydration. Stimulant laxatives should also be avoided by pregnant and lactating women, and by anyone suffering from chronic bowel disorders, such as irritable bowel syndrome, Crohn's disease, or ulcerative colitis.

Nervines enhance the health of the nervous system in one of three ways. Tonic nervines help to strengthen and restore proper nerve function; relaxant nervines help to ease both physical and psychological tension and anxiety; and stimulant nervines directly trigger nerve activity. In recent years, the herbal nervine St. John's wort has become extremely popular for its relaxant and antidepressant properties. Other herbal nervines include balm, celery, chamomile, hops, kava kava, linden, motherwort, nettle, passionflower, skullcap, and valerian.

Stimulants refer to a broad class of herbs that enhance and invigorate physiological and metabolic activity. Herbs that act as stimulants include angelica, bee pollen, bloodroot, cayenne, eucalyptus, ginger, ginkgo biloba, ginseng, guarana, peppermint, prickly ash, spearmint, and wintergreen.

Tonics promote the overall health of the body's various systems and play a major role in the botanical traditions of Ayurveda and traditional Chinese medicine, where they are often employed as preventatives against disease. A number of tonic herbs, such as ginseng and ashwagandha, also act as adaptogens (see above). Other herbal tonics include bearberry, damiana, devil's claw, gotu kola, kava kava, lavender, mugwort, myrrh, rhubarb, sarsaparilla, wild cherry, yarrow, and yerba santa.

CAUTIONS REGARDING THE USE ❧ OF BOTANICAL REMEDIES ❧

Although botanical medicine has a long and culturally diverse history as a natural healing method, herbal remedies need to be used wisely. While most medicinal plants are safe and well suited as self-care approaches for enhancing health, certain herbs can result in adverse side effects and drug interactions. In addition, while certain herbs can be helpful within a certain dosage range, when taken in larger amounts they can prove toxic and even life-threatening. Compounding this issue, herbal potencies can vary widely due to a range of factors, including the climate and geographical region in which herbs are grown, soil conditions, and harvesting and processing methods. Age, sex, weight, genetics, and other unique biochemical traits can also influence how people respond to herbs. If you are considering using botanical remedies for the first time, you should first consult with your physician or a skilled herbalist who can advise you on how best to proceed. The resource organizations listed at the end of this chapter can also assist you in your education process.

While adverse side effects from using herbs properly are rare, caution is still recommended. In particular, people using prescription drugs, pregnant and lactating women, and people susceptible to allergies should be especially careful about using herbal remedies, and should always consult with their physicians before doing so. In addition, a number of herbs should be avoided altogether, due to their potential as health hazards. Among them are comfrey, chaparral, ephedra (also known as Ma huang), herbal laxative and stimulant teas, and kombucha mushrooms. For further information about using herbs wisely, see "Guidelines for Using Botanical Medicine and Selecting an Herbal Practitioner" later in this chapter. 🌿

COMMON HERBS AND THEIR USES

Despite their growing popularity in the United States, herbal remedies should not be used indiscriminately and initially are best explored under the guidance of a holistic physician or trained herbalist. The following herbs, however, are generally safe and can be used to enhance and maintain optimal wellness.

Aloe Vera (Aloe barbadenis, Aloe vulgari). In addition to being widely used as an ingredient in many cosmetic products, the aloe vera plant offers a wide range of health benefits. Applied externally as a gel, aloe promotes healing of burns, cuts, and scrapes due to its zinc and vitamin C and E content, as well as its antimicrobial and anti-inflammatory properties. (Aloe gel is not suitable as a treatment for deep wounds, however, which require immediate medical attention.) The gel also serves as an effective moisturizer. Taken internally as a juice, aloe acts as both a tonic and cleansing agent and can be an effective aid against asthma and for regulating noninsulin-dependent diabetes.

Cayenne (Capsicum annum). Also known as red pepper, cayenne acts as a general tonic and has been shown to improve circulation by increasing blood flow, and to stimulate digestion. Cayenne has anti-inflammatory properties, as well, and can be useful in preventing allergic reactions in people suffering from food allergies or sensitivities. Capsaicin, the primary active ingredient in cayenne, applied as a topical cream or ointment, has also been shown to be a safe and effective means for alleviating pain associated with arthritis and nerve disorders, such as fibromyalgia. Cayenne can safely be used as a seasoning in meals and is also available in capsule form.

Chamomile (Matricaria recutita). Many cultures around the world consume chamomile tea due to its ability to aid digestion. Acting as both an anti-inflammatory and antispasmodic inside the gastrointestinal tract, chamomile is helpful for irritable bowel syndrome and other gastrointestinal conditions, including peptic ulcers, and in Germany it is licensed as an over-the-counter medicine for such ailments. External applications of chamomile teas and extracts can help alleviate mouth and gum conditions and soothe inflammatory skin conditions. It also serves as an effective sedative and mouthwash. In addition to chamomile tea, the herb is available as both a powder and a tincture.

Echinacea (Echinacea angutifolia). Also known as purple coneflower, echinacea is a perennial herb native to the American Great Plains and renowned for its ability to stimulate the immune system. It is also effective as an antimicrobial agent, anti-inflammatory, and wound healer. According to Dr. Morris, echinacea should properly be considered a natural antibiotic. He recommends taking it regularly in order to achieve its full therapeutic benefits. Dr. Morris cautions, however, that tolerance to its benefits can occur if echinacea is taken for longer than three weeks. "In general, I recommend that my patients take echinacea daily until their symptoms are completely gone, and then continue using it for another three or four days to ensure that symptoms don't recur," he explains. "For people who choose to use it for long periods of time, I advice stopping for at least a week between each three-week period of use before resuming again." Widely used as a medicinal plant by Northern Native American cultures, echinacea is available as a tincture or in capsule form.

Garlic (Allium sativum). A member of the lily family, garlic is one of the oldest herbal remedies in the world. A potent antimicrobial, garlic is effective for treating coughs, sinus and lung congestion, poor circulation, and rheumatism, and as a preventive measure for colds and flu, yeast infections, and certain forms of cancer (particularly stomach and colon cancer), due to its ability to boost immune function and increase natural killer (NK) cell activity. Garlic also provides a number of cardiovascular benefits, including its ability to lower blood pressure and reduce platelet aggregation. In Germany, garlic extracts have been approved as over-the-counter medications for reducing serum cholesterol and triglyceride levels and raising healthy HDL cholesterol. The easiest way to enjoy garlic's many health benefits is to eat one fresh clove daily or to include it in meals. A variety of supplements rich in allicin, garlic's primary active ingredient, are also available for those averse to the odor that can be caused by garlic consumption.

Ginger (Zingiber officinalis). A medicinal plant mainstay in China, India, and other regions of Asia and Indonesia since the fourth century

B.C., ginger is an effective remedy for indigestion, flatulence, and overall stimulation of the gastrointestinal tract. It is also useful as an aid in the treatment of nausea, morning sickness, motion sickness, and coughs and asthma related to allergy or inflammation. Like garlic, ginger has also been found to reduce blood platelet aggregation, suggesting that it may be useful in reducing the risk of cardiovascular illness. In addition, ginger helps to increase the activity of other herbs and is therefore included as an ingredient in a number of herbal formulas. Ginger can be eaten raw and added to meals as a seasoning, and is also available as a tea, powder, or in capsule form.

Ginkgo biloba (Ginkgo biloba). Derived from the ginkgo tree, the oldest living tree species in the world (estimated to have originated 200 million years ago), ginkgo biloba is highly regarded by practitioners of traditional Chinese medicine as a treatment for respiratory conditions, and for maintaining and enhancing brain and memory function. Due to its ability to increase blood flow in the brain, ginkgo helps to improve concentration, absentmindnesses, mental fatigue, and lack of energy, and is also helpful in treating dementia and Alzheimer's disease. Vertigo, tinnitus, and dizziness also respond favorably to ginkgo, and it can be used to help peripheral vascular disease, such as Reynaud's syndrome, numbness, tingling, and intermittent, severe calf pain caused by prolonged walking and other forms of exercise. Studies have also found ginkgo to be useful for macular degeneration, asthma, impotence, and certain types of head injury. In recent years, ginkgo has become one of the most widely purchased herbal remedies in the United States.

Ginseng. Herbalists and holistic physicians primarily employ three types of ginseng: Asian (*Panax ginseng*), American (*Panax quinquefolious*), and Siberian (*Eleutherococcus senticosus*). Asian ginseng is one of the world's oldest and most highly regarded tonic and adaptogenic herbs, due to its ability to support and improve adrenal function. It is useful for improving energy levels, alleviating the effects of stress, and for enhancing concentration. It also aids the body in maximizing both oxygen and glycogen use, allowing muscles to operate in an aerobic state longer and more efficiently, thereby improving physical performance and enhancing reaction time. In addition, Asian ginseng helps regulate blood sugar and cholesterol levels, and has been shown to decrease the risk of cancer and to minimize the side effects of chemotherapy and radiation. American ginseng, while less known, has many of the same health properties of Asian ginseng.

Siberian ginseng, also known as Eleuthero, is one of the most effective herbal adaptogens, a fact supported by a wealth of scientific research conducted by scientists in Russia and the former Soviet Union, China, and Japan. Eleuthero is effective in enhancing the body's capacity to endure and resist stress. It also serves as an aid to resisting and recovering from disease, and helps protect against environmental toxins, in addition to supporting conventional cancer treatments.

Like echinacea, ginseng in all its forms is not recommended for long-term use. Typically, three to four weeks of daily use should be followed by a break of one to two weeks, before resuming. Caffeine use should also be avoided when taking ginseng, to avoid overstimulation, and ginseng is not recommended for people suffering from uncontrolled hypertension, or for pregnant and lactating women.

Milk thistle (Silbum marianum). Milk thistle is one of the most effective herbal cholagogues, and has been used in Europe as a liver tonic for over two millennia. Silymarin, milk thistle's primary active ingredient, has been shown to act as a protective and healing agent for a variety of liver and gallbladder conditions, including gallstones, hepatitis, cirrhosis, and liver disease caused by alcohol abuse and a wide range of environmental toxins. Milk thistle also has antioxidant properties and is effective in stimulating cell production of glutathione, a potent protective agent against free-radical damage. Since the liver is one of the most important organs in the body, milk thistle (taken as an extract or capsule standardized to 70 to 80 percent silymarin content) is an excellent choice for daily maintenance of proper liver function and has no known side effects.

Peppermint (Mentha piperita). Peppermint is an excellent digestive aid, as well as a cholagogue that stimulates the flow of bile from the liver into the stomach. Widely used in Europe as a digestive aid, in Germany peppermint oil is approved as an over-the-counter medicinal for treating upper gastrointestinal tract cramps, upper respiratory catarrh, and spastic conditions related to the bile ducts. Taken as an enterically coated capsule, peppermint oil acts as an intestinal antispasmodic, making it useful for irritable bowel syndrome. It is also effective for relieving flatulence, nausea, and gallstones and gallbladder inflammation. The most common form of peppermint is as a tea, which can be consumed during or after meals to enhance digestion. Chewing a sprig of peppermint can also freshen the breath.

St. John's wort (Hypericum perforatum). The popularity of St. John's wort has exploded in recent years, due to its ability to relieve anxiety, depression, and nervous tension. Its primary active ingredient, hypericum, is chemically similar to prescription tricyclic antidepressant drugs, without their potential side effects, explaining why the herb is the most commonly prescribed antidepressant in Germany. St. John's wort's other applications include pain reduction (including pain caused by neuralgia, sciatica, and rheumatism), and its anti-inflammatory and antiviral properties. Most commonly taken in capsule form, St. John's wort can also be made into a lotion and applied topically to speed the healing of wounds and sunburn.

Caution: St. John's wort should not be taken when using prescription antidepressant drugs. Some physicians also advise against using it during pregnancy or lactation.

Saw palmetto (Serenoa repens). Saw palmetto tones and strengthens the male reproductive system and has become increasingly popular over the last decade due to its ability to reduce benign prostatic hypertrophy (BPH) and chronic, nonbacterial prostatitis. Research has shown that saw palmetto is up to six times as effective as prescription drugs for treating BPH, and the herb is also useful for increasing subnormal male sex hormone levels.

CONDITIONS THAT BENEFIT FROM BOTANICAL MEDICINE

As a general rule, practitioners of holistic medicine are not advocates of what Dr. Morris describes as "allopathic herbalism," meaning the substitution of herbal remedies in place of drugs in order to treat disease symptoms. "A good example of this is using St. John's wort to take the place of Prozac or Zoloft to treat mild depression," Dr. Morris explains. "Either method is little more than taking a quick Band-Aid approach that at best only serves to mask or minimize the patient's symptoms. Usually people who are depressed require more than that, including perhaps someone to talk to in order to work out whatever issues may be affecting them. For such people, I don't believe simply prescribing an herb or a drug is of much benefit." The "whole person" treatment approach that Dr. Morris and his holistic colleagues prefer instead does not negate the health benefits and usefulness that herbs have for many disease conditions, however. These include immune enhancement, stress reduction, improved gastrointestinal function, prevention of cancer and cardiovascular disease, relief of anxiety and depression, pain relief, headache and migraine reduction, and improved sleep.

Immunity

The immune system is a key component of overall health. A variety of herbs, including echinacea, ginseng, astragalus, and garlic, have been found to be beneficial to immune function. The subject of over four hundred clinical studies, echinacea acts directly as an antiviral agent for such conditions as colds, flu, upper respiratory infections, and herpes, and has properties similar to interferon, a protein group released by white blood cells to inhibit virus. Echinacea has also been shown to enhance T-cell production, aid antibodies in effectively binding with and destroying invading pathogens, and increase natural killer (NK) cell activity. Echinacea also stimulates the thymus gland, considered the immune system's "master gland," and inhibits hyaluronidase, an enzyme secreted by invading bacteria as they attempt to pass through the protective membranes of skin and mucus.

Both ginseng and astragalus, because of their tonic and adaptogenic properties, can also help boost immune function. One study of Korean (Panax) ginseng involving three groups of twenty healthy participants found that after one month, those given 100 mg of standardized Panax ginseng extract every twelve hours showed increased production of lymphocytes and improved resistance to pathogens, compared to the other groups, who received a placebo or a 100-mg water extract of ginseng. After eight weeks, the improvement in immune status of the group receiving the standardized extract was even more noticeable. Astragalus, a mainstay of traditional Chinese medicine for treating viral conditions, has been found to increase T-cell activity and to reverse T-cell damage caused by chemotherapeutic drugs, radiation, and aging. It has also been shown to increase stem cell production in bone marrow and lymph, stimulating them into active immune cells without immunosuppressive affects, even after long-term use. Astragalus also enhances the body's ability to produce interferon and increases its effectiveness in combating disease.

Garlic enhances immune function by improving T-cell, macrophage, and natural killer (NK) cell activity. In addition, garlic has been shown to aid the body in resisting *Candida albicans* infection (the primary cause of candidiasis, vaginal yeast infections, and oral thrush), as well as acting as an antimicrobial against salmonella and *E. coli*. Other herbs with immune enhancement properties include aloe vera, goldenseal, and shiitake mushrooms.

Stress

Stress, which is estimated to play a role in 85 percent of all illness, diminishes health and saps energy due to the toll it takes on the adrenal glands. One of the best herbs for supporting adrenal gland function, and thereby combating stress, is eleuthero, or Siberian ginseng, which also enhances the activities of the hypothalamus and pituitary glands, both of which affect, and are affected by, the adrenal glands. Asian, or Korean, ginseng can also be helpful during times of stress. Rather than stimulating the adrenal glands directly, ginseng enhances the overall functioning of what is referred to in traditional Chinese medicine as the "hypothalamus-pituitary-adrenal axis," which in turn enables the body to more easily adapt to stress and recover from its effects more quickly.

Gastrointestinal Function

A variety of herbs can aid in improving overall gastrointestinal function. These include milk thistle (silymarin), which protects and improves liver and gallbladder function and stimulates bile flow; chamomile, peppermint, and spearmint, all of which act as digestive aids and help to reduce flatulence; aloe vera, which helps soothe the entire lining of the gastrointestinal tract; and cayenne, which acts as a digestive stimulant and helps minimize reactions due to food sensitivities. In Europe, combination tinctures known as herbal bitters have long been employed as aids for improving digestion. A number of these formulas are now available in American health food stores, as well.

Cancer

While many of the claims regarding the effectiveness of herbal remedies as treatments for cancer are false or, at best, anecdotal, scientific evidence has found that certain herbs do have antitumor and cancer-preventive properties. Some of the most promising herbs in this category are garlic, Asian ginseng, green tea, turmeric, and shiitake and maitake mushrooms.

Garlic has been shown to reduce the risk of colon, stomach, and esophageal cancer. One study involving women between the ages of fifty-five and sixty-nine found that garlic consumption was more effective in reducing colon cancer than vegetables and dietary fiber, and that the risk of developing colon cancer decreased by 35 percent when garlic was consumed at least once a week, and up to 50 percent when garlic was eaten more frequently. Animal studies indicate that garlic may also help reduce the risk of breast, bladder, skin, and lung cancer.

A Korean study indicates that Asian, or Korean (Panax), ginseng, taken in the form of an extract or powder, lowers the overall risk of cancer development, and is especially helpful in reducing the risk of throat, lung, and liver cancers. Test subjects who consumed ginseng for a year reduced their cancer risk by 36 percent, while those who consumed it for five years or more had a 69 percent risk reduction.

Green tea, primarily due to its ability to prevent free-radical damage, has been found to lower the risk of skin, stomach, and esophageal cancer, and to be particularly effective in reducing the incidence of skin cancers caused by chemicals and radiation. The risk of developing cancer of the liver has also been shown to be minimized by green tea consumption.

Turmeric has also been shown to have cancer-inhibiting properties and may provide particular benefit for smokers. One study found that smokers who consumed two 750-mg tablets of turmeric daily had a significant reduction in urinary mutagens (an indication of cell damage caused by smoking) after only one month. Another study showed turmeric was effective in reducing DNA damage following exposure to benzoapryrene, a known carcinogen. Another study involving sixty-two patients with either skin or oral cancer, found that topical application of vaseline mixed with curcumin, turmeric's primary active ingredient, significantly reduced cancerous lesions, as well as patient pain, itching, odor, and drainage.

Shiitake and maitake mushrooms can both provide benefits for people at risk for cancer. Lentinan, an active ingredient in shiitake, has been shown to substantially enhance immune response, suppress chemical and viral carcinogens, and to attack cancers directly. The mushroom has also been shown to reduce the risk of cancer recurrence and metastasis after surgery, and to increase the life span of patients suffering from advanced cancers of the stomach, colon, rectum, and breast. Both shiitake and maitake also increase the antitumor activity of the immune system's natural killer (NK) cells and enhance antibody response. Of the two, maitake has been shown to have the more powerful and more consistent effects in this regard. Both medicinal plants can also help minimize side effects from chemotherapy and radiation treatments.

Cardiovascular Disease

Cardiovascular disease consistently ranks as the leading, disease-related cause of death in the United States, despite overwhelming evidence that shows that most cases of heart disease could be prevented by such measures as a healthy diet, regular exercise, and stress management. A variety of medicinal plants can also play an important role in preventing and managing cardiovascular disease. Among them are garlic, hawthorn berry, and grape seed and pine bark extracts.

Garlic is a particularly versatile herb in relation to heart function, due to its ability to minimize the risk factors associated with atherosclerosis, or hardening of the arteries. Research shows that regular consumption of garlic can reduce unhealthy LDL cholesterol levels, while raising healthy HDL levels; relieve high blood pressure; inhibit platelet aggregation; and help break down blood clots, in addition to its known antioxidant activity. In a study of twenty healthy volunteers and sixty-two patients with coronary heart disease (CHD), healthy subjects who ate garlic daily exhibited a significant reduction in LDL cholesterol after six months, as well as improved HDL levels, compared to a placebo group. Similar results were achieved among the CHD patients after a ten-month period. A meta-analysis of five other studies found that daily consumption of a clove of garlic or its equivalent reduces cholesterol levels by a minimum of 9 percent.

Hawthorn berry is another herb that is well recognized as a strengthener of the heart, due to its ability to improve blood flow and oxygen supply to all areas of the cardiovascular system. This herb can protect the heart during times of low oxygen supply and strengthen it during times of exercise. Hawthorn berry is especially useful in minimizing the effects of congestive heart failure. One study, for instance, found that supplementing with 600 mg of hawthorn extract per day substantially improved symptoms of early-stage congestive heart failure, while another study found that 900 mg of hawthorn extract taken daily reduced symptoms by 50 percent after two months among 132 patients with more advanced cases of the disease.

Grape seed and pine bark (pycnogenol) extracts, both of which are rich in plant flavonoids known as proanthocyanidins, have been shown to have antioxidant effects twenty times greater than vitamin E and fifty times greater than vitamin C. Research indicates that both extracts offer a variety of protective benefits for preventing and treating heart disease and stroke.

Anxiety and Depression

Anxiety and depression are often interconnected, and can manifest as both acute and chronic conditions. While severe or prolonged cases require immediate professional attention, milder cases often respond well to herbal intervention. Particularly useful herbs are kava kava, valerian root, St. John's wort, and ginkgo biloba.

Kava kava is one of the most widely researched herbs, and in Europe kava extracts are approved as an antianxiety medication, due to the clinically verified ability of kavalactone, the plant's primary active compound, to promote feelings of calm and relaxation. Double-blind studies of subjects receiving kava extracts have shown that the herb significantly reduces anxiety symptoms, without the side effects of most popular antianxiety medications, and also improves mood, mental alertness and reaction time. Kava should not be taken continuously for periods longer than four months, however, and is also not recommended for pregnant or lactating women, people suffering from Parkinson's disease, and people taking benzodiazepines (a class of psychotropic drugs, including Xanax and Valium).

Valerian root extract can also be useful for treating cases of anxiety, due to its mild sedative actions. It is completely safe for short-term use, and can be taken both during the day and at night to enhance sleep.

For cases of depression, St. John's wort has been shown by a number of clinical studies to be as effective as standard antidepressant medications, with far fewer side effects. Among the depression-related symptoms St. John's wort has been shown to improve are apathy, insomnia and other sleep disturbances, low self-esteem, and feelings of worthlessness. St. John's wort should not be taken with SSRI medications, such as Prozac, Zoloft, or Paxil, however, and should be avoided until four to six weeks following the start of amino acid supplementation. It can also cause mild stomach irritation.

For older people suffering from depression, ginkgo biloba can also be effective and may enhance the effectiveness of standard antidepressant drugs. One study of patients between the ages of fifty-one and seventy-eight for whom antidepressants had provided little to no relief, found that supplementing with ginkgo biloba extract along with antidepressant medication reduced depression symptoms by 50 percent after four weeks of daily use (3X/day), and by nearly 70 percent after two months. Ginkgo is also a potent antioxidant known to improve cerebral circulation and to protect the neural pathways and receptors of the brain from free-radical damage.

Pain

One of the most useful botanical remedies for pain relief is capsaicin, the principal active ingredient of cayenne pepper. Capsaicin has been shown to be effective for easing pain caused by arthritis and nerve conditions when applied topically as a cream or ointment, or ingested as a capsule or tincture. Capsaicin can also benefit people with fibromyalgia, a condition of chronic, widespread musculoskeletal pain and tenderness, as evidenced by a study that found topical application of capsaicin cream resulted in a noticeable reduction in pain, as well as improved grip strength. (Some people experienced a temporary but insignificant burning sensation following application of the cream.) Capsaicin can also minimize pain related to diabetic neuropathy and outbreaks of shingles (herpes zoster infection).

Other useful herbs for pain relief include witch hazel, turmeric, feverfew, licorice root, and bromelain (derived from pineapples), all of which are effective anti-inflammatories.

Headache and Migraine

The number-one botanical remedy for treating migraine is feverfew, which has been prescribed by European herbalists for such use since the Middle Ages. Feverfew has been shown scientifically to reduce the severity and frequency of the condition, even among cases where no relief resulted from conventional medicine. A number of studies indicate that feverfew acts to prevent and reduce migraine by inhibiting platelet coagulation and the release of prostaglandin related to migraine pain.

Other useful herbs for treating headache pain include willow bark, a natural analgesic from which aspirin is derived; ginseng and chamomile, both of which can reduce headache-related stress; and hawthorn leaf, which tones and soothes cerebral arteries.

Sleep

A variety of botanicals are useful as sleeping aids. Two of the most commonly prescribed herbs for promoting restful sleep are valerian root and passionflower. Having a long history as a sedative among herbalists, valerian was shown in a double-blind study of 128 participants to significantly decrease the time needed to fall asleep and improve overall sleep quality, without causing feelings of drowsiness or "hangover effects" common to conventional sleeping aids. Valerian appears to be most effective for insomniacs, smokers, and chronically irregular sleepers, especially women.

Because of its ability to inhibit the breakdown of serotonin, an important chemical for healthy sleep, passionflower is also a useful botanical aid for sleep. Other useful herbs include chamomile and hops, both of which act as mild sedatives.

❧ HEALING ADHD: A CASE HISTORY ❧

The following example involving one of Dr. Morris's patients illustrates the benefits herbal medicine can provide when employed as part of an overall protocol that "treats the person, not the disease." The patient was an eleven-year-old boy previously diagnosed with ADHD (attention deficit hyperactivity disorder). "When he first came to me, he was already on Ritalin and his parents were considering switching to a more powerful medication due to the fact that his condition was worsening," Dr. Morris says. Rather than accept the boy's diagnosis at face value, Dr. Morris ordered a complete lab analysis performed. "I also worked with him nutritionally and in terms of his diet, taking him off all refined carbohydrates, and using seaweed extracts to stimulate his thyroid, which the lab analysis found to be suboptimal," Dr. Morris recounts. "In addition, I recommended he take kava kava and St. John's wort. But just as importantly, I listened to him and what he wanted to express, and got him on a soccer team and into Tae Kwon Do." As a result of Dr. Morris's intervention, the boy's demeanor significantly improved, and he was able to be completely weaned off of Ritalin. "That was three years ago," Morris says. "Today, he's a productive student who is doing well at school, and his attention span is excellent." ❧

GUIDELINES FOR USING BOTANICAL MEDICINE AND SELECTING AN HERBAL PRACTITIONER

Botanical medicine can offer many benefits for anyone interested in achieving optimal health. The key to such benefits lies in using herbs appropriately. What follow are guidelines to help you do so.

Educate yourself about the herbs you are interested in. Not all of the claims made about herbal remedies are accurate. It is vital that you be able to discern fact from hype before choosing a remedy for use. If possible, seek out a competent holistic practitioner who can guide you in your choices. Most members of the American Holistic Medical Association employ herbal remedies as part of their treatment protocols. Naturopathic physicians (N.D.'s) are also trained in botanical medicine. Working with a knowledgeable herbalist is another alternative. The "Resources" section at the end of this chapter includes organizations that can help you locate such practitioners in your area.

If you are unable to find a skilled practitioner near you, you can still learn a great deal about herbs and their use by doing your own research. Two organizations that can assist you in this process are the American Botanical Council and the Herb Research Foundation (also listed below), both of which have Web sites containing a wealth of good information about medicinal plants, as well as links to other credible resources. The books listed in the "Recommended Reading" section can also assist you in your education process.

Know which form of the herb to use. As mentioned above, herbal remedies are available in a variety of forms. Most herbalists recommend using standardized (see below) herbal extracts or tinctures, due to their greater stability and long-term potency. Herbs that have been freeze-dried and put into capsule form can also be useful, whereas bulk herbs and powdered herbs sold in capsules are likely to be less effective because they are far more apt to be adulterated or made inactive due to exposure to air. Herbal teas, while usually not as effective as extracts, tinctures, or freeze-dried capsules, can still provide soothing relief for certain mild complaints, such as indigestion.

Select standardized products. To ensure potency, reputable manufacturers of herbal products now make standardized extract products that contain guaranteed amounts of the herbs' primary active ingredients. Check labels to be sure the product you are buying is standardized and to determine how much of the active ingredient is contained in each dose. Standardization is not a complete guarantee of product potency, however, since standardization itself is currently done on a voluntary basis by manufacturers, instead of an independent regulatory agency.

Buy from quality manufacturers. Because there is no independent regulatory agency overseeing the standardization process, buying from a quality company with an established reputation is advised. Such companies usually supply written documentation pertaining to their manufacturing standards and the source of their herbs. Their product lines are commonly available at reputable health food stores nationwide. Also look for products with the U.S.P. notation on the label, indicating that the manufacturer adheres to the standards of the United States Pharmacopeia.

Caution: Avoid herbal products sold by multilevel, mail order, and Internet companies unless you can verify that the company is legitimate and has a good reputation.

Proceed with caution. Though herbal remedies overall are generally safe, they still must be used with care. Always follow the recommended dosage on the label or prescribed by your physician. If you experience any adverse reactions, discontinue use of the herb, and be sure to mention the reaction to your physician.

Caution: Do not take herbs if you are currently on medication without first consulting with your physician. Pregnant and lactating women should also first consult with a physician before using herbal remedies.

THE FUTURE OF BOTANICAL MEDICINE

With sales of herbal products continuing to soar in the U.S., it seems certain that interest in botanical medicine will continue to increase, as well. "I believe the future of phytomedicine in the United States is going to mimic the stature of botanical medicine in Europe, which has embraced it for over thirty years," Dr. Morris says. "Interest in herbal remedies is an upward trend, and I think it's only going to get more popular, due to botanical medicine's many benefits and how well it lends itself to self-care. The risks, in comparison, are very low, and they can be alleviated if you do the research and are willing to work with a competent physician who can assist you."

RESOURCES

To learn more about botanical medicine contact the following organizations.

American Botanical Council
P.O. Box 144345
Austin, Texas 78714
Phone: (512) 926-4900
Web site: *www.herbalgram.org*

Herb Research Foundation
1007 Pearl Street

Boulder, Colorado 80302
Phone: (800) 748-2617
Web site: *www.herbs.org*

RECOMMENDED READING

Brown, Donald J. *Herbal Prescriptions for Better Health*. Prima Publishing, 1996.

Ottariano, Steven G. *Medicinal Herbal Therapy: A Pharmacist's Viewpoint*. Nicolin Fields Publishing, 1999.

Weiner, Michael and Janet. *Herbs That Heal*. Quantum Books, 1994.

CHAPTER 9

Bodywork

Touch, the basis of all forms of bodywork, is perhaps the oldest form of healing and an instinctual form of comfort that all of us offer to ourselves and our loved ones in times of pain and suffering. "Touch is both an effective form of healing, and perhaps the most powerful and direct means we have for conveying and receiving love," notes Robert S. Ivker, D.O., past president of the AHMA. "Numerous studies now attest to the healing power of touch, yet we in the United States are a touch-averse society. In order to be healthy, we need to consciously make touch a more frequent occurrence in our lives." Dr. Ivker's recommendation echoes the advice of Hippocrates, the father of Western medicine and an early proponent of massage, the most popular form of bodywork. Instructing his students, he wrote, "The physician must be acquainted with many things, and assuredly with rubbing."

Despite the obvious benefits of touch, however, socially acceptable opportunities for touching are few in the United States, compared to other countries, which perhaps explains the continuing rise in the popularity of bodywork and massage therapies. According to Thomas Claire, author of *Bodywork* and an expert in this field, an estimated 20 million Americans each year receive therapeutic massage, a figure that does not begin to address those exploring the more than one hundred other types of therapies available under the bodywork umbrella. While it is beyond the scope of this chapter to provide an overview of all such therapies, the most common categories and types of bodywork are outlined here.

🌿 FAST FACTS 🌿

Aspects of bodywork are a component of the world's two oldest systems of health care: traditional Chinese medicine and Ayurveda. In the West, the use of massage therapy dates back to ancient Greece and Hippocrates, and the benefits of "laying on of hands," the precursor of modern-day "energy healing," are also espoused in a number of ancient healing and spiritual texts, including the Vedas of India, China's *The Yellow Emperor's Classic of Medicine*, hieroglyphic texts from Egypt's Third Dynasty, and the Christian Bible.

There are an estimated eighty forms of massage therapy alone currently available in the United States. Of these, approximately 75 percent were developed after 1970.

Besides Hippocrates, famous Western practitioners of massage throughout history include the ancient Roman physician Celsus (25 B.C.–A.D. 50), author of the encyclopedia *De Medicinia*; Galen (A.D. 131–200), whose influence on Western medicine rivals that of Hippocrates; Avicenna (980–1037); Ambrose Pare (1510–1590), an early pioneer in the fields of surgery and obstetrics; and William Harvey (1578–1657), the first Western physician to discover that blood circulates in the body.

Within the field as a whole, the number of bodywork practitioners is estimated at approximately 250,000, making it the single largest form of health care in the United States, in terms of availability. Of these, over 150,000 bodyworkers are primarily massage therapists.

A growing number of corporations, including many Fortune 500 companies, now offer on-site massage therapy to their employees as a means of reducing stress, enhancing productivity, and minimizing absenteeism.

In 1997, 27 percent of the $21.2 billion spent on nonconventional health care went toward visits to massage therapists, accounting for 114 million visits per year.

Eighty percent of all Americans considering some form of holistic health care say they would most likely try massage or some other form of bodywork over any other modality.

Fifty-four percent of all primary care physicians and family practitioners state they would encourage their patients to pursue massage therapy as a complement to conventional medical care.

Twenty-eight states and the District of Columbia have licensing requirements for massage therapists, and most cities or counties in unregulated states have their own regulatory ordinances. Education requirements in regulated states range from three hundred to one thousand hours of instruction.

Among the leading advocacy and certifying institutions in the field of bodywork are the Commission for Massage Therapy Accreditation/Approval, the American Massage Therapy Association (AMTA), the National Board for Therapeutic Massage and Bodywork, and Associated Bodywork and Massage Professionals (ABMP). 🌿

HISTORY OF BODYWORK

Bodywork in rudimentary form has been known throughout history, as evidenced by cave paintings from 15,000 B.C. that depict the therapeutic benefits of touch. Since ancient times, bodywork has been practiced in China, India, Japan, Egypt, Persia, Arabia, and Greece, and by the indigenous peoples of the Americas. In ancient Rome, massage was a standard medical practice among the upper classes, including Julius Caesar, who received a massage daily to help control his epileptic seizures. Following the spread of Christianity to Europe, the practice of the laying on of hands also became common and was later adopted by royalty. During the Middle Ages, healers known as "bone-setters" were also popular. Such healers practiced massage in conjunction with spinal manipulation, and their methods remained popular until the nineteenth century, before giving way to modern conventional medicine. Massage therapy, however, continued to be popular and was a standard form of medical treatment in many hospitals in the United States until the 1950s, before declining due to the rising dominance of antibiotics and surgery. The most common form was known as Swedish massage, so named because of its developer, a nineteenth-century Swede named Per Henrik Ling. Impressed by the massage techniques he observed in China, Ling returned to Europe to create his own system of massage based on his observations abroad. Soon it was in use by health practitioners throughout Europe and the United States, where it incorporated physical therapy before that discipline evolved into its own separate branch of bodywork and became the one most commonly used in hospitals today.

It was not until the 1970s, however, that the field of bodywork began to truly flourish, spurred in large part by the growth of the human potential movement and the recognition by Western researchers of the body's importance to overall health and well-being. During this time, interest in massage was rekindled, as was interest in non-Western forms of massage, such as acupressure and shiatsu (see Chapter 13). During this period the work of innovative practitioners such as Ida Rolf, Moshe Feldenkrais, Milton Trager, and others came into prominence, side by side with somatic reeducation therapies developed by other researchers, including Alexander Lowen, Ilana Rubenfeld, and Ron Kurtz. Energetic therapies, such as Therapeutic Touch, developed by Dolores Krieger and Dora Kunz, also began to emerge and gain popularity around this time, leading to further research into the "energy field" that surrounds all living organisms. Today, the field of bodywork continues to grow and diversify, with new techniques and methodologies still emerging as we enter the twenty-first century.

TYPES OF BODYWORK

Although the number of bodywork techniques continues to grow, they fall primarily into the following categories: therapeutic massage, structural bodywork, pressure point techniques, movement reeducation therapies, bioenergetic healing, and somatic psychology. Also included in the field of bodywork are Applied Kinesiology and Polarity Therapy. What follows is an overview of the most popular therapies in each category.

Therapeutic Massage

Massage as a form of health care has been practiced for over five thousand years in various cultures around the world, including China, India, and Mesopotamia. Therapeutic massage refers to modern-day massage techniques recommended by conventional and holistic medical practitioners alike because of their proven ability to soothe pain and promote relaxation in both body and mind. According to a survey commissioned by the American Massage Therapy Association (AMTA), the three most frequently cited reasons reported by consumers for receiving therapeutic massage are relaxation, relief of muscle pain or spasms, and stress reduction. The AMTA survey also found that 76 percent of primary care physicians had a favorable view of massage when discussing its possible benefits with their patients. Because of these many benefits, massage therapy has become an increasingly important component of many physical therapy practices, sports clinics, and a number of nursing practices. Many businesses and other institutions now offer massage in the workplace, as research has shown that fifteen-minute, twice-weekly massage sessions while seated in a chair produce decreases in job-related stress levels and significant increases in worker productivity.

Included in the category of therapeutic massage are Swedish massage, deep-tissue massage, lymphatic massage, sports massage, and neuromuscular massage. Self-massage techniques have also become increasingly popular during the last decade due to the growing acceptance of holistic medicine.

Swedish massage, also known as European or traditional Western massage, is the most common form of massage therapy in the United States. It is used primarily to promote general relaxation, relieve muscle tension, improve circulation, and restore flexibility and range of motion. Depending on the practitioner and the individual's need, sessions can vary from gentle stroking of the body's top, or superficial, layers of musculature, to vigorous kneading of tense muscles, especially those of the shoulders, hips, and thighs. In general, a combination of long strokes, kneading, and friction techniques are employed over the full body. Percussion, or tapping, techniques are also sometimes used.

Stroking, also known as effleurage, is a basic element of all massage techniques, and is used to either relax (slow, long movements) or invigorate (brisk motions), and to promote circulation and stimulate lymph flow. Kneading is done using the fingers and thumbs. By squeezing the flesh in much the same fashion as a baker kneads dough, massage therapists are able to stretch and relax tight muscles, enhance the delivery of nutrients to cell tissues, and promote elimination of tissue waste products. Kneading also helps maintain and invigorate skin tone.

Friction techniques usually involve small, circular movements of the fingers, thumbs, or heels of the hand, and are applied firmly and energetically. Such movements are helpful in dissipating adhesions in muscle fiber, thus alleviating muscle tension and spasms. Percussion techniques are used to stimulate large, fleshy areas of musculature, such as the thighs and buttocks. They are not appropriate over the chest and spine or over areas of broken veins.

Massage therapists often use oils or lotions, and some practitioners also use hydrotherapy, such as sauna, to enhance the effectiveness of their work.

Deep-tissue massage, as the name implies, employs greater pressure than Swedish massage and most often deals with deeper muscle layers. In addition to using fingers and thumbs, therapists may also use their elbows in order to break up chronic muscle tension. Slow strokes, direct pressure, or friction techniques that go against the grain of the muscles are the techniques most often used by deep-tissue massage therapists, and they can sometimes be painful and leave the client feeling sore, especially during initial sessions. This form of massage is often effective for treating habitually tight muscles and for relieving low back pain.

Lymphatic massage focuses on stimulating the flow of lymph through the lymphatic system. A network of vessels and lymph nodes running throughout the body, the lymphatic system removes blood proteins and excess water from the interstitial spaces around the cells, thereby allowing them to receive life-supporting oxygen. When lymph flow becomes sluggish, however, the cells become oxygen-deprived, setting the stage for pain and disease. Lymph fluid is filtered primarily by the lymph nodes in the neck, armpits, and around the groin. These and other areas of the body are lightly stroked by lymphatic massage therapists to stimulate lymph flow and prevent congestion.

Sports massage has become increasingly popular in the United States, moving beyond the province of elite athletes into health clubs and spas nationwide. Incorporating methods of both Swedish and deep-tissue massage, sports massage is used primarily to ease stiff joints and muscle tension and to maintain and restore joint mobility. Many athletes, professional and lay alike, use it before sporting events to enhance their performance and to help prevent injury. After a sporting event or vigorous exercise it is also useful for restoring normal muscle tone and eliminating buildup of lactic acid, which can otherwise cause pain and stiffness. Today, many professional and college athletic teams use sports massage therapists to help keep their athletes healthy and injury-free.

Neuromuscular massage refers to deep massage techniques specifically adapted to treat individual muscles or muscle groups. Neuromuscular massage is useful for reducing pain and muscle spasm, relieving nerve pressure caused by impinging muscle tissue, and enhancing circulation.

In addition to the above forms of massage, other specialized forms have become more popular in recent years. Included in this category are infant massage, which uses gentle strokes to promote overall health in infants and children, including babies born prematurely, and pregnancy massage, which is geared toward meeting the unique needs of expectant mothers. Pregnancy massage therapists sometimes come to the hospital to assist women during labor and afterwards, to improve recovery and provide additional care to the newborn child.

Contraindications: When administered by a properly trained massage therapist, all forms of massage therapy are extremely safe and provide a wide range of physiological and psychological benefits. In certain instances, however, massage therapy is contraindicated. People suffering from blood circulation disorders, such as phlebitis or thrombosis, should avoid massage to avoid the loosening of blood clots. Massage should also not be administered to anyone suffering from excessive fever, diarrhea, vomiting, nausea, varicose veins, jaundice, and bleeding. Open wounds, cuts, sores, tumors, and areas of the body that are bruised, swollen, or infected should not be massaged, nor should areas where a broken bone is suspected. Massage during the first trimester of pregnancy is also not recommended, although its benefits during the last trimester and during labor can be significant.

Structural Bodywork

The best-known bodywork approaches in this category are Rolfing, Hellerwork, Aston-Patterning, and Myofascial Release. These approaches seek to enhance body function by addressing chronic muscular tension and imbalances and improving skeletal alignment.

Rolfing, more properly known as Structural Integration, was developed by Ida Rolf, Ph.D. (1896–1979), whose doctorate in biochemistry and physiology, combined with years of study of other bodywork techniques, led her to conclude that all physiological function is a manifestation of structure. Her belief led her to develop her own system of bodywork as a way to resolve her own health problems, which included spinal arthritis and prediabetes. Rolf spent most of the 1950s and '60s teaching her technique to chiropractors and osteopaths in the United States, Canada, and Europe, before finally founding the Rolf Institute in 1972. Since the institute's inception, it has introduced Rolf's work to a much wider lay audience.

In Rolf's view, a body that is poorly aligned must struggle to maintain balance in the face of gravitational pull. As it does so, the body tends to compensate for areas of imbalance or misalignment in one area through adaptive changes in other areas. Over time, according to Rolfers (as practitioners of Rolfing are called), such compensation leads to an overall weakening of the body's entire structure, resulting in compromised body function. The aim of Rolfing is to restore the body to proper alignment so that all of its sections—head, neck, shoulders, torso, hips, legs, ankles, and feet—correspond and interact correctly with gravity. Rolf maintained that when the body's alignment is restored, all systems of the body are able to operate more efficiently, thereby improving total well-being.

Rolfers accomplish their goal over the course of ten hour-long sessions, usually occurring at weekly intervals. During each session deep pressure is applied to the fascia, layers of connective tissue that hold and support the body's muscles and bones, and cover muscle fibers and internal organs. Due to injury and chronic stress, the fascia can shorten or become overly thick as a result of the body's adaptive coping strategies. Poor posture, disease, and emotional trauma can also contort the fascia. As a consequence, rigidity or oversolidity can occur, leading to habitual body distortion, spinal misalignment, and limited range of motion. Rolfers seek to reestablish proper alignment and improved mobility by loosening and manipulating the fascia, using their fingers, thumbs, and sometimes elbows.

Each Rolfing session builds on the work of the one preceding it and addresses a different section of the body, until all parts of the body have been completely integrated. Each session is conducted with the client in his or her underwear, and no oils or lotions are used. Prior to the first session, and again after the final treatment, Polaroids of the client's front, sides, and back are usually taken, providing tangible evidence of the postural changes that Rolfing can provide. At times Rolfing sessions can be painful, although such effects are not long-lasting. During the course of treatment, some people may also recall previous emotional trauma. Such experiences are usually fleeting but in some cases have resulted in positive life changes beyond improved physical well-being alone. Rolfers are typically not trained to provide psychological guidance for their clients, and if such experiences persist, clients may be referred to psychologists or other types of counselors.

Rolfing, like most forms of bodywork, does not focus on treating specific symptoms. Rather, emphasis is on bringing the body back into alignment with gravity by restoring the fascia to its natural state of elasticity. Although Rolfers make no claims of being able to treat specific disease conditions, Rolfing has been found to be useful for alleviating conditions of chronic pain and muscular tension, including low back pain, and to improve posture. People who undergo Rolfing treatment often experience a greater sense of ease, reduced stress, improved energy levels, better posture, greater ease of breathing, and less anxiety. In some cases, clients also gain a slight increase in height (one inch or less) due to an improvement in their posture. During the course of Rolfing treatment, most Rolfers also provide instruction in how their clients can improve the way they move (see "Movement Reeducation Therapies" later in this chapter), to maximize and maintain the benefits of each session. A course of four advanced Rolfing sessions might also be recommended, usually occurring at least a year after the initial ten sessions, and many clients elect to be Rolfed once or twice a year from that point on, in order to maintain the benefits from their earlier treatments.

Caution: Due to its deep manipulation of tissues, Rolfing is not advised for anyone suffering from acute pain or diseases due to underlying bone weakness, such as osteoporosis or fracture. Patients suffering from organic or inflammatory conditions, such as cancer or rheumatoid arthritis, or from acute skin inflammation, should also forgo Rolfing treatment, as should people suffering from chronic addiction. Those suffering from conditions included in the contraindications for massage cited above should also avoid Rolfing treatments.

Hellerwork was developed by Joseph Heller, one of Ida Rolf's early students and the first president of the Rolf Institute. Although originally a proponent of Rolfing, Heller came to believe that its physiological benefits were of themselves insufficient for making a permanent positive difference in how the body functioned. Besides employing deep touch techniques similar to those used by Rolfers to structurally realign the body, Hellerwork practitioners also seek to give their clients a greater awareness of the relationship between mind and body. To this end, they use movement reeducation techniques and verbal dialogue to address the complex interrelationship between the body's mechanical, psychological, and energetic functioning.

Hellerwork involves eleven sessions, each one of which lasts for ninety minutes and makes use of a thematic approach that is geared toward providing clients with a structure for organizing the emotional aspects of the work. In the first session, for example, treatment focuses on resolving tension and unconscious holding patterns in the chest in order to bring about fuller, more natural respiration. During this session, a Hellerwork practitioner will typically engage clients in a dialogue meant to call attention to attitudes and emotions that might be affecting the breathing process. Instruction in proper movement is also provided in order to train clients in more efficient ways of using their body's energy and minimizing mechanical stress. Clients learn how to stand, sit, walk, run, and lift objects in a manner best suited to their own physiology. Videotaping of a client's movements might also be used, to provide feedback and a clearer understanding of how movement patterns may need to be corrected.

In addition to improving body alignment and flexibility, the most commonly reported benefits of Hellerwork are greater energy, relief of chronic muscle tension and pain, reduced stress, improved emotional clarity, and freedom of expression. Due to its easy adaptability to the specific requirements of each client, Hellerwork is generally safe for most people, although the same cautions listed under Rolfing apply to it, as well.

Aston-Patterning is based on the work of Judith Aston, a former professor of dance and movement and a student of Ida Rolf. After suffering a series of debilitating injuries as a result of back-to-back automobile accidents, Aston sought Rolf out at the recommendation of her physician, when conventional medical treatment failed to help her. Following Rolfing treatment, her condition improved significantly, and she went on to develop the initial movement reeducation system used by Rolfers to help maintain the structural alignment achieved in each session.

After training Rolfers in movement analysis and reeducation techniques for seven years, Aston developed Aston-Patterning, a system of bodywork that integrates massage and soft-tissue bodywork with movement reeducation, fitness training, and suggestions on how each client can redesign his or her environment to best suit their physiology. Practitioners of Aston-Patterning initially observe their clients' movements, posture, and the way they hold and store tension in their bodies. Massage and soft-tissue work is then used to help release such patterns, and to restore functional alignment by alleviating unnecessary tension throughout the body, including restrictions in the bones and joints. Afterwards, clients may again be asked to move about and be taught new ways of moving and standing, so that their weight is more evenly distributed and their movements are lighter and freer. Clients also learn how integrate the principles of Aston-Patterning with specific exercises for strengthening and stretching the body. In addition, they are shown how to modify their physical surroundings, such as the height of their desks and furniture, to maintain the benefits of treatment. To this end, Aston has also developed a line of products, including chair and car seat cushions.

Aston-Patterning is useful for improving posture, balance and coordination, overall physical performance, and mobility. It can also benefit people suffering from painful conditions such as backache, headache, neck pain, and tennis elbow.

Myofascial Release was developed by physical therapist John Barnes as a whole-body healing approach. A term referring to "muscle and fascia," Myofascial Release, like Rolfing, focuses on relieving tension in the fascia, as well as the muscles themselves, in order to improve body structure and mobility, and to relieve chronic body tension and stress.

During a Myofascial Release session, which can range in length from a half hour to ninety minutes, a series of deliberately long, slow, and steady strokes are applied to the body. Each stroke lasts a minimum of ninety seconds and can endure for three minutes or more. Besides using their fingers, practitioners may use the palms of their hands or their elbows to stretch the fascia and release its constriction. Initial sessions are often scheduled only days apart in order to maximize their benefit, with longer intervals between sessions occurring as the client's condition improves.

The primary reported benefits of Myofascial Release include reduced muscle tension and stress, relief of chronic pain, improved body alignment, and speedier recovery from injury. In some cases, as with Rolfing, clients may also experience a cartharsis related to suppressed or unconscious emotions. Of all the therapies in this structural bodywork section, Myofascial Release has by far the largest number of practitioners, having been studied by over twenty thousand health care professionals, including massage therapists, physical therapists, and physicians.

Contraindications: Myofascial Release is not appropriate for people suffering from acute rheumatoid arthritis, aneurysm, or malignant tumors. Areas of bruises, fractures, or wounds should also be avoided during a Myofascial Release session until they have time to fully heal.

Pressure Point Techniques

Pressure point techniques involve the use of applied pressure on specific areas of the body (usually acupoints as defined by acupuncture meridian theory—see Chapter 13) to restore energy flow and relieve pain. The most common pressure point techniques are acupressure, shiatsu, reflexology, myotherapy, jin shin jyutsu, and jin shin do.

Acupressure, often referred to as a needleless form of acupuncture, is actually the older of the two techniques and uses finger and hand pressure to stimulate the body's innate healing abilities. Pressure is applied to specific acupoints, along the meridian (energy) pathways of the body. This results in a release of muscular tension and enhances blood circulation, while promoting the healthy functioning of the body's internal organs via the unrestricted flow of *qi*, or vital energy.

Like practitioners of acupuncture and traditional Chinese medicine in general, acupressurists are trained to accurately locate acupoints and determine which ones to focus on during a treatment session. During a session, gentle, even pressure is applied to the acupoints, generally in the direction in which *qi* is said to flow along the meridians. Pressure is applied to corresponding acupoints on both sides of the body, and sometimes circular rotation of the fingers or thumbs is used to further stimulate *qi* flow.

According to Michael Reed Gach, Ph.D., director of the Acupressure Institute in Berkeley, California, acupressure is also effective in relieving headaches, eyestrain, sinus problems, neck and back pain, stress-related tension, menstrual cramps, indigestion, ulcers, and anxiety. An extremely safe modality, acupressure is easily learned and is well suited as a self-care treatment for a variety of pain- and tension-related conditions, as well as other ailments such as constipation, nausea, and fatigue. One form of self-acupressure that is becoming better known in the United States is called *Do-In*, which incorporates stretching and breathing exercises in addition to manual acupoint and meridian stimulation. Acupressure massage techniques, such as *Tui Na*, which employ rubbing, kneading, and percussive stimulation, are also becoming more widely used in the United States.

Shiatsu, which means "finger pressure," originated in Japan following the introduction of traditional Chinese medicine approximately one thousand years ago. Shiatsu is closely related to acupressure in terms of its overall philosophy and focus on stimulating and rebalancing the efficient flow of *qi* energy (known as *ki* in Japanese) throughout the body. Its techniques for stimulating the body's acupoints and meridians differ from acupressure, however, and in addition to applying pressure with their fingers, thumbs, and hands, shiatsu practitioners may also sometimes use their elbows, knees, and feet. Stretching and movement exercises are sometimes incorporated into a treatment session, as well. Prior to beginning treatment, shiatsu practitioners employ pulse diagnosis, client observation and questioning, and palpation of the abdomen in order to determine which meridians and internal organs are either weak or overstimulated. Sustained, stationary pressure is then applied to the corresponding acupoints in a manner that is both supportive and relaxing, and intended to balance the whole body. Sessions generally last between one hour and ninety minutes.

In the United States, one of the most popular forms of shiatsu is *Ohashiatsu*, developed by Wataru Ohashi. *Amma*, a Japanese form of massage and body manipulation similar to the Chinese practice of *Tui Na* above, is also employed by many shiatsu practitioners. Like acupressure, shiatsu is effective as a self-care technique and for treating a similar range of symptoms.

Caution: While generally safe, shiatsu is not recommended for patients suffering from high fever, infectious disease, cancer, heart disease, and osteoporosis. Areas of wounds, inflammation, and scar tissue should also be avoided during shiatsu treatments, and only gentle techniques are appropriate for elderly or people in frail health.

Reflexology originated in the ancient healing traditions of China, Egypt, and Greece and primarily focuses on reflex points on the feet and, to a lesser extent, the hands and ears. Originally known as Zone Therapy in the United States, modern reflexology techniques were developed by William Fitzgerald, M.D., in the early twentieth century, with further refinements made later by Eunice Ingham, a physical therapist. Fitzgerald theorized that the body consists of ten equal zones extending from the head to the toes. Applying manual pressure to a reflex point (specific nerve ending) within a particular zone, Fitzgerald claimed, would also stimulate other parts of the body within the same zone, including the glands and internal organs. For the most part, Fitzgerald focused on stimulating the reflex points in his patients' hands, often with remarkable results. Ingham built on Fitzgerald's work by developing a "body chart" that mapped out the relationship between the various glands, organs, and other body parts to reflex points in the soles of the feet, hence the name "reflexology."

By applying pressure to these reflex points, reflexologists remove blockages and relieve pain in order to normalize corresponding nerve impulses, thereby relieving stress, tension, and organ congestion throughout each of the ten zones of the body. Although reflexology remains unproven as a viable medical treatment, science has shown that each foot contains over 7,200 nerve endings, each of which is connected through the brain and spinal cord to all areas of the body, directly affecting the glands and organ systems.

A typical reflexology session ranges from thirty minutes to an hour in length, with most reflexologists working only on the feet, using their thumbs and fingers to apply various degrees of pressure and manipulative strokes to the reflex points. Commonly reported benefits of reflexology include improved energy levels; greater relaxation; enhanced digestion; and relief of back pain, headache, stress disorders, hypertension, and symptoms related to PMS.

Caution: Reflexology is not an appropriate treatment for cases of thrombosis, foot injuries, or systemic disease in which heightened circulation is capable of spreading infection.

Myotherapy is an outgrowth of Trigger Point Injection Therapy (TPIT) developed by Janet Travell, M.D., during the 1940s. Travell was the first female physician ever to serve at the White House, during the Kennedy and Johnson administrations, and was instrumental in enabling President Kennedy to cope with back injuries sustained during World War II. Travell's work focused on "trigger points," chronically sore or irritated areas in the muscles caused by physical trauma, stress, disease, structural imbalances, or chronic overuse. In response to such stresses, muscles contract and, over time, settle into a holding pattern that can trigger chronic pain. Via injection of saline or procaine solutions, as well as other means, Travell's TPIT technique is able to release these patterns of contraction, resulting in cessation or lessening of pain symptoms.

In the mid-1970s, Bonnie Prudden, one of the original members of the President's Council on Physical Fitness and Sports in the 1950s, discovered that results similar to those achieved by TPIT could be attained by applying deep pressure to trigger points without the use of often painful injections. Over time, her work became known as Bonnie Prudden's Myotherapy. This noninvasive, hands-on therapy focuses on relieving muscle-related pain quickly and cost-effectively, while training patients how to locate and treat their own major trigger points in order to ensure long-term relief.

An initial Prudden Myotherapy session lasts ninety minutes, and patients must first be cleared for treatment by a physician to rule out pain from anatomical dysfunction requiring medical attention. Follow-up visits last sixty minutes. Pressure is applied to the trigger points for between five- to seven-second intervals, or until the first sign of discomfort. Due to chronic underlying tension, usually several sessions are required to eliminate trigger points and reeducate their related muscles to return to normal function. Once the trigger point releases and the muscle relaxes, patients usually perform gentle stretching exercises to enhance the benefits from each session. Additional benefits include improved circulation, increased strength and flexibility, more energy, and greater coordination, as well as improved sleep and posture. Among the conditions Prudden Myotherapists are able to successfully treat are back pain, headache, carpal tunnel syndrome, and inflammation related to arthritis, fibromyalgia, and multiple sclerosis. Sports-related injuries and injuries caused by accidents also respond well to Prudden Myotherapy.

Trigger Point Myotherapy is another form of myotherapy and focuses primarily on the treatment and relief of myofascial pain and dysfunction (see "Myofascial Release" earlier in this chapter). As with Prudden Myotherapy, medical clearance is usually sought before beginning treatment. Sessions consist of manual pressure applied to trigger points, along with myomassage, stretching, and various corrective exercises designed to restore proper balance and function. Practitioners of Trigger Point Myotherapy rely on patient-therapist interaction, both verbal and nonverbal, during the course of treatment, and they encourage patient self-responsibility. They also make recommendations regarding diet and nutritional intake, stress, postural misalignments, and improper movement.

Both forms of myotherapy are appropriate for conditions resulting from chronic musculoskeletal dysfunction. However, myotherapy is not recommended for patients suffering from organic disease or for people who bruise easily or who have a low threshold for pain.

Jin shin jyutsu, meaning "the art of circulation awakening," is believed to have originated in Japan centuries ago, and was then revived and rescued from obscurity by Jiro Murai in the early 1900s, after he used the technique to cure himself of a life-threatening illness. Murai devoted the rest of his life to further developing and refining jin shin jyutsu, and in the 1950s it was brought to the United States by Mary Burmeister, who began teaching it to others a decade later.

Through the use of twenty-six "safety energy locks" along the body's meridian pathways, practitioners of jin shin jyutsu seek to remove blockages in these pathways and balance the body's energy to promote optimal health in body, mind, and spirit. On average, sessions last for one hour, with the practitioner placing his or her fingertips over specific safety energy locks on the client's body. The touch is generally light and can be used to treat a variety of health problems. A self-care version of jin shin jyutsu can also be learned, serving as a simple yet effective preventive tool.

Jin shin do was developed by psychotherapist Iona Marsaa Teeguarden during the 1980s. Meaning "the way of the compassionate spirit," jin shin do employs gentle, yet deep finger pressure applied over various body acupoints, along with body focusing and emotional processing techniques to alleviate physical and emotional tension. As distinguished from jin shin jyutsu, jin shin do is a synthesis of traditional acupuncture theory and acupressure techniques, Taoist breathing exercises, and Reichian philosophy (see "Somatic Psychology" later in this chapter). During each session, which typically lasts for ninety minutes, the client determines the amount of finger pressure that is used, and over a period of ten or more sessions, emotional armoring (body tension caused by unresolved emotional issues) tends to be progressively resolved in the head, neck, shoulders, chest, abdomen, pelvis, and legs. Sessions occur with the client fully clothed and lying on a massage table, while the practitioner simultaneously applies pressure to acupoints in tension areas and corresponding points further away on the body. This allows for tension and armoring to more readily release, and can result in a pleasurable, trancelike state enabling clients to more fully access emotions that may be related to their physical condition. Following a session, feelings of deep relaxation, and even euphoria, are quite common and tend to endure for longer periods after subsequent sessions.

Movement Reeducation Therapies

Bodywork therapies in this category focus on increasing a person's bodily awareness and sense of movement in order to restore proper alignment and improve balance, mobility, and coordination. The best-known therapies in this category are the Alexander Technique, the Feldenkrais Method, and the Trager Approach.

The Alexander Technique was developed by the Australian Shakespearean actor F. Matthias Alexander between 1890 and 1900 in an attempt to cure himself of vocal problems that were jeopardizing his career. As a result of detailed observations of himself in front of a three-part mirror, Alexander discovered that whenever he lost his voice, he also unconsciously and habitually pulled his head and neck back and downward, creating tension in his larynx and chest and making him hoarse. From this discovery, Alexander became aware that the relationship between his head, neck, and back determined whether his body moved and functioned properly. Over time, Alexander learned how to reeducate himself in the ways he moved and functioned, and he went on not only to fully recover his voice, but also to improve his overall sense of coordination and well-being. By now aware that most people habitually "misuse" their bodies in the way they sit, stand, walk, and speak, Alexander began to instruct others in his methods. His technique enabled those he taught to let go of faulty postures and movement patterns and experience greater range of motion and improved balance and posture. In the early 1900s, Alexander moved to England, where his technique was endorsed by such notables as George Bernard Shaw and the Archbishop of Canterbury. In 1973, Nikolaas Tinbergen, after being awarded the Nobel Prize in physiology, significantly boosted awareness of the Alexander Technique by lauding its benefits during much of his acceptance speech. Alexander's work continues to influence many educators and scientists, and is particularly popular among actors, dancers, and musicians. An increasing number of athletes also use the technique to enhance their performance skills and ease pain. Today, the Alexander Technique is taught in North America, Europe, Israel, Australia, South Africa, and South America.

Instructors of the Alexander Technique train clients in the method over a series of private lessons between thirty and sixty minutes in length, focusing on making them more aware of their habitual movement patterns and reeducating them in ways to move more efficiently and with greater ease. On average, twenty or more sessions are required to master what is taught, with each lesson occurring weekly or biweekly. While being led through a sequence of simple movements accompanied by verbal and manual instructions, students gain a deeper awareness of patterns that interfere with their bodies' ability to function properly, and they learn how to identify and alter such habits. Eventually, students develop a new body image and enhanced sensory awareness that allows them to use their bodies more effectively and reduce tension and pain.

Among the reported benefits of the Alexander Technique are improved posture and spinal alignment, reduced stress and anxiety, greater vitality, relief from hypertension, better digestion, and enhanced circulation and respiration. Because of the gentle nature of the Alexander Technique, it is considered safe for everyone regardless of their health status.

The Feldenkrais Method was developed by physicist and engineer Moshe Feldenkrais after he suffered a serious knee injury. Rather than undergo surgery, Feldenkrais devoted himself to study of the nervous system and human behavior. His research, along with his knowledge of physiology, anatomy, psychology, neurology, and the martial arts, led him to conclude that a person's self-image is crucial to how he or she thinks and functions in the world. As he wrote, "Each one of us speaks, moves, thinks, and feels in a different way, each according to the image of himself that he has built up over the years. In order to change our mode of action we must change the image of ourselves that we carry within us." In Feldenkrais's view, the human organism is a complex system of function and intelligence in which all movement reflects the condition of the nervous system, as well as forming the basis of self-awareness. By learning how to interrupt, and then eliminate, his own habitual negative movement patterns, he found that his body responded with greater ease of motion and he was able to retrain himself to walk without pain. From that point on, he devoted his life to teaching others what he had learned.

Central to the philosophy of the Feldenkrais Method is the belief that the central nervous system can be retrained, resulting in improved patterns of behavior and movement. Feldenkrais also emphasized the importance of proper breathing, viewing the breath as an essential aspect of movement. Poor breathing, he maintained, inhibits the body's ability to properly move and function, while improper movement and functioning interferes with the breathing process. In order to help his students overcome lifetime habits that limited movement and breathing patterns, Feldenkrais developed two teaching methods, Functional Integration and Awareness through Movement.

Functional Integration is taught individually in hour-long sessions tailored to the specific needs of each client. Using gentle manipulation and movement exercises, practitioners guide clients through new, easier, and more efficient ways of moving. According to practitioners, Functional Integration results in a retraining of the nervous system that over time also reprograms the brain, resulting in an improved self-image as well. No attempt is made to alter the client's body structure. Instead, practitioners use touch to help clients discover their own most appropriate movement style.

Awareness through Movement classes, by contrast, are taught in a group setting. Classes average forty-five minutes to an hour in length, during which time students are guided through a series of directed movements. By paying attention to each exercise, students acquire a greater awareness of how they move and of any unnecessary tension their movements may have. The exercises are gentle and often subtle, such as lifting one foot slightly off the floor. They may be performed while sitting or lying on the floor, while standing, or while seated in a chair, and they can be accompanied by verbal cues or imagery designed to facilitate a deeper awareness of how each student moves. All exercises are performed slowly, without straining.

Both aspects of the Feldenkrais Method are intended to enhance movement and body functioning through improved posture and greater self-awareness. Like the Alexander Technique, the Feldenkrais Method has no known contraindications.

The Trager Approach, or Trager Work, was developed by U.S. physician Milton Trager, M.D., a specialist in neuromuscular conditions, and a former boxer, acrobat, and dancer. Trager began to develop his approach in 1927, after healing himself of a congenital back problem; he then spent the next fifty years refining it before he started teaching and certifying others in its practice. A naturally intuitive and gifted healer even as a teenager, Trager recognized that the mind and body are inseparable and theorized that pain and other health conditions could be permanently resolved by bypassing the conscious mind to access the unconscious mind directly. Although different from the Feldenkrais Method, the goals of the Trager Approach are largely the same: releasing chronic and habitual tension in the body by helping clients recognize and interrupt limiting or inefficient movement patterns and correcting poor posture.

The Trager Approach is distinguished by the playful quality of its work, which achieves its goals through gentle, rhythmic touch and movement exercises. During sessions that last between an hour and ninety minutes, Trager practitioners lightly and rhythmically manipulate their clients' joints and limbs, using movements tailored to each person's condition. As the work is performed, the client lies passively on a massage table or flat surface, letting the practitioner guide the movements from a meditative state known as "hook up," which enables the practitioner to more deeply perceive the client's flow of energy. Limbs are lightly cradled and moved about in order to retrain the unconscious, via the nervous system, to move beyond old patterns of restriction and holding into a state of greater flexibility and ease.

Clients normally also receive training in Trager Mentastics (a term Trager coined to describe "mental gymnastics"), a series of exercises designed to reinforce and more deeply integrate the benefits received during each session. The exercises, which are taught in group Mentastics classes, consist of gentle stretches and light, dancelike rocking and shaking movements. Regular practice is said to result in an increased awareness of how the body moves, while helping to keep the body in a light, open state and free of pain.

Commonly reported benefits of the Trager Approach include greater energy, improved relaxation, greater mobility, and a heightened sense of mental clarity and creativity. Many individuals also report feeling "more at peace." Among the conditions the Trager Approach is said to benefit are chronic pain, musculoskeletal and neurological disorders, respiratory conditions, and headache and migraine.

Note: The Trager Approach is safe for most people, but should be avoided in cases of broken bones, fever, blood clotting, problem pregnancies, and certain forms of cancer, where manipulation might contribute to the spread of the disease.

Bioenergetic Healing

Also known as energy healing, bioenergy field therapy, or the laying on of hands, bioenergetic healing techniques are as old as human history and can still be found as part of the healing traditions of many cultures around the world, including China, India, Japan, Australia, the Philippines, Africa, the Amerindian cultures of North, Central and South America, and the Huna tradition of Hawaii and Polynesia. Although treatment methods vary, all therapies within this field are based on the premise that all living organisms are enfolded by a "subtle," "vital," or electromagnetic "energy field" (the bioenergy field) that, while invisible to the naked eye, corresponds to the mental, emotional, and spiritual aspects of the self and is responsible for our health and vitality. This field, or fields (some bioenergetic practitioners and researchers claim that the human body is enveloped by a series of interconnected fields of varying subtleties), is often referred to as the "aura," and is said to extend several inches or more from the body. In addition, bioenergy, variously known as *prana, qi, ki,* or *pneuma,* is said to flow throughout the body via energy channels, known as meridians in traditional Chinese medicine, directly influencing the health of the organs and glands. Seven additional primary energy centers, known as chakras in Ayurvedic and other healing systems, are also said to run along the length of the spine, corresponding to the seven glands of the endocrine system, and governing specific emotions and life issues. By balancing and facilitating the free flow of bioenergy through the chakras and meridians, bioenergetic practitioners claim to be able to enhance health and help their clients develop a deeper awareness of themselves and the subtle levels of their being.

Numerous medical pioneers throughout history have accepted the idea that bioenergy fields exist and play an important role in health. Among them are Hippocrates, René Descartes, William Harvey, Austrian physician Franz Mesmer, Andrew Taylor Still (founder of osteopathy), and Daniel Palmer (founder of chiropractic medicine). The concept of a human bioenergy field has yet to be proven to the satisfaction of many conventional scientists, however. Nonetheless, recent developments in the arena of quantum physics, as well as pioneering experiments by researchers like founding AHMA president C. Norman Shealy, M.D., Ph.D., and Valerie Hunt, Ph.D., professor emeritus at UCLA's department of physiological sciences, do seem to suggest that such a field actually exists. In the United States, the best-known types of bioenergetic healing are Therapeutic Touch, Healing Touch, Healing Science, Quantum Touch, Reiki, Pranic Healing, and *Qigong* and *Taiji* (see Chapter 13).

Therapeutic Touch, developed in 1971 by Dolores Krieger, Ph.D., R.N., professor emeritus of New York University, and clairvoyant healer Dora Kunz, is a modern interpretation of several ancient healing methods, including the laying on of hands. It is offered in over two hundred hospitals nationwide and taught in over one hundred fully accredited colleges and universities in the United States, as well as in over seventy-five other countries, making it one of the most widely accepted holistic healing methods. An estimated forty thousand nurses, doctors, and other health practitioners have also learned Therapeutic Touch and use it in their work, and its effectiveness is described in many nursing textbooks.

According to Krieger, most of the Therapeutic Touch process happens within the vital energy field, beyond the edges of the physical body.

Generally, there is no physical contact between patient and practitioner, although in treating fracture or other bodily injuries some touching may occur. A session begins with the practitioner "going on center," a process said to enable practitioners to connect more deeply and consciously with their patient's needs while guiding the flow of vital energy in the most appropriate direction. While remaining in this centered state throughout the session, the practitioner places his or her hands a few inches or more away from the patient and, using slow, rhythmic motions, probes for blockages in the patient's bioenergy field. Such blockages can result in areas of congested or depleted vital energy, which the practitioner then works to rebalance. The patient might have a variety of responses during a session, ranging from a heightened state of relaxation to a release of suppressed emotions. According to Krieger, Therapeutic Touch is able to induce the "relaxation response" in most people within five minutes or less. It has also been shown to reduce stress and discomfort in pregnant women and is now taught in many Lamaze classes around the country. Many hospitals use the technique with patients before and after surgery to minimize the effects of anesthesia. One of Krieger's early experiments with Therapeutic Touch involved a young woman who was dying as a result of a gallbladder disorder. After only a single treatment, her condition noticeably improved, and she went on to make a full recovery. Other commonly reported benefits of Therapeutic Touch include significant relief of fatigue and pain, reduced stress and anxiety, and an improved sense of overall well-being. Therapeutic Touch has no known contraindications.

Healing Touch, developed in 1981 by Janet Mentgen, R.N., seeks to restore and maintain health at the physical, mental, emotional, and spiritual levels by creating harmony and balance in the bioenergy field. In addition to Therapeutic Touch techniques, practitioners use a variety of other energy-based methods involving four levels of certification. Like Therapeutic Touch, Healing Touch is popular among the nursing community, and in 1989 the Healing Touch training program was adopted by the American Holistic Nurses' Association. Healing Touch is safe for people of all ages regardless of their health status. Its most commonly reported benefits include greater relaxation and pain reduction.

Healing Science was developed in 1978 by Barbara Brennan, a former NASA physicist with a background in psychotherapy. Taught over the course of five years at the Barbara Brennan School of Healing, this form of energy healing focuses on maintaining balance within the bioenergy field itself and between it and a person's external environment. Practitioners of this method are said to be able to enter a state of heightened sense perception to determine specific health dysfunctions and their underlying causes. Using hands-on techniques and other methods, the healer works to clear the client's field of congested energies, while recharging or repairing areas that are drained or imbalanced.

Quantum Touch, developed by Polarity Therapist Richard Gordon (see "Polarity Therapy" later in this chapter), is a hands-on healing method that employs light touch to accelerate the body's innate healing response. Through the use of breath, intention, and various meditative techniques, practitioners seek to raise and direct energy to areas of the body needing to be healed. Through a process of resonance and entrainment, Gordon claims that the energy of the affected area changes its vibration to match that of the practitioner, in much the same way that pendulums of different grandfather clocks, when placed side by side will eventually start swinging in phase with each other. In Gordon's view, healing comes not directly from the practitioner, but rather, from contact with the practitioner's vibrational energy, which enables the body's innate intelligence to do what is necessary for healing to occur. According to C. Norman Shealy, M.D., Ph.D., who conducted experiments with Gordon at the Shealy Institute, Quantum Touch is capable of altering a patient's EEG readings even when the practitioner does not touch the patient's body. Quantum Touch can be effectively combined with a variety of other healing modalities, including other forms of bodywork, chiropractic, and acupuncture. It is also useful as a self-care approach and has been shown to be effective for treating a wide range of health problems, including pain and emotional distress.

Reiki, a Japanese term meaning "the free passage (*rei*) of universal life energy (*ki*)," is a form of energy transference between practitioner and patient that is intended to stimulate the body's innate healing abilities by balancing bioenergy. Said to have evolved as an aspect of Tibetan Buddhism that was handed down from master to student, the principles of reiki were rediscovered in the late 1800s by Japanese Christian minister Dr. Mika Usui, after years of study of ancient Buddhist, Chinese and Sanskrit texts. In 1937, Saichi Takata, one of Usui's students, introduced reiki in the United States. Intended to enhance physical, mental, and spiritual health, reiki treatments generally take place with the client lying prone and fully clothed while the practitioner places his or her hands on specific areas of the body, including the head, chest, abdomen, and back. Treatments vary with each individual according to need, as do results, which can be dramatic or gradual. Reiki energy can also be transmitted without touching.

Practitioner training consists of four degrees or levels, during which time students are initiated by a trained reiki master and learn to attune themselves to four healing symbols said to enable reiki practitioners to transmit healing energy to themselves and others, including from a distance. The term *reiki* itself is generic and does not necessary pertain to the method developed by Usui, which is also known as the Usui system of natural healing and overseen by the Reiki Alliance, an international organization that has adopted professional standards and a code of ethics for recognized reiki practitioners. Although little scientific research has been conducted on reiki, in recent years it has become quite popular as a form of bioenergetic healing, with an estimated 200,000 practitioners around the world. Reiki has no known contraindications.

Pranic Healing is a synthesis of various bioenergetic healing techniques common to Tibet, China, India, and the Philippines. Developed after twenty years of research by Master Choa Kok Sui, Pranic Healing uses vital energy, or *prana*, to correct bioenergetic imbalances said to underlie the majority of physical, psychological, and psychospiritual dysfunctions. Pranic Healers learn how to use their hands to evaluate the overall energetic state of each person's bioenergy field, as well as eleven major, and a variety of corresponding minor, chakras. Depending on their assessment, bioenergy is either replenished or unruffled, with holes or cracks within the biofield sealed off to prevent energy seepage. No physical touch occurs within a Pranic Healing session, and sessions are said to be safe and painless.

Basic Pranic Healing techniques involve seven approaches for treating simple and moderate ailments, while Advanced Pranic Healing specializes in treating more severe conditions. A third method, known as Pranic Psychotherapy, focuses on healing mental and emotional disorders by disintegrating or transmuting negative psychic energies said to underlie such conditions. Basic and advanced certification programs are provided for the practice of Pranic Healing, which is now practiced in over thirty countries worldwide. It is also used as an adjunctive treatment by a growing number of conventional and holistic practitioners.

Somatic Psychology

Bodywork methods in the category of somatic psychology share common ground with therapies in the field of mind-body medicine (see Chapter 10) in that both approaches recognize the interrelationship between the body (soma) and the mind (psyche), as well as how each influences the other to affect overall health. According to Christine Caldwell, Ph.D., founder of the Naropa Institute's Somatic Psychology Program, somatic psychology "draws upon philosophy, medicine, physics, existing psychologies, and countless thousands of hours of human observation and clinical experience to unify human beings into an organic and inseparable whole for the purpose of healing, growth, and transformation."

The concept of the interconnectedness of the body, mind, and emotions is not new and was a basic tenet of many ancient healing traditions around the world, including those of Greece, India, and China. Modern somatic psychology derives primarily from the work of Wilhelm Reich, M.D. (1897–1957), a student of Sigmund Freud. Freud, who began his careeer as a physician, was aware of how the body related to a person's mental and emotional state, and felt that the blockage or discharge of physical energy played an important role in the formation of psychological disorders, but he was more interested in the concepts that led him to develop psychoanalysis. Reich, by contrast, was extremely interested in the movement of energy throughout the body and how and why it became blocked. In his view, psychological disorders were directly due to suppressed energy that, over time, led to the formation of chronic muscular tension and postural misalignments he referred to as "armoring."

Reich developed a system of breathwork and physical touch and manipulation that was able to bring up and release buried emotions and memories. By asking his patients to breathe deeply without pausing, he was able to help them let go of chronic physical tension and pent-up, unconscious feelings. He also paid close attention to his patients' posture and how they moved. During his sessions, he would sometimes apply deep pressure to tense mucles in the face and body, and at times would encourage his patients to move, kick, and hit in order to facilitate the carthartic release he was looking for. His views, which included the belief that orgasm is an important function that is meant to be experienced throughout the body, not just in the genital region, were considered radical and threatening to conservative elements of 1950s America. Eventually, this led to his arrest, and he died in prison. Today, however, Reichian Therapy is experiencing a resurgence, and many bodyworkers, as well as psychotherapists, recognize the value of Reich's work and have integrated his methods into their own practices. One therapy that was directly influenced by Reich's work is Bioenergetics. Other types of somatic psychology bodywork include breathwork therapy, Hakomi, the Rosen Method, and the Rubenfeld Synergy Method.

Bioenergetics was developed by Alexander Lowen, one of Reich's former students. Although its focus is primarily psychotherapeutic, Bioenergetics includes a number of breathing and physical exercises designed to release stress and physical patterns of chronic armoring. Lowen himself defined Bioenergetics as the study of the personality based on the body, and he postulated that there are five distinct armoring patterns that can be determined by observation of a person's physical structure and the way he or she moves.

Bioenergetics focuses on helping people become more aware of their unconscious emotions and beliefs and how they correspond to body tension. During a session, muscular tension is often released as repressed feelings and memories come to the surface as a result of the bodywork process. Various exercises may also be performed, which Lowen developed in order to help clients become conscious of where and how they hold tension in their bodies. Usually, clients are also encouraged to breathe fully and continuously while the exercises are performed in order to generate sufficient energy for releasing such tensions. Massage and deep-tissue pressure can also be applied to facilitate this release, as well as encouraging the client to fully express whatever emotions and memories may surface so that they can be resolved. Treatment is different for each individual, and the length of treatment varies, as well. Commonly reported benefits of Bioenergetics include a renewed sense of self, recovery of past pleasurable memories, reduced stress and anxiety, and resolution of mental and emotional trauma. Certain physical benefits, especially with regard to conditions that can have a mental/emotional cause, such as asthma, headache, migraine, sleep disorders, ulcers, and gastrointestinal disorders, have also been reported. There are no known contraindications for Bioenergetics, but it is recommended that you consult with your physician prior to beginning treatment.

Breathwork therapy refers to various breathing approaches that enable practitioners to learn how to breathe more consciously and freely in order to improve health, increase vitality and deal more effectively with emotional pain. Since breathwork can often result in a healing or resolution of deep-seated psychological issues, it can be considered a form of mind-body medicine, yet is included here as well due to the fact that breathing is primarily a physiological function.

There are many approaches to breathwork, including the breathing techniques that are part of ancient traditions such as *Qigong*, *Taiji*, and yoga (see Chapters 13 and 14). In addition to the breathwork techniques of Reichian Therapy and Bioenergetics, two popular modern-day methods are Rebirthing, developed by breathwork pioneer Leonard Orr, and Holotropic Breathwork, developed by Stanislav Grof. All forms of breathwork therapy focus on the breath and its ability to move energy through the body. Connecting with and resolving suppressed emotions and limiting beliefs are additional components of both Orr's and Grof's work.

Most breathwork therapies use the technique of connected breathing, a major component of the Rebirthing process, in which there is no pause between each inhalation and exhalation. Orr and others in the breathwork field observed that most people breathe unconsciously and shallowly, usually pausing between the inhale and the exhale. By breathing in a connected fashion, Orr claims it is possible to significantly resolve bodily tension and heal long-standing trauma and emotional issues that might otherwise remain suppressed and interfere with a person's ability to freely and positively function in the present. Although Orr does not view Rebirthing as a treatment for physical illness, a number of clients have reported spontaneous healing of a variety of disease conditions, including cancer.

The pattern of respiration employed by breathwork therapists varies according to method. Sometimes it is rapid; other times it is deep, slow, and full. In addition, some approaches recommend breathing in and out through the mouth, instead of the nose, and both abdominal and chest breathing can be used. During Rebirthing, sometimes the therapy is performed in a tub or under water, with the use of a snorkel, although typically such sessions do not take place until clients have had a number of "dry" connected breathing sessions and have become comfortable with the movement of energy and integration of emotions that commonly result from this Rebirthing process. Once learned, the Rebirthing method of connected breathing can serve as a powerful self-healing technique that can be performed on a daily basis.

In Rebirthing, the client normally remains still. Other breathwork methods sometimes employ stretches and movement, directing the breath into specific areas of the body that are tense or exhibiting patterns of emotional armoring. In Holotropic Breathwork, rapid deep breathing is combined with specific types of music played at high volume and chosen to help evoke the unconscious. Sessions are usually scheduled as weekend workshops in which clients pair off, each of them undergoing the process on different days while the other partner attends to the needs of the person doing the breathing. Bodywork applied to areas of tension can also be applied at the client's request. Afterwards, clients are asked to draw mandalas to further process their experience, and group sharing may also occur.

Caution: Because of the emotional release that often results from performing breathwork techniques, it is recommended that they initially be learned and performed under the direction of a skilled breathwork therapist. Certain forms, including Holotropic Breathing, are not recommended for people with a history of mental illness, pregnant women, people with cardiovascular conditions, or people prone to epileptic seizure.

Hakomi is a Hopi term meaning "Who are you?" and "How do you stand in relation to these many realms?" It is also a somatic form of psychotherapy developed by Ron Kurtz that blends a variety of Western body-centered psychological methods with Taoist and Buddhist concepts of awareness, mindfulness, and nonviolence. Kurtz founded the Hakomi Institute in 1979 after twenty years of studying both Western and Eastern approaches to philosophy, psychotherapy, and systems theory. Emphasizing nonforceful approaches to growth and healing, Hakomi incorporates touch, massage, structural alignment, movement exercises, and energy work while clients maintain an awareness of themselves and their bodies.

During Hakomi sessions, clients are instructed in how to enter a mindful state of awareness that results in a heightened sense of openness and vulnerability. While in this state, the practitioner makes positive statements, known as "probes," that are capable of eliciting emotions, memories, and insights relating to the client's personal history and life issues. As such experiences are evoked, the habitual defensive patterns that the client uses to manage them, such as muscular armoring, postural contraction, or covering one's face, also become apparent. In contrast with other methods that might seek to interrupt these defensive measures, Hakomi practitioners encourage them through a process known as "taking over," in which they verbally or physically support the pattern. If a client covers his face, for instance, the practitioner, after asking permission, may also place her hands over the client's face. As a result, according to Kurtz, clients typically relax their managing strategies, leading to feelings of safety and deeper insights about themselves.

In addition to the above techniques, clients are also taught how to read their bodies to discover clues to their psychological history and makeup. Core beliefs can be discovered by paying attention to posture and body structure, movement, breathing patterns, facial expressions, and tone of voice, allowing the beliefs to be examined and, if appropriate, transformed into something more positive. Hakomi is a gentle process that is characterized by its compassionate, even spiritual, approach to healing, and there are no known contraindications for its use.

The Rosen Method was developed by German physical therapist Marion Rosen. It incorporates massage, breathing exercises, relaxation techniques, and aspects of psychotherapy in order to assist clients to uncover and release limiting unconscious beliefs and memories stored in the body as chronic tension. Practitioners of the Rosen Method are encouraged to act on their observations and intuitive insights regarding their clients. Using light, gentle touch to detect areas of chronic tension, the practitioner also pays attention to changes in musculature and respiration. As such conditions are detected, the practitioner will often verbalize them and encourage clients to voice any thoughts or emotions they may have regarding them. In this way, clients often become aware of unconscious patterns that have been contributing to their conditions and learn how to release them and achieve a greater state of relaxation. Sessions last one hour, with clients lying on a massage table, stripped to their underwear and covered with a warm blanket. Movement and stretching exercises, known as the Rosen Method of Movement and usually taught in a group setting, can also be employed to retain the benefits gained during the individual bodywork sessions.

Commonly reported benefits of the Rosen Method include greater self-awareness, reduced stress and anxiety, less bodily tension, and improved circulation. The Rosen Method has also been found to be useful for a number of chronic health conditions, including age-related conditions such as joint immobility and dementia. In addition, because of its ability to help clients heal emotional issues, a number of psychiatrists and psychotherapists now use the Rosen Method as an adjunct to their own work. It is considered a safe therapy for all people regardless of their health status.

The Rubenfeld Synergy Method was developed by Ilana Rubenfeld and integrates touch and movement with verbal expression in order to promote greater levels of well-being in body, mind, and spirit. A former instructor of the Alexander Technique and Feldenkrais Method (see earlier in this chapter), as well as Gestalt therapy and Eriksonian hypnosis, Rubenfeld is considered a pioneer in the field of somatic psychology and has been refining Rubenfeld Synergy for nearly forty years.

The underlying philosophy of Rubenfeld Synergy consists of eighteen principles, many of which also inform a number of other therapies included in this section. The principles are:

1. Each individual is unique.
2. The body, mind, emotions, and spirit are part of a dynamically interrelated whole.
3. Awareness is the first key to change.
4. Change occurs in the present moment.
5. The ultimate responsibility for change rests with the client.
6. People have a natural capacity for self-healing and self-regulation.
7. The body's life force and energy field can be sensed.
8. Touch is a viable, accurate system of communication.
9. The body is a metaphor.
10. The body tells the truth.
11. The body is the sanctuary of the soul.
12. Pleasure needs to be supported to balance pain.
13. Humor can heal and lighten.
14. Reflecting clients' verbal expressions validates their experience.
15. Confusion facilitates change.
16. Altered states of consciousness can enhance healing.
17. Integration is necessary for lasting results.
18. Self-care is the first step to client care.

Abiding by these principles, the Synergist, as practitioners are called, uses gentle touch techniques to discover areas of the body that are holding tension. As these areas are detected, the Synergist may ask questions or otherwise engage the client in conversation in order to help him or her become more aware of the tension's cause. Attention may be given to the client's breathing and movement patterns, as well, along with visualization and Gestalt techniques that help resolve whatever underlying issues may also be present. Overall, Rubenfeld Synergy is a gradual process that is primarily focused on helping clients become more self-aware while integrating their physical, mental, emotional, and spiritual energies to become more whole. Sessions last forty-five minutes, and treatment can range from six weeks to several years. Rubenfeld Synergy workshops are also available for those interested in learning more about this healing method. There are no known contraindications for the Rubenfeld Synergy Method, and commonly reported benefits include increased relaxation, reduction of physical symptoms, and greater self-esteem and self-confidence.

Applied Kinesiolgy

Applied Kinesiology (AK) was developed in 1964 by George Goodheart, D.C., arising from his observation that distortions in posture, when not due to skeletal deformities, were often the result of muscle dysfunction. Rather than focusing on tight muscles to correct such imbalances, Goodheart experimented with strengthening muscles that were weakened. Originally using manual muscle tests developed at Johns Hopkins University in the 1940s, Goodheart went on to develop an entire system of noninvasive techniques for both testing neuromuscular function and strengthening and correcting neuromuscular imbalances. In 1980, he also became the first non-M.D. to serve as a member of the U.S. Sports Medical Committee of the U.S. Olympic Team during the Lake Placid Winter Games.

Muscle weakness can occur for a variety of reasons. These include nerve interference between muscles and the spine, reduced blood supply, congested lymph flow, organ or gland dysfunction, chemical imbalances, or abnormal pressure in the cerebrospinal fluid. As a result of muscle weakness, the bones the muscle supports can become misaligned, inflamed, or prematurely degenerate. Among the techniques employed by AK practitioners to restore proper neuromuscular function are muscle testing (often in conjunction with standard conventional tests), spinal manipulation, massage, and stimulation of the body's reflex and acupoints. Attention is given to posture, muscle strength, range of motion, how a patient walks, and possible joint misalignment. A patient's history, including diet and lifestyle, is also assessed. Following such diagnosis, the AK practitioner works to correct indicated imbalances in the body, as well as to restore full range of motion and improve the patient's gait.

Many practitioners in the bodywork field use Applied Kinesiology for its ability to correct structural and musculoskeletal problems and joint dysfunction, as do many chiropractors, osteopathic physicians, and naturopaths, as well as podiatrists and a number of M.D.'s. A growing number of sports therapists also use AK in order to prevent and treat sports injury.

Caution: Since the advent of Applied Kinesiology, a number of other muscle-testing and kinesiology-based techniques have arisen, many of which are geared for use by laypersons. The International College of Applied Kinesiology warns, however, that there are definite limitations to the diagnostic conclusions made by someone not properly trained in manual muscle testing, and recommends that the practice of AK be limited to trained health care professionals.

Polarity Therapy

Polarity Therapy was developed by Randolph Stone, D.O., D.C., N.D., an Austrian-born healer who spent many years investigating a wide range of healing modalities, including traditional Chinese medicine (TCM), Ayurveda, botanical medicine, and esoteric Egyptian and Hermetic traditions. As a result of his studies, Stone came to believe that all individuals are spiritual beings, and that health and personal fulfillment were dependent on the free flow of vital energy throughout the body. This belief, combined with his background as both a chiropractor and an osteopathic physician (see Chapters 6 and 7), enabled Stone to merge Eastern energetic healing approaches with Western approaches to bodywork and structural manipulation.

To a large extent, Polarity Therapy's core philosophy is derived from the principles of Ayurveda (see Chapter 12) and to a lesser extent the TCM concepts of *qi* and yin-yang (see Chapter 13). Stone shared the view of Ayurveda and TCM that illness is primarily the result of energy blockages, either within the body itself or on subtler energetic levels in the body's surrounding biofield (see "Bioenergetic Healing" earlier in this chapter), and that energy itself has both positive and negative qualities. In Stone's view, life energies pulsate outward during their positive, expansive phase, and pulsate inward during their negative, contractive phase. He called this pulsation between the two opposite poles the Polarity Principle and maintained that it formed the basis of all life. Polarity Therapy's primary goal, therefore, is to restore and maintain the flow of energy between the positive and negative poles in the body.

To accomplish this goal, Polarity Therapists employ bodywork approaches such as pressure point techniques, joint massage, and reflexology, along with stretching exercises known as polar energetics and a simple holding technique in which both hands (one being positive, the other negative) are held over various pressure points to release energy blockages. In addition, the therapist will work with the client to create an overall wellness program that addresses any mental or emotional blockages that may also be present, and provides counseling to help clients achieve a deeper understanding of themselves in order to resolve limiting, stress-producing beliefs and attidues. Dietary and nutritional recommendations (also based on Ayurvedic theory) may also be made in order to cleanse and rebuild the body's cells and internal organs. Breathing exercises may be employed, as well. Throughout the course of treatment, the primary focus is on stimulating and rebalancing the body's energy fields, while emphasizing patient self-responsibility. While not a treatment for symptoms per se, commonly reported benefits of Polarity Therapy include reduced pain, improved range of motion, diminished stress and anxiety, enhanced digestion and respiratory function, reduction in the incidence of headache and back pain, and greater self-awareness.

CONDITIONS THAT BENEFIT FROM BODYWORK

The health benefits of bodywork are many and varied and continue to be widely acknowledged due to ongoing research. While bodywork is not intended as a substitute for conventional medical care, properly trained and certified bodyworkers can play an important adjunctive role in the treatment of a number of disease conditions, as well as restoring structural balance, which in turn has been shown to improve respiration and enhance one's overall sense of well-being. Bodywork's obvious ability to relieve muscle tension and promote relaxation is well known and recognized by conventional and holistic practitioners alike, as well as increasing numbers of the general public.

Therapeutic massage is perhaps the most researched form of bodywork, offering a broad range of scientifically validated benefits. These include relief for muscle pain and spasms, spinal curvatures such as scoliosis and lordosis, pain due to injury or stress, headache, whiplash, tension-related respiratory conditions (including asthma, bronchitis, and emphysema), cardiovascular conditions, and temporomandibular joint syndrome (TMJ). Massage has also been shown to be effective for correcting body posture and relieving musculoskeletal disorders, improving range of motion, eliminating toxins from the body, and reducing swelling. Other studies reveal that massage helps promote recovery from fatigue due to physical exertion, helps reduce swelling caused by fractures, increases blood circulation, aids in relieving constipation and promoting overall elimination, and can help reduce scar tissue and adhesions. In addition, massage helps to relieve sinus and lung congestion and has a soothing effect on the nervous system. Massage can also be effective in relieving anxiety and depression, including anxiety and depression due to chronic fatigue syndrome, and to cancer and cancer-related pain.

Massage also provides benefits for people suffering from rheumatoid arthritis and fibromyalgia. One study conducted in 1997, for example, found that children suffering from juvenile rheumatoid arthritis who were massaged for fifteen minutes a day by their parents had greater improvement in symptoms and lower stress hormone levels after thirty days than did children in a control group who were instructed in relaxation therapy techniques. Another study of patients suffering with fibromyalgia compared the benefits of Swedish massage versus TENS (transcutaneous electrical nerve stimulation) treatment. After five weeks of daily treatments, patients showed a marked reduction in symptoms, as well as lowered cortisol levels immediately after receiving a massage throughout the study period. By contrast, those who received TENS treatment did not experience similar benefits until the final day of the study.

Another area in which massage therapy shows promise of providing significant benefits involves babies born prematurely. A number of studies indicate that premature babies receiving daily massage following their birth exhibit nearly a 50 percent improvement in weight gain, are more attentive and active, and are able to leave the hospital an average of six days earlier, compared to premature babies receiving only standard hospital care. In addition, one study of thirty premature infants born of mothers who used cocaine experienced a 28 percent greater weight gain after only ten days of thrice-daily massage, compared to similarly born babies receiving standard care. The massaged group also exhibited less stress and greater motor skills and had fewer medical problems.

Therapeutic Touch has been widely studied, and findings from such studies are often cited to substantiate other bioenergetic therapies. The first study of Therapeutic Touch was conducted by its originator, Dr. Dolores Krieger, who examined its effects on hemoglobin levels among patients. Krieger's findings revealed that patients receiving Therapeutic Touch had significantly increased hemoglobin levels, compared to patients in the control group. (In a study conducted in the late 1980s, reiki was also shown to noticeably increase hemoglobin levels.) Krieger's findings were subsequently borne out by one of the earliest studies conducted by the National Institutes of Health's Office of Alternative Medicine (now known as the National Center for Complementary and Alternative Medicine), which revealed that blood samples of people who received Therapeutic Touch over a three-day period had significantly higher levels of immunoglobulins, an indication of increased immune function. Further research has shown that Therapeutic Touch reduces stress and anxiety, promotes the relaxation response, decreases pain, and can provide relief for problems due to dysfunctions of the autonomic nervous system. It has also been shown to be capable of significantly reducing headache pain, as well as reducing pain following surgery, and to ease fever, inflammation, and respiratory conditions such as asthma. In addition, Therapeutic Touch can accelerate the healing of wounds due at least in part to its ability to alter enzyme activity.

There has been less research conducted on most of the other bodywork therapies included in this chapter with regard to specific health conditions. (Two exceptions are acupressure and shiatsu, which have been shown to produce many of the same health benefits as acupuncture, highlighted in Chapter 13.) One reason for this is that treating disease conditions is not the primary focus of these modalities, which focus more on improving overall body structure and function or, in the case of somatic psychology, emotional and mental well-being. As these therapies become more widely known, however, research will most likely increase as well, especially given the wide body of anecdotal evidence suggesting the range of health conditions for which the therapies may be effective. What follows are the results of some studies that have already been conducted for some of the modalities.

Rolfing has been shown to reduce chronic stress and enhance neurological functioning through its ability to positively impact body structure, and to be effective for minimizing spine curvatures from conditions such as lordosis. Rolfing may also be useful for reducing anxiety, as indicated by a five-week study of forty-eight college students that compared the benefits of Rolfing to various relaxation and movement exercises. Students who underwent Rolfing showed significant reduction in anxiety levels, compared to students who performed the exercises. Studies on Rolfing's kinesiological effects have also shown that Rolfing is able to produce body movements that are smoother, more energetic, and less constrained, while resulting in a more erect carriage that can be maintained with less strain. *Hellerwork* has produced benefits similar to those of Rolfing, particularly with regard to back pain. One study found that workers who underwent Hellerwork also reported improvements in their job performance and work relationships, as well as an increased ability to communicate. *Aston-Patterning* is also effective for treating back pain, as well as neck pain and general postural dysfunctions.

Myotherapy has been found to be extremely effective for relieving most cases of pain caused by muscle tension, especially back pain. Bonnie Prudden Myotherapy is also useful for treating headache, migraine, muscle spasm, sprains and dislocations, and pains of the neck, shoulders, chests, abdomen, arms, and legs. Hemorrhoids, impotence, and incontinence due to muscle tension or spasm in the pelvic region also respond well to Bonnie Prudden Myotherapy, as do certain cases of arthritis, lupus, and multiple sclerosis.

Reflexology, besides relieving tension and stress, is also effective for reducing low blood pressure and certain types of body pain. It is also capable of dramatically reducing symptoms of premenstrual syndrome (PMS).

In addition to producing greater relaxation and improved posture, range of motion, and overall flexibility, movement reeducation therapies have also been found to be useful for dealing with specific health conditions. *The Feldenkrais Method*, for example, can be useful for people with low back pain or those recovering from neurological disorders, including stroke. It also shows promise as a pain management measure, and for enhancing recuperation from spinal injuries. Improved breathing patterns are another direct result of the Feldenkrais Method and Awareness through Movement exercises, due to the emphasis both modalities place on becoming aware of the breath.

The Trager Approach can also be useful for improving respiration and overall lung function. One uncontrolled study of patients suffering from chronic lung disease revealed increased chest movement and improved lung function after only two weeks of Trager therapy. Anecdotal reports also suggest its usefulness for chronic pain conditions, muscle spasm, sprains, and injury, and Dr. Trager himself was particularly interested in how his approach could benefit patients suffering from neuromuscular disorders, including polio, cerebral palsy, multiple sclerosis, and muscular dystrophy.

Improved chest mobility and lung function among healthy adults has also been shown to result from training in the *Alexander Technique*. A variety of chronic pain conditions have responded favorably to the Alexander Technique, and a recent study revealed that it was capable of improving balance and overall range of motion among elderly women.

YOUR FIRST SESSION

Your experience with bodywork will vary according to the type of bodywork therapy you choose to explore. Before beginning treatment, expect to be asked about any preexisting health conditions or pains you may have. You may also be asked to fill out an intake form to provide your practitioner with a better understanding of your reasons for being there. During this time, be sure to share what your goals for treatment are, and express whatever concerns you may have regarding disrobing.

With the exception of movement reeducation therapies, most forms of bodywork occur with the client lying on a massage table. For therapeutic massage sessions and certain forms of structural bodywork, such as Rolfing, typically you will be asked to strip down to your underwear. The parts of your body that aren't being worked on will be covered by a sheet or blanket. Massage oils may also be used, depending on the type of treatment you select. For most other therapies, you will most likely remain clothed except for your footwear.

Session length also varies according to treatment, usually ranging from thirty to ninety minutes. Some therapies, such as Rolfing and Hellerwork, require a specific number of treatment sessions typically spaced a week apart. Others vary in number according to the specific needs of each client. Although at times during a session you may experience pain, especially with deep-tissue therapies, such experiences should quickly resolve themselves, leading to greater relaxation and improved energy. If you feel your practitioner is hurting you, or if your pain becomes too intense, speak up at once. Body temperature can also change during a bodywork session. If you become cold, request additional covering. Due to its restful nature, some clients fall asleep while receiving bodywork. At other times, feelings of sorrow or other unexpressed emotions may well up for release. Such occurrences are normal and not a cause for alarm. Counseling may be recommended for emotional issues that remain troubling, however.

To get the most from bodywork, you should avoid eating for at least an hour before and after each session. Also remove belts, eyewear, and jewelry, and be aware of any areas of tension in your body as the session progresses. Be aware of your breath as well. Full, relaxed breaths can significantly help release tension and enhance the effects of your session.

SELECTING A PRACTITIONER

Before selecting a practitioner, focus on what your goals are. If you are more interested in relieving physical tension and muscle pain, therapeutic massage, deep-tissue therapy, structural bodywork, or bioenergetic therapy might best suit your needs, while movement reeducation therapies or somatic psychology might be more appropriate for persons interested in improving overall well-being. After you have decided what form of bodywork you wish to explore, the following guidelines are recommended for choosing a practitioner.

Choose a practitioner who is properly trained and certified. While many of the therapies within the field of bodywork do not require licensing, most competent practitioners are affiliated with at least one professional organization, such as the American Massage Therapy Association (AMTA) or Associated Bodywork and Massage Professionals (ABMP), or the various associations that oversee the specific therapies themselves (see the "Resources" section on the following page). Many practitioners can also be located through physician referrals, health clubs, or spas, as well as through the many massage and bodywork schools around the nation. Recommendations from satisfied customers you know and trust are also a good criterion for choosing a practitioner. If you have any doubts about a practitioner's qualifications, don't hesitate to ask for information about his or her background.

Before beginning treatment, also ask about fees and whether your insurance policy will cover them. Costs vary widely in the bodywork field, ranging from $30 to $75 a session, to as much as $150 or more. Certain forms of massage and bodywork therapies may be covered by your insurance plan, especially if they are prescribed by your physician. Usually, however, such coverage will be limited to a certain number of treatments. In general, you should expect to pay for your treatments out-of-pocket.

THE FUTURE OF BODYWORK

For many decades conventional medicine ignored the physiological and psychological benefits of touch, focusing instead on prescription drugs and surgical techniques. In recent years, however, the medical establishment has shown an increasing interest in, and acceptance of, bodywork techniques, with a number of hospitals now employing massage therapists on staff. This trend is likely to continue in the future in light of further research that is currently underway regarding the bodywork field in general. The growing interest in bodywork therapies by the general public also bodes well for this particular subset of holistic medicine.

In the years ahead, it is likely that there will also be an increasing shift toward multidisciplinary approaches to bodywork, such that practitioners will be competent in a variety of bodywork techniques and able to provide a greater range of health benefits, both physical and psychological. This trend is already underway in many of the nation's massage and bodywork schools. As advances in science continue to broaden our understanding of the human body's bioenergetic field and its relationship to health, bioenergetic therapies are also likely to grow in popularity.

Finally, given the growing body of research devoted to fully mapping out the connection between the body in relation to health and psychological states, as well as the burgeoning interest within the fields of psychiatry and psychology in body-centered forms of therapy, a wider acceptance of somatic psychology is also likely to occur in the early part of the twenty-first century. In fact, Jack Rosenberg, a pioneer in this field, predicts that before long "it will be considered unethical to do therapy without a somatic perspective." If he is correct, bodywork may soon play a pivotal role in healing the schism between body and psyche that for so long has been a part of conventional Western medicine.

RESOURCES

To learn more about the bodywork therapies discussed in this chapter, or to locate a bodywork practitioner near you, contact the following organizations.

Associated Bodywork and Massage Professionals
28677 Buffalo Park Road
Evergreen, Colorado 80349
Phone: (800) 458-2267
Fax: (303) 674-0859
Web site: *www.abmp.com*

American Massage Therapy Association
820 Davis Street, Suite 100
Evanston, Illinois 60201
Phone: (847) 864-0123
Fax: (847) 864-1178
Web site: *www.amtamassage.org*

The International Alliance of Healthcare Educators (IAHE)
11211 Prosperity Farms Road, Suite D-325
Palm Beach Gardens, Florida 33410
Phone: (800) 311-9204
Fax: (561) 622-4771
Web site: *www.iahe.com*

RECOMMENDED READING

General

Claire, Thomas. *Bodywork.* Quill/William Morrow, 1995.
Dychtwald, Ken. *Bodymind.* Pantheon Books, 1977.

Murphy, Michael. *The Future of the Body*. Tarcher/Putnam 1992.

Acupressure and Shiatsu

Gach, Michael R. *Acupressure's Potent Points*. Bantam Books, 1990.
Namikoshi, Toru. *The Complete Book of Shiatsu Therapy*. Japan Publications, 1981.

Alexander Technique

Barlow, Wilford. *The Alexander Technique*. Alfred Knopf, 1991.

Applied Kinesiology

Goodheart, George, Jr. *You'll Be Better: The Story of Applied Kinesiology*. AK Printing, 1989.
Valentine, Tom and Carol. *Applied Kinesiology: Muscle Response in Diagnosis, Therapy and Preventive Medicine*. Inner Traditions, 1989.

Breathwork

Hendricks, Gay. *Conscious Breathing*. Bantam, 1995.
Orr, Leonard. *Breaking the Death Habit: The Science of Everlasting Life*. North Atlantic Books, 1998.

The Feldenkrais Method

Feldenkrais, Moshe. *Awareness through Movement: Health Exercises for Personal Growth*. Harper & Row, 1972.
Feldenkrais, Moshe. *The Potent Self: A Guide to Spontaneity*. Harper & Row, 1992.

Hakomi Method

Kurz, Ron. *Body-Centered Psychotherapy: The Hakomi Method*. LifeRhythm, 1990.

Hellerwork

Heller, Joseph, and William Henkin. *Bodywise*. Wingbow Press, 1991.

Massage Therapy

Downing, George. *The Massage Book*. Random House, 1972.

Myotherapy

Prudden, Bonnie. *Myotherapy*. Ballantine Books, 1985.
Prudden, Bonnie. *Pain Erasure*. Ballantine Books, 1985.

Polarity Therapy

Stone, Randolph. *Polarity Therapy: The Complete and Collected Works*, Vols. 1–2. CRCS Publications, 1987.

Pranic Healing

Sui, Choa Kok. *Pranic Healing*. Samuel Weiser, Inc., 1990.

Quantum Touch

Gordon, Richard. *Quantum Touch: The Power to Heal*. North Atlantic Books, 1999.

Reflexology

Byers, Dwight. *Better Health with Foot Reflexology*. Ingham Publishing, 1987.
Kunz, Barbara and Kevin. *Hand and Foot Reflexology*. Simon and Schuster, 1987.

Reiki

Baginski, Bodo, and Shalila Sharamon. *Reiki: Universal Life Energy*. LifeRhythm Publishing, 1988.

Rolfing

Rolf, Ida P. *Rolfing: The Integration of Human Structures*. Harper & Row, 1977.

Somatic Psychology

Caldwell, Christine, ed. *Getting in Touch: The Guide to New Body-Centered Therapies.* Quest Books, 1997.

Hanna, Thomas. *Bodies in Revolt: A Primer in Somatic Thinking.* Freeperson Press, 1970.

Therapeutic Touch

Krieger, Dolores. *Accepting Your Power to Heal.* Bear and Company, 1993.

Tragerwork

Trager, Milton, and Cathy Guadano. *Trager Mentastics: Movement as a Way to Agelessness.* Station Hill Press, 1987.

CHAPTER 10

Naturopathic Medicine

Naturopathic medicine is a primary health care system that closely approximates the model of holistic medicine espoused by the American Holistic Medical Association (AHMA), in that it employs a comprehensive, multifactorial approach for the diagnosis, treatment, and prevention of disease, with an emphasis on treating the whole person. According to the American Association of Naturopathic Physicians (AANP), the nonprofit organization that represents naturopathic physicians (N.D.'s) across the United States, naturopathic medicine is further distinguished by its underlying principles (see "How Naturopathic Medicine Works" later in this chapter), which are "based upon the objective observation of the nature of health and disease, and are continually reexamined in the light of scientific advances." The treatment methods employed by N.D.'s. are drawn from a wide-ranging repertoire of therapies that recognize the body's innate healing mechanisms and take into account each patient's individuality.

Because of the effectiveness of naturopathic medicine in treating both acute and chronic illness, in 1983 the World Health Organization recommended that this approach, also known as naturopathy ("nature cure"), be integrated into conventional health care systems worldwide. After being largely unrecognized for most of the twentieth century despite its more than one-hundred-year history, naturopathic medicine has, since the 1980s, enjoyed a resurgence in popularity. Because of this resurgence, however, a number of correspondence schools now offer N.D. degrees that in no way match the rigorous medical degree programs offered by the three naturopathic colleges currently accredited in the United States (see "Fast Facts" on the following page). Because of this discrepancy, the AANP is actively involved in working to ensure that practitioners who call themselves naturopathic physicians meet the standards of these colleges, while working to gain licensing for N.D.'s in all fifty states. All N.D.'s endorsed by the AANP attend a four-year graduate-level program and are educated in all of the same basic sciences as conventional M.D.'s, while also trained in the use of holistic and nontoxic medical approaches, with a strong emphasis on disease prevention and helping patients achieve optimal wellness. Before beginning their medical practice, all N.D.'s sanctioned by the AANP must also pass professional board exams before they can be licensed by a state or other jurisdiction as primary care general practice physicians. N.D.'s who meet the standards established by the AANP are also eligible for associate membership in the AHMA.

❦ FAST FACTS ❦

The term *physician* is derived from the Greek root word *phu-sis*, which means "nature."

The term *naturopathy* was first used in 1895 by New York City physician John Scheel. Scheel coined the term by combining the Latin word *natura* with the Greek word *pathos*, to signify a method of healing that was natural in scope. Seven years later, the core curriculum of naturopathic physicians was first organized in the United States. Subsequently, naturopathic practices were employed by as many as 20 percent of all U.S. physicians until the 1930s, at which time its practice significantly waned, due to the emergence of antibiotic drugs and the wholesale subsidy of medical schools by the chemical and pharmaceutical industries.

Currently, eleven states and five Canadian provinces license N.D.'s as primary care physicians. These states are Alaska, Arizona, Connecticut, Florida, Hawaii, Maine, Montana, New Hampshire, Oregon, Utah, and Washington. Naturopathic medicine has also been licensed in Puerto Rico since 1998. All states and provinces that license naturopathic medicine require N.D. candidates to complete at least four years of residency training and 4,100 hours of study from an institution recognized by the State Examining Board. Additionally, N.D. candidates must pass the Naturopathic Physicians Licensing Exam, which includes basic sciences, diagnostic and therapeutic subjects, and clinical sciences.

Due to its proven effectiveness and cost-efficiency as a primary system of health care, in Germany conventional physicians and pharmacists are now required by the German government to be trained in naturopathic methods.

Currently, there are approximately one thousand licensed N.D.'s who meet the standards of the AANP, with an estimated additional one thousand N.D. candidates entering naturopathic college each year. Accredited three- to four-year naturopathic medical training programs are now available in Australia, New Zealand, Israel, and South Africa, as well.

At present, there are three accredited naturopathic colleges in the United States, and one in Canada. All three accredited colleges in the United States require more hours of study in basic and clinical medical science than do the medical schools at Stanford and Yale universities. In addition, graduates of accredited naturopathic colleges have more formal training in clinical nutrition than M.D.'s, osteopathic physicians (D.O.'s), or registered dieticians. The three accredited U.S. institutions are Bastyr University in Seattle, Washington; National College of Naturopathic Medicine, in Portland, Oregon; and Southwest College of Naturopathic Medicine and Health Sciences in Tempe, Arizona.

The whole foods diet now promoted by the National Cancer Institute as a preventive measure for cancer first appeared in a naturopathic medical textbook published in the 1940s. ❦

THE HISTORY OF NATUROPATHIC MEDICINE

Naturopathic medicine has roots in ancient medical practice and draws upon the healing traditions of many cultures, including the Ayurvedic tradition of India and traditional Chinese medicine (see Chapters 12 and 13). In many respects, however, Hippocrates, the father of Western medicine, can most accurately be considered naturopathic physicians' earliest predecessor. A firm advocate of natural healing methods, Hippocrates was also the first person to articulate two of the guiding principles of naturopathic medicine (see "Principles of Naturopathic Medicine" later in this chapter), teaching his students to "first do no harm" and to recognize that all healing occurs through the healing power of nature. His healing philosophy has been followed by indigenous healers in cultures worldwide for centuries, all of whom employed foods, water, fasting, botanical remedies, and various bodywork methods to bring about healing.

Hydrotherapy, or "water cure," a staple therapy in naturopathy's healing repertoire, has also been a common health practice for millennia in many different cultures, including those of ancient Assyria, Babylon, China, Egypt, Greece, India, Israel, Persia, and the native peoples of the Americas. An early European chronicle of water therapy was compiled in 1697 by John Floyer in his book *The History of Hot and Cold Bathing*. Later in Europe, a form of hydrotherapy known as "taking the cure" became popular at spas located near natural mineral springs. One of the first modern-day records of water therapy is *Primitive Physick*, written in 1747 by Reverend John Wesley, the founder of the Methodist religion. In 1816, the Austrian physician Vincent Priessnitz established a systematic use of hydrotherapy after using water wraps to speed the healing of his sprained wrist. As a result, he went on to explore a broader range of applications for hydrotherapy, eventually developing over fifty cold-water hydrotherapy approaches, including the "Priessnitz compress," which is still discussed in medical texts today. In 1830, Priessnitz received authorization by the government of Austria to use it to treat patients. He went on to treat over forty thousand patients suffering from a wide range of disease conditions.

In 1842, another Austrian, Sebastian Kneipp, after being rejected for priesthood in the Catholic church because he suffered from tuberculosis, used hydrotherapy to cure himself. After being accepted into the priesthood, Father Kneipp used hydrotherapy to tend to his sick parishioners. Over time, he developed some 120 hot- and cold-water hydrotherapy applications, as well various herbal and other bath additives, all of which were intended to fortify the immune system. During a cholera epidemic, he earned the nickname "the cholera vicar" after saving the lives of many of his parishioners using hydrotherapy during an epidemic. His activities were frowned upon by his superiors, however, who transferred him to a remote village. But even there, hundreds of thousands of patients across Europe traveled to see him because of his reputation as a healer. Father Kniepp rarely charged a fee for his services and sold gifts donated from his patients to establish several sanitariums. He wrote twenty-two books on health and hydrotherapy and was also a master herbalist.

In 1892, twenty-year-old Benedict Lust, M.D., D.O., after being cured by Father Kneipp of his own tuberculosis, accepted the priest's commission to introduce hydrotherapy to the United States. Lust (pronounced "Loost") is considered the modern-day founder of naturopathy, even though the term itself was coined by fellow physician John Scheel. Scheel sold the term and all rights associated with it to Lust in 1900. Originally focused on promoting Father Kneipp's water cure, Lust eventually combined water therapy and eclectic medical approaches of his time with a variety of other natural healing methods that had been used throughout recorded history. In 1894, he founded the Naturopathic Society of America, which was later renamed the American Naturopathic Association and incorporated in Washington, D.C., in 1919. In 1902, Lust founded the first U.S. naturopathic medical school in New York City, which began as a two-year postgraduate program, but soon evolved into a four-year residential program on a par with the accepted standards of the day for conventional medical education. Included in its curriculum were diet, nutritional and herbal therapies, homeopathy, spinal manipulation, exercise, hydrotherapy, and stress reduction techniques.

Due largely to Lust's efforts, as well as the work of other early naturopaths such as Michigan's John Kellogg, founder of the Battle Creek Sanitarium, naturopathic medicine flourished until the 1930s. By that time, there were twenty-nine naturopathic medical schools in the United States, with naturopathic physicians licensed to practice in eighteen states. At that point, however, naturopathy, along with most other forms of holistic healing, all but disappeared throughout most of the country, because of three major developments: the advent of a new class of antibiotic drugs, such as penicillin; the subsidy of medical schools by pharmaceutical interests; and the passage of legislation nationwide that greatly restricted the practice of all non-allopathic forms of medicine, a result of political pressure from the conventional medical profession. Were it not for the efforts of naturopaths from Canada and the Pacific Northwest, who established Oregon's National College of Naturopathic Medicine in 1956, the use of naturopathic medicine in the United States might have vanished altogether.

In the 1970s, this trend reversed itself, however, as increasing numbers of Americans began to express disenchantment with conventional medicine's high costs and clinical limitations. Recognizing this shift, in 1978, Joseph Pizzorno, Jr., N.D., along with fellow N.D.'s Les Griffith and Bill Mitchell, founded Bastyr College of Naturopathic Medicine (now Bastyr University) in Seattle, Washington, named after their teacher, the well-known Seattle naturopath John Bastyr. Since that time, Dr. Pizzorno, who served as Bastyr's founding president, has been at the forefront of the naturopathic physicians, educators, and researchers who have overseen the continued resurgence of naturopathic medicine.

In 1992, the value of naturopathic medicine was recognized by the National Institutes of Health's Office of Alternative Medicine, when it invited leading naturopaths to serve on key federal advisory panels and to help define priorities and design protocols for researching the various therapies of holistic medicine. In 1994, Bastyr's status as a leading institution of its kind was further recognized by the NIH when it designated the university as the national center for research on alternative treatments for AIDS and HIV, granting it $1 million in funding for this purpose. Government recognition of naturopathic medicine's value continued in 1996, when King County, Washington's Department of Public Health funded Bastyr's Natural Medicine Clinic in Kent, Washington, making it the first natural medicine facility in the United States to have its operating expenses and service to the community paid for by tax dollars. Two other events, both occurring in 1999, have left naturopathic medicine poised to become an increasingly popular form of health care during the twenty-first century. In July of that year, AANP members Konrad Kail, N.D., and Leanna Standish, N.D., Ph.D., were appointed by Donna Shalala, secretary of health and human services (HHS), to four-year terms on the National Advisory Council for Complementary Alternative Medicine. In addition, King County's Harborview Medical Center made Jane Guiltinan, N.D., dean of clinical affairs at Bastyr University, the first U.S. naturopathic physician ever appointed to a county hospital's board of trustees.

HOW NATUROPATHIC MEDICINE WORKS

According to the philosophy of naturopathic medicine, disease is a manifestation of the body's attempt to heal itself from underlying imbalances. Unless a disease is life-threatening, rather than suppress its symptoms, naturopathic physicians seek to address their cause while helping the body to restore itself to optimal health. All naturopaths sanctioned by the AANP are trained to treat patients in all phases of primary, nonemergency health care. They employ a clinical approach that combines the model used by conventional physicians (patient medical history, physical examination, laboratory testing, and other conventional diagnostic measures) with a broad range of natural diagnostic and treatment methods, depending on patient need and each naturopath's particular orientation. After determining the nature of their patients' conditions, naturopaths devise an appropriate course of treatment, working closely with their patients and advising them on how they can most effectively assist themselves in the healing process. Often it is necessary for patients to make lifestyle or dietary changes during this process, and to resolve mental, emotional, social, or spiritual issues that might be contributing to their illness. Naturopaths can play an important role in helping their patients discover the most appropriate course of action. As treatment progresses, they also use standard medical monitoring methods, as well as follow-up exams, to assess outcome and continue guiding their patients along the road to optimal health.

Principles of Naturopathic Medicine

Throughout the course of their patients' treatment, naturopaths are guided by seven underlying principles.

Primum no nocere (first, do no harm). This central tenet of the Hippocratic Oath is underscored by the safe and effective natural therapies that naturopathic physicians use to treat disease. These therapies work to help each patient's innate healing mechanisms restore them to health without burdening them with unwanted and potentially dangerous side effects. To further minimize the risk of side effects, naturopaths apply the lowest possible amount of intervention necessary to diagnose and treat illness.

Vis medicatrix naturae (through the healing power of nature). Like Hippocrates, naturopaths recognize that the body is designed to heal itself. The diagnostic methods and natural, nontoxic therapies used by naturopaths help to facilitate and enhance this process as much as possible, both by identifying and removing obstacles to health, and by supporting the creation of a healthy internal and external environment for each of their patients.

Tolle causam (identify and treat the cause). Like holistic physicians in general, naturopathic physicians focus on the cause of disease rather than its symptoms. As a result, they avoid suppressing disease symptoms unless they are life-threatening, viewing them as manifestations of the healing process. Instead, they seek to determine and resolve all underlying imbalances that are at the root of their patients' illnesses, recognizing that such causes can be physical, environmental, mental, emotional, social, or spiritual.

Treat the whole person. This central tenet of all holistic therapies results in the multifactorial approach taken by naturopaths as they treat their patients. Each patient is recognized as a complex individual with unique needs, both inner and outer. Optimal health encompasses spiritual health and healthy relationships, and N.D.'s. encourage their patients to pursue their social and spiritual well-being. This perspective also enables naturopaths to view serious illness as not automatically incurable, due to their ability to ferret out underlying causes that symptom-oriented treatment approaches are more likely to miss or ignore.

The physician is a teacher. The Latin root for "doctor" is *docere*, meaning "to teach." In the same way that teaching people to feed themselves is a more effective long-term strategy than temporarily feeding them, teaching patients how they can proactively meet their individual health care needs is better than simply treating them without such education. Naturopathic physicians accomplish this by motivating their patients to assume greater responsibility for their health by empowering them with more effective dietary and lifestyle habits and encouraging healthier attitudes.

Prevention is the best cure. Because of their comprehensive training, naturopathic physicians are specialists in preventive health care. They educate their patients on how to adopt lifestyle habits that support health and prevent disease, as well as assessing patient risk factors and genetic predispositions to disease.

Establish health and wellness. The ultimate goal of naturopathic medicine is to help patients achieve and maintain optimal health and wellness. Naturopaths regard health as a state of optimal well-being in body, mind, and spirit, while defining "wellness" as a state of positive thoughts, attitudes, beliefs, and emotions. According to Dr. Pizzorno, naturopathic physicians strive to increase their patients' wellness levels regardless of their state of health or disease since, even in cases of severe illness, a positive mental/emotional outlook can be an important aspect of healing.

Therapies of Naturopathic Medicine

Naturopathic physicians are trained in a wide range of therapeutic methods in order to most comprehensively and effectively meet their patients' needs. Included in their repertoire is training in all conventional clinical and diagnostic techniques, including diagnostic radiology and other imaging approaches. Naturopaths also have backgrounds in diet and clinical nutrition (nutritional medicine), botanical medicine, acupuncture and traditional Chinese medicine (TCM), homeopathy, hydrotherapy, minor surgery, naturopathic physical medicine, obstetrics (natural childbirth), and counseling and psychotherapy. In certain states where naturopathic physicians are licensed, such as Oregon and Washington, N.D.'s also have prescription privileges for naturally derived prescription items, including vitamins, minerals, hormones, pancreatin, bile acids, antibiotics, and plant-based drugs such as belladonna and scopolamine. By its very nature, however, naturopathic medicine excludes major surgery and the use of most synthetic drugs, and when such measures are necessary, N.D.'s will make the appropriate referrals for proper conventional medical or surgical care.

Botanical medicine, homeopathy, and acupuncture and TCM are covered elsewhere in this book (see Chapters 8, 11, and 13). The remaining therapies used by naturopaths are covered below.

Clinical Nutrition. Naturopaths have viewed proper diet and nutrition as fundamental aspects of health since naturopathy's inception, whereas only in the last few decades have conventional physicians and researchers begun to emphasize the role nutrition plays in health. Naturopathic physicians sanctioned by the AANP receive more formal training in clinical nutrition than M.D.'s, osteopathic physicians (D.O.'s), or registered dieticians. During the course of their education, N.D.'s receive an average of 200 total hours of training in basic nutrition, nutritional assessment, and the therapeutic use of diet to treat disease, compared to an average of only 21 hours by M.D.'s. They also undertake an average of 1,300 hours of internship related to diet and disease, whereas M.D.'s receive no such additional training. This difference in expertise makes N.D.'s eminently qualified to treat their patients using dietary intervention and proper nutritional supplementation.

Regardless of their patients' conditions, it is standard practice for naturopathic physicians to assess nutrient status and check for digestive disturbances that can contribute to disease. Once this assessment is made, patients are provided with a healthy eating plan specific to their needs, along with whatever nutritional supplements are required to restore nutritional imbalances. Many times, this simple step alone can result in major improvements in a patient's health status. (For more on the use of diet and nutritional supplements to treat disease, see Chapter 3.)

Hydrotherapy. Hydrotherapy is one of the oldest healing methods in the world and is another important cornerstone of naturopathic medicine. Naturopathic physicians employ a variety of hydrotherapy approaches in treating and preventing disease, including hot- and cold-water baths and showers, foot baths, sitz baths (immersion of the pelvic region in hot or cold water), ice, steam (sauna), and the use of compresses and poultices. Hydrotherapy can be employed as both a primary and an adjunctive therapy. It improves blood and lymph circulation, stimulates immune function, and is useful for treating strains and sprains. It can also be of benefit for arthritis, colds and flu, digestive problems, headache, respiratory conditions, and other disorders, including use as an adjunctive method for relieving symptoms of serious and terminal illness.

Constitutional hydrotherapy is one of the most common types of hydrotherapy performed by naturopaths. In this method, towels are soaked in hot water, then squeezed and placed over the patient's front torso. After five minutes, the hot towels are replaced with towels soaked in cold water for an additional ten minutes. This process is then repeated on the patient's back torso. Variations of this procedure can also be used. The alternation of hot and cold towels helps to dilate and constrict blood vessels and eliminate stored body toxins, while enhancing the delivery of needed nutrients to the bloodstream.

Minor Surgery. While major surgical procedures are beyond the scope of naturopathic training, many naturopaths are trained to perform minor surgical procedures. These include suturing surface wounds; removing warts, moles, cysts, and other undesirable surface masses using local anesthesia; circumcisions; setting fractures; and hemorrhoid surgery.

Naturopathic Physical Medicine. Depending on patient need, naturopathic physicians often employ a variety of physical therapies in their practice. These include therapeutic exercise, massage, bodywork, joint mobilization and immobilization techniques, and soft-tissue and musculoskeletal manipulation techniques known as naturopathic manipulative therapy. Similar to osteopathic and chiropractic techniques (see Chapters 6 and 7), naturopathic manipulative therapy is employed to return bones and joints to their correct positions and to correct misalignment of spinal vertebrae.

Also included under the heading of naturopathic physical medicine are physiotherapy approaches such as ultrasound, diathermy (the therapeutic use of high-frequency current to generate heat and increase blood flow to specific areas or the body), and other electromagnetic energy techniques to relieve pain and stimulate improved biological function.

Obstetrics (Natural Childbirth). In states where naturopathic medicine is licensed, increasing numbers of women are choosing natural childbirth over conventional childbirth approaches. As a result, many naturopaths offer natural childbirth in home or clinical settings, having been trained in a variety of natural, noninvasive pre-, peri-, and postnatal methods. As part of their approach to natural childbirth, N.D.'s will typically screen both mother and child to ensure that the pregnancy proceeds with minimal risk. Additionally, they take care to assess a pregnant woman's diet and nutritional status, making sure that she receives the optimum supply of nutrients necessary to give birth to a healthy, normal child. A number of N.D.'s also work with midwives throughout the pregnancy.

Counseling and Psychotherapy. N.D.'s recognize that their patients' psychological state plays an important role in their overall health and ability to recover from disease. During the course of their medical training, they receive an average of 150 hours in counseling and psychotherapeutic intervention, compared to zero hours in the training curriculum of most M.D.'s. Included in this training are stress management techniques, family therapy approaches, hypnosis, and guided imagery. AANP-sanctioned N.D.'s are also formally trained in proper interview, response, and active listening methods, as well as other contact and body language skills in order to work most effectively with patients to uncover and heal unresolved mental, emotional, or spiritual issues. They are also trained to recognize and deal with their patients' prevalent development problems, abnormal behavior patterns, addictions, sexual issues, stress, and other psychological concerns, and to clinically assess any underlying organic factors, such as nutritional imbalances, that might negatively affect mental and emotional health.

Because of the diversity and depth of training that N.D.'s receive, even when naturopathic medicine is not appropriate as a form of primary health care, it is often useful as a complement to conventional medicine. According to Dr. Pizzorno, this is especially true for severe conditions that may require pharmacological or surgical intervention, such as cancer or cardiovascular disease. Both of these conditions have been shown to benefit from the appropriate use of nutrients and botanical medicine, yet for the most part conventional M.D.'s lack the necessary training to properly provide such substances to their patients. By working in conjunction with N.D.s, M.D.'s can offer patients suffering from such serious conditions a more integrated spectrum of treatment options.

CONDITIONS THAT BENEFIT FROM NATUROPATHIC MEDICINE

Naturopathic medicine is an effective treatment approach for most cases of chronic and degenerative disease, either as a form of primary care or in conjunction with other therapeutic approaches. It is also ideally suited as a primary form of preventive medicine. Naturopathic medicine is not recommended for cases of acute or severe trauma, emergency childbirth, or orthopedic conditions requiring corrective surgery, however, although it can be beneficial during the recovery phase of such situations.

Because naturopathic medicine encompasses a variety of diagnostic and therapeutic approaches (see "Therapies of Naturopathic Medicine" earlier in this chapter), research regarding its effectiveness has tended to focus on each therapy separately. Today, however, a wealth of research substantiates the value of many of the therapies N.D.'s employ, such as diet, nutritional and botanical medicine, acupuncture, and homeopathy, for treating a wide range of both acute and chronic disease conditions. Scientific evidence supporting each of these therapies is provided elsewhere in this book.

According to the National Institutes of Health (NIH), naturopathic medicine is an appropriate and effective choice for treating ear infections, female health conditions, infectious disease, and respiratory conditions. Clinical research, for instance, has shown that naturopathic medical formulas are an effective alternative to conventional hormone replacement therapy for women. In another study involving forty-three women with abnormal Pap smears (cervical dysplasia), thirty-eight of them had normal Pap smear and tissue biopsy readings after being treating with naturopathic medicine. Naturopathic childbirth has also been shown to minimize the risks of birth-related complications and result in a significantly lower incidence of cesarean-section births than is experienced with conventional birthing approaches.

Statistics also show that naturopathic medicine is an effective, non-surgical approach for treating cases of middle-ear infection (otitis media), which affects approximately 30 percent of all U.S. children under the age of six. By incorporating diet, clinical nutrition, homeopathy, hydrotherapy, and physical therapies, N.D.'s are able to successfully treat over 80 percent of otitis media cases without surgery, thus avoiding side effects such as permanent scarring of ear tissue that can occur following conventional treatment. Moreover, naturopathic treatment is more cost-effective, with an average cost of between $200 and $700, whereas conventional treatment can exceed $7,000 and has a median cost of approximately $1,100.

In 1994, the NIH's Office of Alternative Medicine acknowledged the role that naturopathic medicine can play in treating degenerative illness by awarding a $1 million grant to Bastyr University's department of Natural Health Sciences to research naturopathic approaches for treating AIDS and HIV. The grant was awarded based on previous studies overseen by

Bastyr's Leanna Standish, N.D., Ph.D., in 1988 and 1989, known as the Healing AIDS Research Project (HARP). As part of the HARP study, participants diagnosed with HIV were given baths in hot water heated to 102 degrees Fahrenheit, since research shows that HIV is heat-sensitive and becomes progressively inactive during extended periods above normal body temperature. This form of hydrotherapy was administered for forty minutes twice a week for three weeks at a time, over a twelve-month period. According to Dr. Standish, initial results of the HARP program resulted in enhanced immune response and a decrease in HIV progression among participants who underwent the hydrotherapy treatments, compared with a control group who received conventional care.

In addition to being effective as a primary treatment option, one of naturopathic medicine's other primary values lies in its ability to prevent illness from occurring in the first place. N.D.'s sanctioned by the AANP are trained both to accurately assess their patients' risk for disease and to work with them to implement preventive strategies that minimize all controllable risk factors. They also spend considerable time and effort in patient education, guiding them in dietary, lifestyle and attitudinal choices that enhance health and diminish stress. Studies have shown that the benefits of such patient wellness programs not only reduce the incidence of illness and the need for hospitalized care, but also can reduce health care costs by as much as 76 percent. This emphasis on wellness and prevention explains why naturopathic medicine has one of the highest rates of patient satisfaction within the holistic health care field.

HEALING THE IMMUNE SYSTEM: ❦ A CASE HISTORY ❦

The following case history, recounted by Dr. Joseph Pizzorno in his book *Total Wellness*, illustrates the health benefits that naturopathic medicine can provide. The case involved a three-year-old girl who suffered from chronic ear infections and impaired immune function. On an average of every six to eight weeks, the girl experienced colds that usually led to ear infections. In the eighteen months before first seeing Dr. Pizzorno, the girl had suffered eight such infections, and received eleven courses of antibiotic treatments, and her pediatrician was now recommending myringotomy (the surgical insertion of ear tubes to allow drainage), fearing that otherwise the girl's hearing would become permanently impaired.

During his initial consultation, Dr. Pizzorno immediately noticed the girl was overweight and suffered from a runny nose, and that her eyes were red, with dark circles beneath them. During the consultation, he was also told that she regularly ate foods that were high in sugar and unhealthy fats, and low in vitamins and minerals. Further evaluation revealed that the girl's primary problem was not the continued incidence of bacterial growth in her ears, but a compromised immune system due to poor diet, dairy food allergies, and deficiencies of zinc and vitamins A and C. Reacting to her food allergies, which until her visit to Dr. Pizzorno had not been diagnosed, the girl's eustachian tubes would swell closed, thus inhibiting her ears' normal drainage mechanisms and turning the ear canals into breeding grounds for bacteria.

Dr. Pizzorno's treatment approach was simple and noninvasive. He took her off all dairy products, substantially limited her sugar intake, and worked with her mother to create a healthy eating plan that included fresh fruits, vegetables, and whole grains rich in the three nutrients the girl was lacking. He also briefly recommended daily supplements of all three nutrients. As a result, the girl's health soon noticeably improved, and within four months her weight had normalized and the dark circles under her eyes disappeared. Over the next year, her resistance to colds dramatically improved, and she only had one further ear infection, which Dr. Pizzorno treated with hot packs over her ears, along with the botanical remedies echinacea and goldenseal. ❦

YOUR FIRST SESSION

When visiting a licensed naturopathic physician for the first time, expect to receive a comprehensive evaluation of your overall health status. This evaluation might include a physical exam, X-rays, and conventional lab testing, such as blood tests. In states that license N.D.'s, such testing can be conducted or ordered by the N.D.'s themselves. In all other states, N.D.'s are required to send patients to other physicians for lab testing. In addition, your consultation will address the nature of your specific health complaints, as well as your diet, nutritional status, lifestyle, stress levels, and possible exposure to food or environmental allergies. Given the training N.D.'s receive as counselors, you may also be asked about, and encouraged to discuss, any mental, emotional, or spiritual concerns that might be affecting your health. Typically, your initial consultation will last for an hour or more and serve as the beginning of a proactive relationship with your N.D. as he or she prepares an individualized treatment and lifestyle regimen to restore you to optimal health.

In addition to the various therapeutic approaches that might be employed (see "Therapies of Naturopathic Medicine" earlier in this chapter), you will receive guidance about the foods and nutritional supplements most appropriate for you, information about exercises and stress reduction techniques tailored to meet your specific needs, and instruction in how you can best go about reversing any lifestyle choices or habits you need to change. Throughout the course of your treatment, you will be encouraged to assume greater responsibility for your health while learning to recognize the factors, both internal and external, that serve as indicators of your progress. Follow-up sessions will be scheduled as necessary, with your treatment plan adjusted as appropriate, according to your specific needs.

In general, fees charged by licensed N.D.'s are on par with those of conventional M.D.'s. More than one hundred health insurance companies nationwide also offer full or partial coverage for naturopathic care.

SELECTING A PRACTITIONER

Since many people purporting to be naturopathic physicians possess only mail-order or correspondence degrees, one of the most important steps anyone can take in choosing to explore naturopathic medicine is to work only with a licensed practitioner who is also a member of the AANP. (To locate AANP-sanctioned N.D.s, see the "Resources" section on the following page.) All states that license N.D.'s recognize them as primary care physicians who are qualified to both diagnose and treat disease. If you live in one of the states that do not provide licensing, ask where the naturopaths you interview received their training. Currently, only the three colleges listed in this chapter offer accredited naturopathic doctorate degree programs.

Though the practice of naturopathic medicine encompasses a variety of therapeutic methods, most N.D.'s tend to specialize in certain methods over others. Not all N.D.'s, for instance, offer natural childbirth services. If you have a preference for particular therapies, ask if the N.D.'s you are considering use them.

Finally, make sure that you feel comfortable with the practitioner you select. Your practitioner should be a good listener who takes time to explain the rationale behind the treatment protocols he or she recommends for you, as well as providing you with the information you need to make an educated choice about your treatment options. To help you in your selection process, seek referrals to N.D.'s from people whose opinions you respect and trust.

THE FUTURE OF NATUROPATHIC MEDICINE

After decades spent in obscurity in the United States, naturopathic medicine's continued resurgence now seems assured, especially given the acceptance it has recently received from such government organizations as the National Institutes of Health and the appointment of naturopathic physicians to advisory positions in both areas of government-sponsored health research and within conventional hospitals and health clinics. In tandem with such trends is the fact that additional states are now considering licensing N.D.'s, with a number or them likely to grant such licensing in the near future. Eventually, the AANP hopes to see licensing offered to N.D.'s in all fifty states.

One of the challenges facing the naturopathic profession is the creation of universal standards applicable to all health care practitioners who call themselves N.D.'s. In order for this to be achieved, the disparity of training received by N.D. candidates in accredited naturopathic colleges and those who receive their degrees from mail-order and correspondence courses must be fully addressed. This is a situation that the AANP is actively working to rectify. Such standardization is likely to become a reality as ongoing research continues to validate naturopathic medicine as a primary health care system.

RESOURCES

To learn more about naturopathic medicine, or to locate an AANP-sanctioned N.D. near you, contact the AANP at:

American Association of Naturopathic Physicians
8201 Greensboro Drive, Suite 300
McLean, Virginia 22102
Phone: (703) 610-9037
E-mail: webmaster@naturopathic.org
Web site: *www.naturopathic.org*

Further information is also available by contacting the following accredited naturopathic colleges:

Bastyr University
14500 Juanita Dr. NE
Kenmore, Washington 98028-4966
Phone: (425) 823-1300
Fax: (425) 823-6222
Web site: *www.bastyr.edu*

National College of Naturopathic Medicine
49 S.W. Porter
Portland, Oregon 97201
Phone: (503) 499-4343
Fax: (503) 499-0027
Web site: *www.ncnm.edu*

Southwest College of Naturopathic Medicine and Health Sciences
2140 East Broadway Road
Tempe, Arizona 85282
Phone: (480) 858-9100
Fax: (480) 858-9116
Web site: *www.scnm.edu*

Canadian College of Naturopathic Medicine
1255 Sheppard Avenue East
North York, Ontario, Canada M2K 1E2
Phone: (416) 498-1255
Fax: (416) 498-1576
Web site: *www.ccnm.edu*

RECOMMENDED READING

Murray, Michael, N.D., and Joseph Pizzorno, N.D. *Encyclopedia of Natural Medicine*. 2d ed., rev. Prima Publishing, 1998.
Pizzorno, Joseph, N.D. *Total Wellness*. Prima Publishing, 1996.

CHAPTER 11

Homeopathy

"Homeopathy is a holistic practice of medicine that works by stimulating the body's inherent ability to heal itself," says Kathleen K. Fry, M.D., president of the American Holistic Medical Association, who employs homeopathy as an integral part of her medical practice. Derived from the Greek words *homoios* and *pathos*, meaning "similar suffering," homeopathy was developed by the German physician and chemist Samuel Hahnemann (1755–1843) in 1796, and is today a popular form of medicine in Europe, India, Mexico, South America, and other parts of the world. In the United States, however, it remains poorly understood and underutilized, despite the fact that at the beginning of the twentieth century as many as one in five physicians incorporated homeopathy as part of their practice. Nonetheless, homeopathy is currently undergoing a resurgence in this country due to its effectiveness in treating a wide range of chronic disease conditions for which conventional medicine offers little more than symptom relief. In addition, homeopathic remedies are officially recognized as drugs by the Food and Drug Administration (FDA), which also regulates how they are manufactured and dispensed, in accordance with the guidelines of the *Homeopathic Pharmacopoeia of the United States*, which was first published in 1897.

🌿 FAST FACTS 🌿

In addition to inventing the word *homeopathy* to explain his approach to treating disease, Hahnemann also coined the word *allopathy* ("other suffering") to describe the medical approaches of his day, from which the term *allopathic medicine* is derived.

An estimated 500 million people worldwide use homeopathic remedies to treat their health conditions, and homeopathy has been officially recognized by the World Health Organization as a system of medicine that should be used to meet the global health care needs of the twenty-first century.

During the early 1900s, the practice of homeopathy was commonplace in the United States. At that time, there were more than a hundred homeopathic hospitals nationwide, and twenty-two homeopathic medical schools. Homeopathic formulas were also quite popular as treatments for the various infectious epidemics common during this period, including typhoid, cholera, and scarlet fever. Moreover, homeopathic hospitals experienced death rates that were 50 to 88 percent lower than those in hospitals that relied primarily on conventional medical treatments during the outbreak of such epidemics. The decline in homeopathy's popularity in the United States was largely due to the publication of the Flexnor Report in 1910, a report that was biased against all alternative healing methods and resulted in the closing of most homeopathic colleges. Homeopathy's popularity was further eroded by the advent of antibiotics and other so-called miracle drugs.

Elsewhere around the world, acceptance of homeopathy has been greater. In Germany, homeopathy is a required discipline for all medical students and is used by 20 percent of all German physicians. In France, approximately 40 percent of physicians use homeopathic remedies, and in India there are over one hundred thousand homeopathic physicians and 120 homeopathic medical schools. Homeopathy is particularly well accepted in England, where it has been recognized as a postgraduate medical specialty in an act of Parliament. Over 40 percent of British physicians either use homeopathic remedies or refer their patients to homeopathic physicians. In addition, homeopathic hospitals and outpatient facilities are part of the British national health care system, and homeopathy has been used for most of the twentieth century by England's royal family.

In the United States, there are an estimated three thousand homeopathic physicians, with licensing programs varying from state to state. Many other health practitioners employ homeopathic remedies, as well, including M.D.'s, osteopaths, chiropractors, acupuncturists, naturopaths, nurse practitioners, and veterinarians. In recent years, there has also been a rise in the number of lay practitioners around the country. ❧

HISTORY OF HOMEOPATHY

In the West, the Greek physician Hippocrates, during the fifth century B.C., first articulated the concept that substances that when taken in large doses produce disease symptoms, will cure those same diseases when taken in smaller doses. In the East, this same principle informed the medical philosophies of Ayurveda and traditional Chinese medicine many centuries earlier (see Chapters 12 and 13). In homeopathy, this concept of "like cures like" is known as the Law of Similars and was one of the original tenets proposed by Samuel Hahnemann, based on the experiments he conducted that led him to develop homeopathy.

During his lifetime, Hahnemann was a highly regarded physician, chemist, botanist, and author, at a time when medical theory held that all illnesses were due to imbalances in what were known as the four humors. "This was before the microscope and the concept that microbes caused disease," Dr. Fry explains. "When people got sick, physicians attempted to restore balance by bloodletting and the use of leeches, followed with purgatives and cathartics like arsenic and mercury, which often had effects far worse than the original disease themselves." Hahnemann was appalled by such practices and convinced they did not work in view of the rampant diseases in his day. He also was one of the first European physicians to stress the importance of diet and good hygiene in relation to good health, but his advice was little heeded. Disillusioned, Hahnemann eventually gave up his practice, turning to supporting his family by translating medical texts into German. Among the works he translated were those of Hippocrates and Paracelsus. As he read them, he came to realize that other scientific disciplines had strict, immutable universal laws that governed them, whereas the medical practices of his time were not founded on any similarly firm principles. Convinced that proper medical treatment must abide by corresponding principles, he set out to discover what they might be, and began to read whatever texts he could find relating to the theory and practice of medicine.

In 1789, while translating *A Treatise on Materia Medica* by the eminent Scottish physician Dr. William Cullen, Hahnemann became intrigued by a passage in which Cullen postulated that the ability of the Peruvian bark cinchona to cure malaria was due to its bitter, astringent qualities. As a chemist, Hahnemann knew that there were other substances with even greater bitter and astringent properties than cinchona that were ineffective in treating malaria, so he doubted Cullen's explanation. In order to discover the actual reason that cinchona reversed malaria, he repeatedly ingested doses of the bark while recording his reactions to it. After a few days, he started to manifest all of the symptoms of malaria, even though he knew he was not suffering from the disease. His symptoms abated when he stopped taking cinchona, yet each time he took another dose, his symptoms recurred, causing Hahnemann to suspect that cinchona was effective as a treatment for malaria precisely because of its ability to *cause* the same symptoms. In order to verify his theory, Hahnemann gave doses of cinchona to others, including members of his family, all of whom developed similar symptoms. Based on these experiments, which he called "provings," Hahnemann developed his theory of the Law of Similars. To further substantiate it, he did other provings of other substances and, in the process, discovered the "symptom signature" of many diseases common to his time. "Ultimately, Hahnemann was responsible for proving over a hundred remedies," Dr. Fry says. "He did this by meticulously writing down every single symptom that he and his test subjects experienced in the process of taking each substance."

Hahnemann continued his proving experiments for twenty years, cataloging each symptom picture according to the substance that elicited it. In the process, he discovered that individuals varied both in the severity of the symptoms they experienced and in how they healed from them. In addition, he found that the more closely he could match a remedy to each patient's symptom picture, the more successful the treatment would be. In order to achieve this most effectively, Hahnemann not only gave his patients a physical examination, he also inquired about their health history, lifestyle, personal likes and dislikes, and any factors that they felt made their symptoms better or worse. Based on his research, the foundation for homeopathy's *materia medica* was laid.

In 1796, Hahnemann published his first writings on homeopathy. These were followed in 1810 by the first complete homeopathic textbook, known as the *Organon of Rational Medical Science*, which was revised and published in 1819 as the *Organon of the Art of Healing*. This book went through six editions, the last being published in 1921, nearly eighty years after Hahnemann's death.

Despite the fact that the *Organon* was one of the first medical texts to outline the principles governing health and disease based on scientific reasoning and experimentation, Hahnemann's theory was strongly opposed by many of the physicians and pharmacists of his time, in large part because the system of medicine he advocated posed a serious threat to their livelihood. In 1820, while living in Leipzig, Germany, he was arrested and convicted of administering his own medicines to patients, and banished from the city. Due to a special dispensation from Grand Duke Ferdinand, he was allowed to continue to practice and teach homeopathy in the town of Köthen. Following the cholera epidemic that swept through Europe in 1832, however, acceptance of homeopathy became more widespread, as cholera patients who were administered homeopathic remedies had a much higher rate of recovery than patients who received allopathic medicine. In fact, in Paris, the demand for homeopathic remedies to treat cholera was said to have increased their price one hundredfold, due to their effectiveness. And in Russia, the mortality rate of patients receiving homeopathic care during the epidemic was less than 10 percent, compared to 60 to 70 percent among patients receiving conventional care. At the time of Hahnemann's death, homeopathy had spread to every European country except Sweden and Norway and was also being practiced in Russia, Mexico, Cuba, and the United States. By the mid-1800s, it had also spread to South America and India.

When cholera next struck Europe in 1854, the London Homeopathic Hospital exclusively treated cholera victims, achieving a mortality rate of less than 17 percent, compared to nearly 52 percent among patients treated in allopathic hospitals. When these figures were submitted by the British Medical Council for inclusion in their Blue Book of Statistics, however, they were purposely omitted for fear that they would unjustifiably sanction homeopathy as an empirical practice. Only after a great deal of protest were the figures finally produced one hundred years later.

In the United States during this time, homeopathy also enjoyed growing popularity, due primarily to the efforts of Dr. Constantine Hering, a student of Hahnemann, who, in 1835, established the first U.S. homeopathic medical school in Allentown, Pennsylvania. Known as "the father of American homeopathy," Hering is best known for his contributions to the theory of isopathy, which holds that all disease conditions contain within themselves their own remedy and the means by which they can be prevented, and his experiments with pathogenic excretions and secretions from humans and animals, which he termed *nosodes*. Hering developed the first nosodic homeopathic remedy, *Lachesis*, derived from the venom of the bushmaster snake, which furthered the understanding of how homeopathy could work and also resulted in the development of many other homeopathic remedies. Hering is also known for his theory Hering's Law of Cure, a guiding principle in the use of homeopathic remedies.

As a result of Hering's efforts, the number of homeopathic practitioners in the United States continued to grow, leading, in 1844, to the formation of the American Institute of Homeopathy, the first national medical association ever founded in the United States. In response, conventional physicians formed the American Medical Association (AMA) two years later, in large part to denounce homeopathy as a fraudulent health care practice. To this end, using tactics similar to what they would employ against chiropractic a century later (see Chapter 7), the AMA forbade its members to associate with homeopathic physicians professionally and socially, and prevented any physician who incorporated homeopathy in his or her practice from joining the AMA. Despite the AMA's efforts, however, homeopathy continued to gain a following throughout the rest of the nineteenth century, again largely due to outbreaks of epidemic diseases. In 1849, when a cholera outbreak swept through Cincinnati, Ohio, patients treated with homeopathy experienced a mortality rate of only 3 percent, compared to death rates of between 40 to 70 percent among patients treated with conventional medicine. Thirty years later, during an outbreak of yellow fever in New Orleans, fewer than 6 percent of 1,945 patients who received homeopathic treatment died, compared to 16 percent of patients who received conventional care. Due to its greater success rate, homeopathy soon attracted the support of a number of influential Americans, including Samuel Clemens (Mark Twain), Thomas Edison, and John D. Rockefeller.

Another influential American homeopath was James Tyler Kent (1849–1916), whose passion for homeopathy began when his wife made a dramatic recovery from a prolonged period of anemia, anxiety, and insomnia following treatment by a homeopathic physician. Since previous conventional and eclectic treatments (botanically based, symptom-specific medicine popular in the nineteenth century) had failed to help his wife, Kent gave up his practice as an eclectic physician in order to study with the homeopath who had cured her. He went on to serve as a professor at a number of leading homeopathic colleges and, by the time of his death, was regarded as one of the leading homeopathic physicians and educators in the United States. Kent is most famous for his *Repertory* and his emphasis on simultaneously treating not just a patient's physical body, but the emotional, mental, and spiritual factors, as well. To do so most effectively, he advocated the use of single remedies of high-dose potencies. He also contributed to the homeopathic theory of "constitutional types" of patients, a concept that has been further developed throughout the twentieth century.

At the start of the twentieth century, an estimated 15 to 20 percent of all physicians in the United States practiced homeopathy, and there were twenty-two homeopathic medical schools and one hundred homeopathic hospitals around the country. By 1910, however, following the publication of the AMA-sponsored Flexnor Report, which disparaged all forms of nonconventional medicine, homeopathy's popularity began to decline and was further eroded by the advent of penicillin and other antibiotic drugs, along with modern medicine's increasing focus on surgical procedures and pharmaceutical treatment of symptoms. Despite this decline, homeopathy's nearly three thousand remedies have, since 1938, been officially recognized as valid medicinal formulas by U.S. statute, and since the 1970s its popularity as an effective alternative to conventional medical treatment has once again steadily increased, both in the United States and abroad.

HOW HOMEOPATHY WORKS

Like other holistic practitioners, homeopaths are concerned with treating the whole person, not just their patients' disease conditions. In doing so, they abide by three principles first formulated by Hahnemann that have guided the practice of homeopathy ever since. These principles are the Law of Similars ("like cures like"), the Law of the Minimum Dose, and prescribing for the individual, which recognizes that illness is specific to each patient and must therefore be treated accordingly. Hering's Law of Cure also influences the type of homeopathic treatment given, as does the question of whether the patient is treated according to the principles of classical homeopathy or with combination remedies (polypharmacy).

The Law of Similars

This first principle of homeopathy holds that substances that in larger doses cause illness in healthy people, will provoke healing in people suffering from the same or similar symptoms. It was first taught in the West by Hippocrates, who wrote, "An illness is caused by similar means, and similar means cure man of illness." Hahnemann further developed this concept through the many provings of substances he conducted using healthy volunteers. He found that a substance that most nearly produced symptoms similar to those of a specific disease was the one best suited to treat such conditions when administered as a single remedy. A homeopathic example of the Law of Similars can be found in the remedy *Coffee cruda*, which can be effective in treating conditions of insomnia and hyperactivity, both of which can occur when too much coffee, from which the formula is derived, is consumed.

For the most part, the Law of Similars is the antithesis of the approach taken by conventional physicians, who predominantly treat disease by evoking the opposite of their patients' symptom pictures, such as treating diarrhea by using medications that temporarily cause constipation. The Law of Similars is not entirely foreign to allopathic medicine, however. Both vaccinations, which employ trace elements of various pathogens to bolster the body's immune response to the diseases the pathogens cause, and allergy desensitization, which treats allergy by injecting small amounts of suspected allergens into the body, are based on the principle of the Law of Similars, which also influenced the work of medical pioneers such as Louis Pasteur and Jonas Salk.

The Law of the Minimum Dose

As Hahnemann began using homeopathic remedies to treat his patients' health problems, he observed that their symptoms often worsened before their conditions improved. Seeking to minimize such reactions, he discovered that he could achieve better results, with far less likelihood of side effects, by using smaller, more dilute doses of the remedies. Over time, he found that the more diluted a substance was, the greater its potency. This led him to formulate the Law of the Minimum (or Infinitesimal) Dose, which states that a remedy's healing properties are enhanced in direct proportion to the degree that it is diluted. This dilution process, known as potentization, is achieved by progressively diluting a substance in pure water or alcohol, and then vigorously shaking it after each dilution (known as succussion). During this process, the original substance is soaked in alcohol, after which a drop of this "mother tincture" is added to ten, one hundred, or one thousand parts of water. The diluted solution is then added to neutral milk sugar pills. Dilutions of a ratio of 1:10 are known as "X" potencies, while those of 1:100 and 1:1,000 are known respectively as "C" and "M" potencies.

This potentization process is the source of the most controversy regarding homeopathy's effectiveness, since remedies of potencies 24X (or 12C) or greater (meaning they have undergone 24 or more successive dilutions and succussions) contain no chemical trace of their original substances. "The explanation as to how potentization works lies in the fact that everything in nature has both a material and an energetic component," Dr. Fry explains. "As you dilute and succuss a remedy, you lessen its material component while strengthening its energetic component." Although the theory has yet to be proven, proponents of homeopathy postulate that the potentization process imprints the energetic signature, or frequency, of the original substance onto the water or alcohol solution, which in turn stimulates each patient's "vital force" or bioenergy field to activate the body's natural healing response.

Research conducted in the 1960s of twenty-three homeopathic remedies using nuclear magnetic resonance imaging seems to support the theory of homeopathy's bioenergetic efficacy. All of the remedies displayed distinctive readings of subatomic activity, while various placebo substances did not. Additional research by German biophysicist Wolfgang Ludwig indicates that homeopathic remedies emit dominant, measurable electromagnetic frequencies. Dr. Ludwig's findings, along with those of Italian physicist Emilio del Giudici, who theorizes that water molecules are capable of storing minute electromagnetic frequencies, help to further explain how homeopathy works. Most recently, a study conducted by Italian chemistry professors Vittorio Elia and Marcella Niccoli suggests that homeopathic remedies do indeed contain active properties, even when all molecules of their original substances have been diluted out. Drs. Elia and Niccoli measured the amount of heat given off by double-distilled water alone compared to double-distilled water in which various substances, including salt and vinegar, were placed. Both the control water and the treated water were consecutively diluted and succussed from one to thirty times, after which the researchers conducted more than five hundred experiments on both liquids. Their findings showed that 92 percent of the treated solutions in which base substances had been added emitted higher-than-expected heat signatures, compared to the untreated water. Commenting on his research, Dr. Elia said, "We are setting the basis for a new science, the physics-chemistry of homeopathic water. These results make for a strong support to the hypothesis of the existence of a memory of water."

Prescribing for the Individual

According to homeopathic theory, disease does not occur randomly or in isolation but is a direct reflection of each patient's overall state of being.

Therefore, rather than focus on treating patient symptoms, homeopaths treat their patients on an individual basis, taking note of factors such as each patient's medical history, temperament, personality traits, mental and emotional states, dietary preferences, sleeping patterns, and personal likes and dislikes. Attention is also given to each patient's symptom picture, which includes any factors that either improve or worsen their conditions, as well as how the condition may alter throughout the day. Homeopathic remedies are also based on the patient's constitution, which includes both inherited and acquired characteristics. Only after this individual and constitutional profile has been compiled will a remedy be prescribed, matched to the patient's total symptom picture.

Hering's Law of Cure

Originally formulated by Constantine Hering, this principle has three basic tenets: healing begins from the top of the body, downward; it progresses from the inside out, and from major to minor organs; and symptoms resolve themselves in reverse chronological order from their original appearance. Unlike conventional medicine, which treats disease symptoms by attempting to suppress them, the goal of homeopathy is to reverse any suppression that may be present in order to free up the patient's vital energies so that healing can occur. Like holistic practitioners in general, homeopaths regard symptoms as attempts by the body to maintain balance and restore vitality. Ignoring or suppressing initial symptoms often results in more serious complications later. According to Hering's Law of Cure, as symptoms progress, they can also move into more important areas of the body. "Consider a child born with eczema," Dr. Fry explains. "Due to her condition, which manifests as skin rash, a conventional physician might prescribe steroids. As a result, the eczema might go away, but because the underlying cause of the eczema was ignored, later a more serious complication, such as asthma, can occur, affecting the lungs. The skin is a relatively innocuous organ, whereas the lungs, on a hierarchical level, are more important to health. Since the original disturbance in the child's vital force was not addressed, it grew stronger. As a result, her body, in a sense, has to produce a bigger symptom picture to match the strength of whatever factors caused her initial disease, as well as the suppressive action of the steroid prescribed."

Dr. Fry likens the healing process to peeling an onion. "The body has a hierarchy of organs, and in its wisdom tries to do the least amount of damage as it attempts to maintain balance when the vital force becomes depleted," she says. "If the initial depletion is minor, you may develop symptoms such as skin rash, but if the symptoms are suppressed and the underlying cause of the depletion is not addressed, you may develop problems in the bones and joints, and then in the internal organs, or in the mental sphere, such as depression or hyperactivity. In cases of chronic illness, the symptom picture is usually multilayered, and according to Hering's Law, those you've developed most recently will resolve themselves first, and those that you've had the longest will be the last to go away."

For this reason, once a homeopathic remedy is prescribed, changes and reactions on the part of the patient are carefully noted to determine how healing is progressing. In the process, patients, especially those suffering from chronic disease conditions, may initially experience a worsening of symptoms. At times, such an experience, known to homeopaths as "symptom aggravation" or a "healing crisis," can be dramatic, yet also usually only temporary. Moreover, to homeopaths, such an aggravation is an indication that the selected remedy is working. As initial symptoms abate, often previous symptoms from a patient's past will manifest, at which time a new remedy may be chosen, with this process repeating itself until the original symptom cause is healed.

Due to the way homeopathy works, treatment for long-term conditions may require time, although in many cases healing can occur quickly, sometimes with as few as one or two office visits. For the most part, however, Dr. Fry cautions that patients suffering from chronic conditions should undertand that they may "have to suffer with symptoms" as the healing process unfolds. Based on her clinical experience, Dr. Fry reports that most patients have far less symptomatic aggravation when they are started on a remedy given as a low potency that is then gradually increased over time.

Classical Homeopathy versus Polypharmacy

Until the twentieth century, homeopathy was primarily practiced according to the principles of classical homeopathy, which is based on Hahnemann's belief that each patient's total symptom picture best determines the specific remedy to use, not the name of his or her disease. According to Dr. Fry, practitioners of classical homeopathy employ "one remedy at a time, at the right time, and in the right potency." Classical homeopathy is the form of homeopathy predominantly practiced in Great Britain, India, and South America.

In Germany and France, a more recent approach, known as polypharmacy, is more the norm. This form of homeopathy uses a mixture of remedies (often called combination remedies), which are usually prepared as low-potency formulations. In contrast to classical homeopathic remedies, combination remedies are often cataloged according to disease condition, and are sold as over-the-counter treatments for conditions such as cold and flu, headache, respiratory conditions, and yeast infections. The most popular combination remedy is *Oscillococcinum*, which is the best-selling cold and flu formula in France.

In the United States, both forms of homeopathy are practiced, with classical remedies usually employed by homeopaths, and combination remedies more commonly used by other practitioners who use homeopathy as an adjunct to other healing modalities. While polypharmacological remedies can provide benefit for certain acute, nonserious conditions, classical homeopathy is better suited for treating chronic and more serious diseases, because of its emphasis on matching a remedy to each patient's specific symptom picture, including subtle factors related to the patient's personality and mental/emotional disposition. The results achieved by classical homeopathy also tend to be longer-lasting and more significant, compared to combination remedies, which, because of their less precise nature, tend to act more superficially. A number of classical homeopaths, including Dr. Fry, believe that combination remedies are suppressive and more dangerous than conventional drugs, because they are capable of disrupting the body's vital force, which conventional drugs, being more crude, don't touch. "Combination remedies are a short-cut approach that uses homeopathic remedies in an allopathic manner," Dr. Fry says, who acknowledges that her view is at the heart of the controversy between practitioners of classical and polypharmacological homeopathy.

While *how* homeopathy works has yet to be explained to the satisfaction of homeopathy's critics, that it *does* work is becoming increasingly difficult to dispute. This fact was made clearer in 1991, when the *British Medical Journal* published the result of a meta-analysis conducted by research physicians in Holland involving all human clinical trials of homeopathy published in credible medical journals from around the world between 1966 and 1990. In all, 107 trials were examined, with 81 (77 percent) of them demonstrating homeopathy's effectiveness in treating a variety of disease conditions, including cardiovascular disease, respiratory conditions, headache, gastrointestinal disorders, hay fever, psychological disorders, physical trauma and sprains, and postoperative infections and other aftereffects. Based on a careful evaluation of how the trials were performed, the researchers concluded that the vast majority of them were scientifically on a par with conventional medical standards and, in fact, more rigorous than studies in which pharmaceutical companies had a vested financial interest. Based on their analysis, the researchers stated that they accepted homeopathy as an effective medical treatment even though they still had trouble grasping its mechanism of action.

HOW HOMEOPATHIC REMEDIES ARE USED

Homeopathic remedies are taken one at a time and can change as symptoms clear or alter. Most remedies are in pellet form, but they can also be taken as tablets, powder, or liquid. Because of their energetic nature, it is recommended that remedies not be touched by hand. They can either be placed into the cap of their container, or onto a spoon, and then taken sublingually (beneath the tongue) thirty minutes before or after meals or drinking water. Depending on each patient's specific needs, the nature of his or her illness, and potency selected, remedies can be taken throughout the day, or at intervals ranging from once a day to once a week or longer.

When not being used, remedies should be stored in a cool, dark place, in a closed container, and kept away from substances such as air fresheners, perfumes, household cleaners, scented cosmetic products, and essential oils, all of which can neutralize, or antidote, the remedies' effectiveness. Other substances that can counteract homeopathic remedies include coffee, alcohol, tobacco, drugs, and products containing, or flavored with, mint.

CONDITIONS THAT BENEFIT
FROM HOMEOPATHY

Based on its ability to match remedies to patients' complete "symptom picture," homeopathy can be effective as either a primary or adjunctive treatment for almost any type of disease condition, both chronic and acute, including those of a psychological nature. In addition to the conditions cited in the meta-analysis of homeopathic clinical trials above, other published studies have found that homeopathy is an effective treatment for sinusitis, bronchitis, motion sickness, vertigo, varicose veins, the flu, attention deficit hyperactivity disorder, and acute otitis media (ear infection) among children. Research published in the *European Journal of*

Pharmacology also showed that the homeopathic remedy *Silicea* is capable of boosting immune function by stimulating macrophage (essential cells of the immune system) activity, while published research in Germany indicates that homeopathy can be helpful in treating Parkinson's disease. Other conditions for which homeopathy has been found to be useful are listed later in this chapter.

DISCOUNTING THE PLACEBO EFFECT: ❧ HOMEOPATHY AND ANIMALS ❧

Critics of homeopathy often attribute cures or relief of symptoms achieved by homeopathy to the placebo effect, meaning that reported improvements are merely the result of patients' beliefs and expectations. This argument loses considerable weight, however, when one considers the many benefits reported by veterinarians who use homeopathy to treat animals.

The first use of homeopathic remedies on animals was conducted by Joseph Wilhelm Lux in the early 1800s after he became familiar with Hahnemann's published work. As a result of Lux's work, the use of homeopathy as a treatment for animal conditions spread throughout France and Germany. Today, homeopathy is widely used by veterinarians throughout Europe and is becoming increasingly popular in the United States, as well, where an estimated 75 percent of holistic veterinarians use homeopathic remedies as part of their practice. The primary reason given for their use of homeopathy is that it is both safer and more effective than previous conventional treatments they employed. Since animals are unable to reason whether or not a treatment will work, placebo remedies do not have the same psychological effects that they exhibit among humans. Therefore, placebo cannot be used to explain homeopathy's success in treating animals.

One of the most dramatic trials demonstrating the value of veterinary homeopathy was a controlled study involving a herd of pig sows having a high rate of miscarriage and stillbirth. After a group of sows received homeopathic treatments, their miscarriage rate dropped by 50 percent, compared to the control group. As a result, the entire herd received the same remedy, whereupon its newborn mortality rate decreased from 20 percent to 2.6 percent. After the treatment was discontinued, however, the rate climbed back to approximately 15 percent, before dropping back to less than 2 percent once the remedy was resumed.

A recent meta-analysis of 186 homeopathic studies published in *Lancet* in 1997 further discounts the placebo effect of homeopathy in humans. After pooling and assessing the data from all of the studies, the authors of the study found that patients who used homeopathic remedies were 2.45 times as likely to receive therapeutic benefit compared to patients given a placebo. ❦

Rheumatoid Arthritis

In 1978, researchers at Scotland's Glasgow Homeopathic Hospital conducted a double-blind study comparing homeopathic remedies to both conventional pain relievers and placebo for the treatment of rheumatoid arthritis. Forty-six patients were involved in the study. Patients given homeopathic remedies that matched each patient's individual symptom picture showed an 82 percent improvement in symptoms compared to only 21 percent improvement in patients who received pain relievers or placebo. In addition, within a year, 42 percent of patients receiving the homeopathic remedies were able to discontinue all treatment without a return of symptoms. A follow-up study conducted in 1980 involving twenty-three people with rheumatoid arthritis produced similar results, with patients receiving homeopathic remedies showing significantly greater improvement compared to the control group. In the same study, the homeopathic remedies were also determined to be safer than conventional arthritis formulas.

Asthma

A 1994 *Lancet* study involving twenty-eight patients suffering from severe asthma showed that homeopathic treatment can significantly improve the efficacy of conventional care. All twenty-eight patients required daily administration of bronchodilators, and twenty-one also required daily steroid treatment. Throughout the study, all participants in the study continued to receive their conventional treatment while receiving placebo for four weeks. In the fifth week, the patients were randomly divided into two groups, one continuing to receive placebo, the other receiving homeopathic remedies consisting of the allergens to which they were primarily allergic. Within one week, all patients who received homeopathic care reported far greater improvement of symptoms and exhibited enhanced bronchial and overall respiratory function, compared to the placebo group.

Migraine

A randomized, double-blind study of sixty patients suffering from migraine found that homeopathy can significantly decrease the incidence of migraine and improve overall migraine symptoms. In the study, patients were divided into two groups. The first received one biweekly dose of a homeopathic remedy matched to their individual symptom picture, while the other group received a placebo. After eight weeks, the placebo group averaged 7.9 migraine attacks per month, compared to 9.9 attacks at the beginning of the study. In comparison, those who received homeopathic remedies went from an average of 10 attacks per month to only 3, and two months later, their incidence of migraine had dropped to only 1.8 attacks per month and were of far less intensity than at the onset of the study.

Homeopathy's effectiveness in treating migraine was further established in a case history documented in the *Journal of Alternative and Complementary Medicine*. The case involved a fifty-five-year-old male who suffered from severe migraine headaches that lasted an average of twelve hours in length and were accompanied by throbbing pain, nausea, and hourly attacks of vomiting. After three years of unsuccessful results using conventional medical treatment, the man was referred to a homeopathic physician at Glasgow Homeopathic Hospital. After conducting a complete medical history, the physician prescribed the homeopathic remedy *Bryonia*, which the patient took twelve times over a period of three weeks. At the end of the three-week period, the man was completely migraine-free and had experienced no recurrence of his condition during the three years leading up to his case's publication.

Diarrhea

Diarrhea has long been a condition for which homeopathy has shown benefit, and today homeopathic antidiarrheal remedies are commonly used by travelers as a preventive measure when visiting foreign countries. One randomized, double-blind study, published in *Pediatrics* in 1994, involved eighty-one children in Nicaragua between the ages of six months and five years who suffered from acute diarrhea. The children were divided into two groups, with the first group receiving homeopathic remedies specific to their overall constitutions and symptom pictures, and the other group receiving placebo treatments. Both groups also received standard oral rehydration treatment. After only seventy-two hours, the children who received homeopathic remedies experienced a notable decrease in both the intensity and duration of their diarrhea symptoms, compared to the placebo group.

Fibromyalgia

A double-blind study published in the *British Medical Journal* in 1989 showed that the homeopathic remedy *Rhus toxicondendron*, given to patients as a match for their symptom pictures, resulted in a 25 percent reduction of pain symptoms, compared to patients in the placebo group, indicating that homeopathy may play a role in the treatment of this disease, for which conventional medicine has so far proven to be ineffective.

Pain

In a double-blind study headed up by C. Norman Shealy, M.D., Ph.D., founding president of the AHMA, and published in 1998 in the *American Journal of Pain Management*, homeopathy was found to be "at least as effective" as the pain reliever acetaminophen for the treatment of pain related to osteoarthritis. The study involved 65 patients. Fifty-five percent of those who received homeopathic remedies experienced measurable relief of their pain symptoms, compared to only 38 percent among patients who were given acetaminophen. Moreover, the study showed that homeopathic remedies lacked the potential side effects of the pain reliever, which can include possible liver and kidney damage. In addition, many of the patients who received homeopathic treatment asked to continue it after the study was concluded.

Research has also shown that homeopathy can ease pain symptoms following tooth extraction. In one study, cases of acute pain in localized lesions due to extraction were shown to resolve themselves after as little as one homeopathic treatment, and 76 percent of test subjects experienced pain relief overall, compared to only 40 percent who were given a placebo.

In another study involving sixty-nine patients suffering from sprained ankles, application of the homeopathic ointment *Traumeel* resulted in twenty-four of thirty-three patients being completely pain free after ten days, compared to only thirteen of thirty-six patients on placebo. In a different study, the same remedy, administered as an injection, was shown to provide pain relief and reduce healing time among patients suffering from hemarthrosis (a condition wherein blood or other body fluids seep into joints or body cavities).

Another double-blind study involving *Arnica*, a popular homeopathic remedy for pain relief, and the active ingredient for *Traumeel*, found that when the remedy was given to patients suffering from prolonged venous perfusion (a condition of spreading blood that commonly results in phlebitis in the veins), it not only reduced pain symptoms and inflammation, but also lowered the risk of hematoma formation, improved blood flow, and increased coagulation and platelet aggregation.

Childbirth

Homeopathic remedies taken throughout the course of pregancy have been shown to reduce the duration of labor and lower the incidence of difficult labor, according to a French study conducted in 1987. Other published studies conducted in 1993 and 1994 found that the homeopathic remedy *Caulophyllum*, administered after labor was underway, is capable of significantly reducing the duration of labor and also reducing labor-associated pains. According to Dr. Fry, it can also initiate labor and improve contractions.

Hay Fever

Another double-blind study conducted at Glasgow Homeopathic Hospital involved 144 patients suffering from active hay fever symptoms. The study, published in *Lancet* in 1986, found that a homeopathic preparation of mixed grass pollens implicated in hay fever was able to substantially reduce symptoms in those who received it, compared to those who did not. The decrease in symptoms was observed both clinically and by patient self-assessment.

Cancer

One of the more intriguing aspects of homeopathy has to do with its potential as a treatment against cancer. While no research suggests that homeopathy is effective against cancerous tumors directly, two published reports indicate that it may have worth as an immune booster, particularly for cancer patients with accompanying psychological problems. One study published in 1990 reports that two patients suffering from leukemia (acute myoblastic and chronic leukemia, respectively) who refused all other forms of treatment, went into full remission and remained cancer-free throughout three years of follow-up care and diagnoses after receiving classical homeopathic treatment. In the first case, treatment lasted for twenty-two months, with the homeopathic remedies changing over time in accordance with changes in the patient's symptom picture. Within the first six months of treatments, however, hematocrit values (percentage of total blood volume consisting of mature red blood cells) returned to normal, and after one year all aspects of the patient's health were at normal levels. In the second case, treatment lasted twenty-one months, with all clinical and laboratory data reverting to normal in the fifth month. As in the first case, the remedies used changed over time as the patient progressed. In both cases, the initial consultation revealed that the patients were also suffering from major psychological upset due both to their inherent emotional sensitivities and their reaction to their diagnoses. These problems resolved themselves early on as their treatment unfolded, and did not return.

❦ HEALING GRIEF: A CASE HISTORY ❦

The following case history involving one of Dr. Fry's patients illustrates how homeopathy treats the whole person, not simply disease symptoms. The patient was a forty-four-year-old woman who came to Dr. Fry for routine gynecological care. As Dr. Fry took the woman's medical history, however, she burst into tears, revealing that she was getting a divorce. "She was the mother of two teenaged children, worked part-time, and was scared to death about what would happen to her and her children," Dr. Fry says. "She told me that she cried all the time, even over Hallmark commercials, and had no idea how she was going to be able to carry on. At one point, she said, 'All I've ever known is being a wife and a mother. How will I survive?'"

The woman's medical history also revealed that she was suffering from profound fatigue and insomnia and had no appetite. Dr. Fry prescribed *Ignatia*, a very common homeopathic remedy for grief. "Since she was taking allergy medication and had never used a homeopathic remedy before, I started her on a dose of LM1 taken in water," Dr. Fry explains. "This has the advantage of being a high potency while still acting gently like a low potency since it is given in water."

On her next follow-up visit, the woman reported that her crying had stopped "almost immediately," and that by the end of the week she was again sleeping normally. As she continued to improve, Dr. Fry increased the potency of her remedy over the next five months, during which time her fatigue went away and her emotions continued to stabilize. "At her final visit she hugged me, telling me she couldn't thank me enough," Dr. Fry relates. "She said, 'I feel so strong inside now, like I can handle whatever life brings me.' Even though her divorce was still not finalized, she told me she wasn't worried any longer, being confident that both she and her children would be just fine."

YOUR FIRST SESSION

In order to select the most effective remedy for their patients, homeopathic practitioners conduct an extensive initial consultation, which can range in length from one to two hours. During this time, you and your practitioner will work together to compile a detailed symptom picture upon which your specific remedy will be based. You will be asked to provide as much information as possible about your background and present characteristics. In addition to a complete medical history, you will likely be asked about your educational background, occupational and marital status, lifestyle, daily routine (including eating habits), and any mental or emotional concerns that may be a factor in your illness. Other personal data can be included, as well, such as information about your childhood development, personal and dietary likes and dislikes, sleep patterns, the nature of your dreams (including any recurring dreams or nightmares), sexual status, possible financial problems, and how you react to changes in various conditions, including weather, temperature, and environment. A detailed description of your primary health complaint will also be compiled. You will be asked to fully describe the nature of your complaint, including your symptoms, how they began, what areas of your body were first affected by them, how they may have spread, and what circumstances, both physical and emotional, you were experiencing just before you became ill. Attention will also be given to any accompanying secondary symptoms you may be experiencing, as well as any conditions or actions that either ease or aggravate your condition.

Some homeopaths use questionnaires to gather the above information, while others, such as Dr. Fry, simply let their patients talk and listen to what they say. "I pay attention not only to what my patients tell me, but also how they say it," Dr. Fry says. "Some patients will talk throughout the entire consultation, without me having to ask a question. In homeopathy, we call that loquaciousness, so I know I am looking for a loquacious remedy. Other patients tend to be closed up and private, not wanting to share much, so obviously they have a different remedy state."

Once your symptom picture is completed, the remedy and potency that most closely matches it will be selected, and you will be instructed in how to use it. Remedies can be derived from plant, animal, mineral, and other sources, and are completely safe and nontoxic. They are also inexpensive, usually costing no more than four to six dollars per bottle, which usually contains seventy-five doses. If your practitioner is a classical homeopath, you will typically be given a single remedy that will often have to be repeated, with follow-up remedies given, if needed, based on how your body responds. Depending on the nature of your condition, your next session might be scheduled a few days or a week later, or not occur for another month. In the interim, you will be asked to note any changes in your condition that you experience, so that your practitioner will be able to most effectively evaluate your progress. In cases of acute conditions, results can be swift and dramatic when the correct remedy is prescribed, whereas chronic conditions may take longer to resolve themselves. If your symptoms persist, a different remedy may be prescribed, and the waiting and observation process repeated. Once your symptoms cease and your vitality is restored, usually your remedy will be discontinued.

The average cost of an initial homeopathic consultation is approximately $150, with follow-up visits averaging between $50 and $60, although higher fees are possible. A number of insurance companies now reimburse for visits to homeopathic physicians (not including the cost for remedies), although few HMO-based health care plans do.

SELECTING A PRACTITIONER

State licensing of homeopaths varies from state to state, with only Arizona, Connecticut, and Nevada offering separate homeopathic licensure to physicians. Because of this variance, finding a competent practitioner in your area may require a bit of time and effort. Both the National Center for Homeopathy and the International Foundation for Homeopathy (see the "Resources" section at the end of this chapter) can provide referrals. It's also important to note that not all homeopaths are physicians. Most who are have studied homeopathy as a postgraduate discipline for a period of four to five years. The primary physicians who practice homeopathy in the United States are M.D.'s and naturopathic physicians (N.D.'s), and those who are board-certified in its practice are known as Diplomates (D.Hom.). Other practitioners can carry the designation "CCH," which means they are certified in classical homeopathy.

When choosing a homeopath, Dr. Fry offers the following guidelines: Choose someone who has been practicing homeopathy for some time, and find out where they were trained and if they are cerified. Ask to speak to their patients so that you can gain a better understanding of how they practice and the level of patient satisfaction they have achieved. For the most effective results, Dr. Fry also recommends working with someone who practices classical homeopathy rather than polypharmacy. "For the best results, you want to work with a homeopath who is capable of prescribing the right remedy in the right potency, at the right time," she advises. Dr. Fry also points out that a practitioner does not necessarily have to be a physician in order to be an effective homeopath. "What matters most is whether he or she has the skills, knowledge base, and experience needed to choose the right remedy," she says. "When homeopathy fails to work, it is always due to selection of the incorrect remedy or because the remedy has been antidoted."

THE FUTURE OF HOMEOPATHY

Interest in homeopathy continues to grow, both in the United States, and worldwide. This trend is supported by the rise in training programs in homeopathy, which in the United States has grown from only three in 1990, to more than twenty by 1997. In addition, a survey of physicians belonging to the American Medical Association conducted in 1997 found that nearly 50 percent of them were interested in receiving training in homeopathy.

"I think homeopathy's future is very bright," Dr. Fry states. "Both in the United States and abroad, it's on an upsurge. More people are studying it all the time, and more patients are investigating it, as well, due to the fact that our regular health care system has such a poor track record in safely and inexpensively treating chronic disease." According to Dr. Fry, the biggest problem currently facing homeopathy is the fact that there aren't enough well-trained homeopaths to meet the demand for it. But with the continued growth in medical conferences devoted to its application, as well as the higher standards in homeopathic training and education that are now resulting from the rise in its popularity, it appears likely that homeopathy will soon be accepted by greater numbers of health care practitioners and patients alike.

RESOURCES

For more information about homeopathy, and referrals to homeopathic practitioners in your area, contact:

National Center for Homeopathy
801 North Fairfax, Suite 306
Alexandria, Virginia 22314
Phone: (703) 548-7790
Fax: (703) 548-7792
Web site: *www.homeopathic.org*
E-mail: info@homeopathic.org

North American Society of Homeopaths (NASH)
1122 East Pike Street, Suite 1122
Seattle, Washington 98122
Phone: (206) 720-7000
Fax: (206) 329-5684
Web site: *www.homeopathy.org*
E-mail: nashinfo@aol.com

For books, tapes, software, and other information about homeopathy, contact:

American Institute of Homeopathy (AIH)
P.O. Box 80178
Valley Forge, Pennsylvania 19484
Phone: (610) 296-3131
(The AIH is the oldest national medical organization in the United States and is comprised of medical doctors, osteopathic physicians, and dentists, all of whom use homeopathy as part of their practice.)

Homeopathic Educational Services
2124B Kittredge Street
Berkeley, California 94704
Phone: (510) 649-0294
Fax: (510) 649-1955

Email: mail@homeopathic.com
Web site: *www.homeopathic.com*

To find a veterinarian who uses homeopathy, contact:

Academy of Veterinary Homeopathy
751 NE 168th Street N
Miami Beach, Florida 33162
Ph: (305) 652-5372 or (305) 652-1590
Fax: (305) 653-7244
Web site: *www.AcadVetHom.org*
E-mail: avh@naturalholistic.com

Additional online resources:

www.homeopathyonline.com
www.lyghtforce.com

RECOMMENDED READING

Bellavite, Paolo, and Andrea Signorini. *Homeopathy: A Frontier in Medical Science.* North Atlantic Books, 1995.

CHAPTER 12

Ayurveda

Ayurvedic medicine, or Ayurveda, along with traditional Chinese medicine, represents one of the oldest complete medical systems in the world. A Sanskrit term meaning "science of life," Ayurveda is indigenous to India, where it has been widely practiced for over five thousand years. According to Vasant Lad, B.A.M.S., M.A.Sc., director of the Ayurvedic Institute in Albuquerque, New Mexico, and one of the foremost exponents of Ayurveda in the United States, the origins of Ayurveda lie in the Vedas, considered by most scholars to be the world's oldest surviving body of literature. "Ayurveda views both health and ill health in holistic terms, combining both medical and metaphysical approaches to promote perfect health and happiness in the life of the individual," Dr. Lad says. "It teaches that every individual is an indivisible, total, unique expression of cosmic consciousness, a microcosm of nature. If a person knows his or her unique nature through studying the teachings of Ayurveda, he or she can establish a balance between body, mind, and consciousness in order to live in harmony and and achieve self-healing."

Each person's capacity for self-healing is basic to Ayurveda's core tenets, which teach that all of humanity is ultimately a manifestation of one Absolute source (*Paramatman*, or pure consciousness). From this perspective, disease is seen as the result of man's ignorance about his essential self, coupled with disharmony between the individual and the laws of nature (*Prakiti*). Ayurvedic care involves far more than merely treating symptoms, offering a treatment protocol that encompasses science, philosophy, and patients' religious beliefs. "Just as everyone has a unique fingerprint, each person has a particular pattern of energy comprised of unique physical, mental, and emotional characteristics which together comprise their own constitution," Dr. Lad explains. "Ayurveda enables one to understand how to create balance within this energy pattern according to one's individual constitution, and provides the tools to make the lifestyle changes necessary to bring about and maintain this balance." This is achieved by various Ayurvedic practices, including *tridosha* (dietary and lifestyle counseling based on one's individual constitution), *pancha karma* (detoxification therapy), meditation, *pranayama* (breathwork), and yoga (see "The Therapies of Ayurvedic Medicine" later in this chapter).

❦ FAST FACTS ❦

Ayurveda is often referred to as "the mother of all healing systems" since it encompasses many of the branches of both conventional and alternative medicine. The disciplines of pediatrics, toxicology, surgery, psychiatry, geriatrics, internal medicine, eugenics, ophthalmology, otolaryngology, and gynecology and obstetrics are all referred to in ancient Ayurvedic texts, as are the principles of diet and nutrition, herbology, bodywork and massage, mind-body medicine, and color and gem therapy.

In addition to being widely practiced in India, Ayurveda is now receiving considerable attention in the United States, Europe, Japan, Russia, South America, and South Africa.

Ayurveda is recognized by the World Health Organization (WHO), which supports research and integration of Ayurveda as part of a comprehensive modern medical approach to health.

In India, there are over a hundred Ayurvedic colleges that grant degrees after five years of training.

Over 300,000 Ayurvedic physicians are represented by the All India Ayur-Veda Congress, India's leading advocacy organization for Ayurvedic medicine.

A number of leading Western research organizations, including the National Institutes of Health and the National Cancer Institute, are now conducting studies on Ayurveda's potential to provide both preventive and therapeutic benefits for a variety of disease conditions, including stress, cancer, premature aging, and cardiovascular disease.

In the United States, the most popular form of Ayurvedic medicine is Maharishi Ayurveda, introduced by Maharishi Mahesh Yogi, founder of the Transcendental Meditation movement. In recent years, however, traditional Ayurveda has also gained increased stature as more Westerners have come to recognize the value of this ancient health care system. 🔥

HISTORY AND ORIGIN
OF AYURVEDIC MEDICINE

According to Dr. Lad, Ayurveda is an all-inclusive system of philosophy, science, and medicine that is primarily based on the *Samkya* (literally meaning "to know truth") philosophy, which elaborates step by step the journey of consciousness into matter and was adhered to by India's ancient spiritually realized seers, known as *rishis*. "Ayurveda evolved from the *rishis'* practical, philosophical, and religious illumination, which was rooted in their understanding of creation," Lad says. "Through intensive meditation and other disciplines, they manifested truth in their daily lives by perceiving how cosmic energy manifests in all living and nonliving things. They also realized that the source of all existence is pure, or cosmic consciousness, which manifests as masculine and feminine energy, called *Shiva* and *Shakti*. For thousands of years, the teachings of the *rishis* were orally passed down from teacher to disciple, before being finally set down in Sanskrit verse, many of which still survive to this day."

The earliest recorded mention of Ayurveda occurs in the Vedas (primarily the Rig and the Atharva Veda), India's most sacred literature, as well as the Upanishads, a body of extensive commentaries that deal with all aspects of human existence. Other Sanskrit texts that mention Ayurveda include the Mahabarata, the Puranas, the Tantras, and the Yoga Shastras. All of these works are held in high regard by followers of Hinduism. Over time, Ayurveda spread beyond its Hindu roots to be used by Buddhists, Jains, and Sikhs, and it is said to form the basis of Tibetan medicine, as well. Many modern-day yogic masters known to the West, including Paramahansa Yogananda, Sri Aurobindo, and Swami Sivananda, have also stressed the value of Ayurveda to their students.

The earliest written specific body of Ayurvedic literature came into being largely due to two physician-sages, Charaka and Sushruta, whose written records became the first textbooks devoted to Ayurvedic principles. These textbooks are still used by students, practitioners, and teachers in Ayurvedic medical schools and colleges throughout India.

Charaka, who taught approximately three thousand years ago, is credited with the discovery that all substances, both organic and inorganic, as well as thoughts and actions, have definite potential or kinetic attributes.

Careful observation led Charaka to categorize twenty basic attributes into ten opposite pairs that function together, such as hot and cold, wet and dry, slow and fast, and so forth. Charaka further taught that the universe as a whole is formed by the interaction of the two most basic opposites, male and female energy, a philosophy much akin to the yin-yang theory that is an essential component of traditional Chinese medicine (see Chapter 13).

Charaka can also be considered one of the earliest proponents of mind-body medicine, due to his insight that thoughts and emotion could directly affect physical health. In prescribing proper care for the heart, for instance, he wrote: "One who wishes to protect the heart, circulatory system and the vital essence should avoid, above all else, the causes leading to mental stress and instability. One should regularly adopt measures that support the heart and vital essence, cleanse the blood vessels, increase knowledge and calm the mind." In advising physicians, he said, "A physician, though well versed in the knowledge and treatment of disease, who does not enter into the heart of the patient with the virtue of light and love, will not be able to heal the patient." Such concepts as these have only become accepted by Western medical science during the last three decades.

Charaka's writings are known as the *Charaka Samhita*. In them Charaka makes clear that illness is usually natural in origin and that the Ayurvedic physician requires great skill, knowledge, and experience in order to make a diagnosis and provide proper treatment. Among the treatment methods Charaka recommended were diet, herbal medicine, and physical manipulation. He also listed over seven hundred plants and their medicinal properties.

Sushruta, who practiced nearly one thousand years after Charaka, is best known for writing Ayurveda's classic text on surgery, the *Sushruta Samhita*. "In his writings, Sushruta anticipated much of modern medicine," Dr. Lad says. "Among the topics that he treated in detail were surgical procedures for knitting broken bones and curing blood-borne disorders, the deleterious effects external trauma can have on vital organs, postmortem dissection, and even techniques of plastic surgery."

Due to the prohibition Hinduism placed on dissecting dead bodies, only a partial understanding of human anatomy existed during Sushruta's time. Even so, during his lifetime over 120 surgical instruments were being employed by Ayurvedic physicians for a variety of operations, and India continued to lead the world in plastic surgery techniques until the late 1700s.

Both the *Charaka Samhita* and the *Sushruta Samhita* continued to be interpreted and revised by later Ayurvedic teachers, but their core teachings remain unaltered to this day. Eventually additional commentaries and supportive texts built on Charaka's and Sushruta's work, including the writings of Madhava and Vagbhata, two other notable Ayurvedic teachers. In all of these works, the goal of medicine is to promote healthy longevity, with emphasis on the lifestyle and diet suited to each person's unique constitution.

Ayurveda's growth in India paralleled the spread and evolution of Hinduism, then began to lose influence following India's subjugation by the British Empire. Today, while numerous Ayurvedic schools still exist in India, the majority of the country's Ayurvedic physicians practice primarily in the villages, due to a lack of government funding and an opposition to Ayurveda by the many Indian physicians trained in allopathic medicine. Ironically, this trend is now starting to be reversed, and an interest in Ayurveda is being rekindled in India, thanks to the growing interest in Ayurveda in the West. As a result, a modern-day version of Ayurveda, including upscale treatment facilities, is now appearing on the subcontinent in tandem with the spread of similar facilities and treatment centers in the United States, Japan, and Europe. According to David Frawley, O.M.D., an American expert in Ayurveda and founder of the American Institute of Vedic Studies, "The interest in the West is helping to revive Ayurveda in India and make it more respectable as an important medical system in its own right, not just a poor alternative for those who do not have access to modern medicine." As research into Ayurveda's ability to treat disease continues around the world, this trend is likely to continue.

THE THERAPIES OF AYURVEDIC MEDICINE

Ayurveda achieves its goals through an integrated healing approach that takes into consideration all aspects of a patient's life. Among the therapies used by Ayurvedic physicians are *pancha karma* (detoxification therapy), *rasayana* (rejuvenation therapy), diet therapy, botanical medicine, yoga, meditation, massage, *pranayama* (breathwork), and *satvajaya* (mental and spiritual hygiene). Used in conjunction with each other, and in the appropriate sequence, the therapies work to improve health by restoring balance, enhancing energy, promoting mental and emotional equanimity, and facilitating greater patient self-awareness.

Pancha Karma *(Detoxification Therapy)*

According to Dr. Lad, Ayurvedic theory holds that beginning any form of treatment without first eliminating the toxins in the patient's system serves only to push the toxins deeper into the body's tissues. "Symptomatic relief of the disease process may result from superficial treatment," he states. "However, if the toxins are not dealt with first, the fundamental cause of the patient's illness will not be affected and therefore the problem will manifest again, either in the same form or perhaps as something more serious." Eliminating and neutralizing toxins is the goal of *pancha karma* (literally "the five karmas" or "actions"). An internal and external preoperative program, known as *purva karma*, or oleation, usually precedes *pancha karma* in order to prepare the body to let go of toxins. "Internal oleation typically lasts three to five days but can continue for longer periods, depending on the patient's individual circumstances," Dr. Lad explains. "Most patients will be asked to drink a small quantity of ghee, or clarified butter, during this time. Ghee creates a thin film that lubricates the inside of the body, allowing toxins lodged in the deep connective tissues to pass freely to the gastrointestinal tract for elimination." Dr. Lad points out that for some patients, such as those with high cholesterol, triglycerides, or blood sugar, ghee is inappropriate, in which case flaxseed oil can be substituted.

Following internal oleation, the patient undergoes a few more days of external oleation in the form of oil massage and induced sweating. "Oil is applied to the entire body with a specific type of massage that helps toxins move toward the gastrointestinal tract, while also softening both the superficial and deep tissues to relieve stress and nourish the nervous system," Dr. Lad explains. "Then the patient spends time in a steam bath to further loosen the toxins and increase their movement toward the GI tract. After three to seven days of these procedures, the patient is ready for the procedures of *pancha karma* itself."

There are five basic components to *pancha karma: vamana, virechana, basti, nasya,* and *rakta moksha.* Depending on the patient's need and constitution, one or more of them will be used to complete the detoxification process. When there is congestion in the lungs or toxins in the stomach, *vamana,* or therapeutic vomiting, may be prescribed to eliminate mucus. Patients may drink one or two glasses of salt water upon arising, or teas made from licorice or calamus root, and then rub their tongues to induce vomiting. "Once the mucus is released, the patient will feel instantly relieved," Dr. Lad notes. "Congestion, wheezing, and breathlessness will disappear and the sinuses will become clear." According to Dr. Lad, therapeutic vomiting is also effective for treating skin disease, chronic asthma, chronic indigestion, diabetes, chronic cold, edema, epilepsy (between attacks), and tonsillitis.

Virechana, or laxative therapy, is used to relieve congestion and eliminate toxins in the small intestine, stomach, spleen, liver, kidneys, and colon. A number of herbs grown in the United States, such as senna leaf taken as a tea, are effective as mild laxatives, as is hot milk to which two tablespoons of ghee have been added. "This aspect of *pancha karma* should be avoided for persons with low digestive fire, acute fever, diarrhea, severe constipation, or bleeding from the rectum or lung cavities," Dr. Lad cautions. "Nor should laxatives be administered in cases of emaciation or weakness, or when the patient suffers from a prolapsed rectum."

Basti, or medicated enema therapy, helps to remove toxins from the colon. Sesame oil, calamus oil, or herbs decocted in liquid are administered in the form of an enema and then retained for a minimum of half an hour before the bowels are evacuated. "*Basti* alleviates constipation, distention, low backache, chronic fever, the common cold, sexual disorders, kidney stones, vomiting, arthritis, gout, hyperacidity, and neck pain, among other conditions," Dr. Lad says.

Nasya, or nasal administration of medication, is used to expel residual toxins in the throat, nose, and sinus cavity, and to improve breathing. Oils, ghee, aloe vera juice, warm milk, or dry herbal powders, such as ginger, gotu kola, calamus powder, or cayenne, are inserted into the nostrils and then slowly massaged, using the little finger. "Nasal massage helps to relax the deeper tissues and can be done every day or anytime a person is under stress," Dr. Lad says. Nasal irrigation with salt water is another form of *nasya* that can be helpful in flushing out congested sinuses.

Rakta moksha, or bloodletting, is the final aspect of *pancha karma*, and is used to purify toxins that have been absorbed in the bloodstream. "Traditionally *rakta moksha* is performed by extracting a small amount of blood from the veins, which helps stimulate detoxification of the blood," Dr. Lad explains. "In the United States, however, this procedure is illegal, so blood-purifying herbs, such as burdock root, aloe vera, or neem are used instead."

In addition to the above procedures, emotional release is also employed as part of the detoxification process. "Ayurveda teaches that we should allow ourselves to let go of all of our emotions, including anger, fear, anxiety, nervousness, jealousy, and greed," Dr. Lad says. "When such emotions are repressed, they cause imbalances that result in disease-causing toxins. Repressed fear, for example, affects the kidneys, while anger affects the liver, and greed and possessiveness affect the heart and spleen. Instead of repressing these emotions, Ayurveda recommends dealing with them by observation and release. When anger appears, for instance, one should be completely aware of it, observing as it unfolds from its beginning to its end. From such observation, one learns more about the nature of anger and therefore becomes better able to release it whenever it arises. All negative emotions can be dealt with in this way. Learning to do so can significantly enhance the physical effects of *pancha karma.*"

Caution: *Pancha karma* is a powerful procedure that requires the guidance of a properly trained Ayurvedic medical staff. It requires close observation and supervision at every stage, including the period after the final stage is completed. "Anyone considering *pancha karma* treatment should be certain that they receive it from someone who is a truly competent Ayurvedic practitioner," Dr. Lad advises, "not just someone with a modest amount of training."

Rasayana *(Rejuvenation Therapy)*

Following the completion of *pancha karma*, the emphasis shifts to patient rejuvenation, known as *rasayana*. As Dr. Lad explains, "*Pancha karma* purifies the body, and *rasayana* then strengthens it by bringing renewal and longevity to the cells. Through *rasayana* therapy the body becomes more robust, and vitality and immune function increase." Like all aspects of Ayurvedic medicine, *rasayana* treats the entire person—body, mind, and spirit. In addition to its physiological benefits, rejuvenation therapy also helps promote increased mental calm and improved spiritual focus and detachment. During this process, which can last from a few days to a month or more, patients are advised to get plenty of rest and to spend time daily practicing meditative or contemplative techniques, as well as following specific dietary and exercise protocols. Usually rejuvenative preparations are also used, such as *ashwagandha, chyavanprash,* or *shatavari.*

Diet Therapy

Like Hippocrates, the father of Western medicine, and practitioners of traditional Chinese medicine, Ayurvedic practitioners regard proper diet as a primary medical therapy. Ayurveda's dietary approach is distinguished by the emphasis placed on matching foods to each person's individual constitution, known as *prakruti*, which is formed by a combination of three basic energies, or *doshas* (see "How Ayurvedic Medicine Works" later in this chapter). "If one understands the constitution and its relationship to the qualities of various foods, then it is possible to select a proper diet," Dr. Lad explains. In this selection process, consideration is given to six categories of taste (sweet, sour, salty, pungent, bitter, and astringent), as well as whether the food is heavy or light, oily or dry, liquid or solid, and hot- or cold-producing. Seasonal dietary recommendations are also made, with each season also characterized by a specific *dosha*. Food quality and freshness are also considered, as is food combining, to prevent meals of foods that are incompatible when eaten together.

Another important consideration is each person's *agni*, or "digestive fire," which Dr. Lad states is necessary for healthy digestion. "In addition, the subtle energy of *agni* transforms the lifeless molecules of food, water, and air into the consciousness of the cell," he says. "For this reason, Ayurveda says that each person is as old as his or her *agni*."

Traditional Ayurvedic texts recognized that diet is dependent on the individual's current needs. While spiritual aspirants are often advised to follow a vegetarian diet regardless of their *dosha*, for others poultry, meats, and fish are allowed, within certain prescribed limits. Many patients experience noticeable improvement in their health simply from adhering to the dietary recommendations appropriate for their *dosha*, and diet therapy is an essential part of all overall Ayurvedic treatment programs.

Botanical Medicine

The use of herbs and herbal tonics is another important aspect of Ayurveda, with botanical medicine comprising a large part of the Ayurvedic pharmacopoeia. A number of herbs valued by Ayurveda for their medicinal properties are also quite common here in the West, including ginger, alfalfa, aloe vera, cardamom, cinnamon, cloves, cayenne pepper, coriander, cumin, licorice, nutmeg, onion, and garlic. Like foods and liquids, Ayurveda classifies herbs according to their *doshic* qualities. They can be used internally as teas, seasonings, tinctures, and tonics, or when appropriate, applied as poultices and pastes.

Caution: Certain Ayurvedic herbal tonics include small amounts of metals, such as silver, based on centuries-old traditions regarding their preparation. Proponents of such formulations stress that the metals are processed in a manner that makes them nontoxic, enhancing the tonics' efficacy. Occasionally, however, cases of metal poisoning following use of such tonics and herbal tablets have occurred, usually from visitors traveling to India. Therefore, if you are considering using Ayurvedic herbal remedies, be sure to purchase them from a reputable supplier. (See the "Resources" section at the end of this chapter.)

Yoga

Perhaps the best-known component of Ayurveda in the West, yoga is a very effective means of maintaining good health and longevity due to its ability to naturally regulate the nervous system, improve muscle tone and flexibility, and enhance respiration. As such, Ayurvedic practitioners regard yoga as an important preventive measure for ensuring optimal health. The most popular form of yoga in the West is known as *hatha yoga*, a system of physical exercises and postures. By combining Ayurvedic principles with yoga, Ayurvedic practitioners are able to prescribe yoga exercises best suited to each individual's constitution, thus improving their effectiveness. (For more on yoga, see Chapter 14.)

Meditation

Dr. Lad describes meditation as "the art of bringing harmony to body, mind, and consciousness. Life with meditation is a flowering of bliss and beauty. Life without it is stress, confusion, and illness." An integral practice to many traditions in the East and Middle East for centuries, the value of meditation has, comparatively speaking, only recently been recognized in the West, where a substantial body of scientific research now attests to its many physiological benefits. As with yoga, there are a variety of meditative techniques that can be practiced. For those unfamiliar with meditation, Dr. Lad suggests the following exercise, which should ideally be performed in the morning prior to the start of your daily activities.

Sit quietly, keeping your spine erect and relaxed. Spend a few moments allowing your eyes to survey your surroundings, listening to any sounds that may be present. As you do so, relax your muscles. After a few moments more, close your eyes and bring your attention inward. Notice the movements of your thoughts, desires, and emotions, without judging them, or attempting to stop or change them. Simply observe their movements as you breathe in a relaxed manner. Try to perform this exercise daily for at least twenty minutes. "Through this internal observation, you become cleansed of distractions," Dr. Lad explains. "You will begin to enjoy increased relaxation, and storehouses of energy will unlock within you." (For more on meditation, see Chapter 5.)

Massage

From the perspective of Ayurveda, the purpose of massage is to help move energy throughout the body and to create and maintain balance among the *doshas*. Typically, Ayurvedic massage is given using various oils that, after being absorbed by the skin, help to remove toxins (see *"Pancha Karma"* earlier in this chapter). Both the massage process and the type of oil used is determined by each person's specific constitution, as well as any disorders that may also be present. Commonly used oils include sesame, sunflower, sandalwood, corn, and calamus root oils. Specific times of day for massage can also be suggested, depending on a person's individual makeup. (For more on massage, see Chapter 9.)

Pranayama *(Breathwork)*

Meaning "to control the breath," *pranayama* refers to various yogic exercises that are intended to promote mental calm and enhance physical energy. "Ayurveda says that breathing is the physical part of thinking and thinking is the psychological part of breathing," Dr. Lad explains. "Every thought changes the rhythm of breath, and every breath changes the rhythm of thinking. When one is happy, blissful, and silent, breathing is rhythmic. If one is disturbed with anxiety, fear, or nervousness, breathing is irregular and interrupted."

According to Dr. Lad, *pranayama* has many healing benefits, including purification of the lungs, heart, and other organs. It is also said to stimulate creativity. Dr. Lad cautions, however, that *pranayama* should not be practiced without the guidance of a trained instructor, since it can create imbalance and contribute to disease if it is done improperly. Different forms of *pranayama* are also suited for individuals of different constitutions.

Satvajaya *(Mental and Spiritual Hygiene)*

Recognizing the connection between physical health and disease to mental, emotional, and spiritual functioning, Ayurvedic treatment also includes techniques for releasing emotional and psychological stress, and healing unconscious, negative beliefs. In addition to meditation (see above), other *satvajaya* methods include *mantram*, a type of sound therapy in which a Sanskrit word or phrase is chanted aloud and then inwardly in order to achieve mental equanimity; *yantra*, a technique in which geometrical images are concentrated upon in order to move beyond ordinary modes of thought; and the use of various gems, metals, and crystals for their subtle vibratory healing properties. Regular practice of *satvajaya* techniques can result in a lessening of habitual prejudices, negative emotions, and limiting thought patterns and beliefs, all of which have been shown to diminish physical health and contribute to disease (see Chapter 5).

HOW AYURVEDIC MEDICINE WORKS

The underlying philosophy of Ayurvedic medicine holds that all of creation is a manifestation of divine or cosmic consciousness and is made up of male and female energies, known respectively as *Purusha* and *Prakruti*. Such concepts are similar to the principles of Tao and yin-yang espoused by traditional Chinese medicine (see Chapter 13). Also like TCM, Ayurveda holds that each of us is a microcosm of the universe, and we share all of the qualities of the cosmos, including the five basic elements present in all matter: space, air, fire, water, and earth. "According to Ayurveda, the five elements manifest sequentially, beginning with space, from the pure, unified, unmanifested cosmic consciousness that is the source of all life," Dr. Lad explains. "Our psychological tendencies, as well as our five senses and the various aspects of how our body functions, are all directly related to these five elements."

Space, which is also referred to as "ether," is associated with sound and hearing, according to Dr. Lad, and manifests in the body in the spaces of the mouth, nose, respiratory and gastrointestinal tracts, abdomen, and thorax. "All of us need space in order to live, move, grow, and communicate," Dr. Lad says. "For this reason, psychologically, space is said to provide freedom, peace, and expansion of consciousness. It is also responsible for love and compassion, as well as feelings of separation, isolation, emptiness, insecurity, anxiety, and fear."

Air represents the principle of movement and controls sensory and neural impulses, the pulsation of the heart, the breathing mechanism of the lungs, the ingestion of food, and the elimination of waste products. "Thought, desire, and will are all governed by the air principle, which is associated with happiness, joy, and excitation," Dr. Lad says. "Along with space, air is also responsible for fear, anxiety, insecurity, and nervousness."

Fire is active and changeable and is produced by the friction caused by air's movement. Mirroring the sun in the solar system, our biological fire resides in the solar plexus and regulates body temperature and metabolism. According to Dr. Lad, fire also corresponds to intelligence and is associated with light and vision. "Attention, comprehension, appreciation, recognition, and understanding are all governed by the fire principle, as are anger, hatred, envy, criticism, ambition, and competitiveness," he says.

Water is associated with the qualities of fluidity, heaviness, softness, viscosity, density, cohesiveness, and coldness. In the body, it exists as plasma, cytoplasm, serum, saliva, cerebrospinal fluid, sweat, urine, and nasal secretion. It also governs thirst and taste, and acts as a universal chemical solvent, while emotionally being associated with contentment, love, and compassion.

Earth, the final and most solid of the five elements, corresponds to physical energy, and gives the body its strength, structure, and stamina. "All of the body's solid structures, such as the bones, cartilage, hair, nails, teeth, and skin, are derived from the earth element," Dr. Lad says. Governing the sense of smell, the earth principle fosters forgiveness, support, growth, and the feeling of being grounded, as well as attachment, greed, and depression.

"Both internally and within our external environment, the proportion and balance of these five elements is forever shifting, changing with the seasons, the weather, the time of day, and the stages of our lives," Dr. Lad says. "In order to be healthy, we have to continuously accommodate ourselves to these changes through what we eat, what we wear, where we live, and so on. Ayurveda provides the tools for understanding and properly responding to this balancing act, which plays the elements against each other, so that health and longevity are assured."

The Three Doshas

According to Ayurveda, the five elements above form three basic energies, or humors, that are present in varying degrees in all living things. Known as the three *doshas* (or *tridosha*)—*vata, pitta,* and *kapha*—these elements govern all human physiological and psychological functions and must be maintained in a proper state of balance in order for health to be present. The concept of the three *doshas* is a unique aspect of Ayurvedic theory. "The *doshas* are responsible for the huge variety of individual differences and preferences, and influence all we are and do, from the foods we like to how we relate to others," Dr. Lad explains. "In addition, they regulate the creation, maintenance, and destruction of bodily tissue, and the elimination of waste products, and also govern our emotions."

Ayurvedic theory holds that each person's individual constitution, or *prakruti*, is based on the particular pattern of *doshic* qualities he or she is born with. Generally speaking, there are seven Ayurvedic constitutional types: *vata, pitta, kapha, vata-pitta, pitta-kapha, vata-kapha*, and *vata-pitta-kapha*, with numerous subtler variations that are determined by the percentage of each *dosha* that each person has. "All three *doshas* are present in each human being," Dr. Lad says, "but one of them is usually primary, one secondary, and the third least prominent. Thus, each person has a particular pattern of energy and an individual combination of physical, mental, and emotional characteristics that make up his or her constitution. Health depends on maintaining this proportion in balance."

Vata, which is formed by the elements of space and air, relates to the energy of movement and each person's vital life essence, known in Ayurveda as *prana*. As such, *vata* is said to regulate all physiological and psychological activites, including respiration, heartbeat, and all movement within the cytoplasm and cell membranes. On the emotional level, *vata* in balance enhances creativity and promotes feelings of happiness and joy, while *vata* out of balance contributes to fear, nervousness, and anxiety.

Pitta is formed by the elements fire and water and generates the energy of metabolism, governing all of the body's biochemical changes, such as digestion, absorption, assimilation, and body temperature, as well as promoting appetite and vitality. "*Pitta* governs not only our physical metabolism, but also the way we process, or digest, every outside impression that we encounter," Dr. Lad says. "Thus, when in balance, *pitta* promotes intelligence and understanding and is crucial for learning. But when *pitta* is out of balance it can arouse the fiery emotions, such as anger, hatred, criticism, and jealousy."

Kapha, which is formed by water and earth, is the energy of structure, forming the body and holding its cells together, and proper fluid balance. *Kapha* maintains immunity and provides strength and physiological stability, and supplies the liquid necessary for the proper functioning of all of the body's systems. According to Dr. Lad, when *kapha* is in balance, it is expressed as love, calmness, and forgiveness, while an imbalance can result in attachment, lust, envy, and greed.

"The three *doshas*, acting together, govern all of the body's metabolic activities," Dr. Lad explains. "*Kapha* promotes anabolic activities, which include the growth and creation of new cells as well as cell repair. *Pitta* regulates metabolism by governing digestion and absorption, and *vata* triggers the catabolic process that is necessary for breaking down larger molecules into smaller ones. Since *vata* is the principle of movement, it acts on both *pitta* and *kapha*, which are both otherwise immobile. Therefore, when *vata* is out of balance, it influences and disturbs the other *doshas*, which is why the majority of all illnesses have aggravated *vata* at their source."

Ayurveda also divides the human life span into three *doshic* sections, with birth to age sixteen called the age of *kapha*, the years from sixteen to fifty called the age of *pitta*, and the years from fifty and beyond known as the age of *vata*. "Childhood is the time of the greatest physical growth and structuring of the body, which are *kapha*, or anabolic, processes," Dr. Lad says. "In the prime of adulthood, the *pitta* traits of activity and vitality are most apparent, while in old age, the *vata*, or catabolic, processes of deterioration start to take hold."

By determining their patients' *doshic* constitution and providing guidelines for keeping each *dosha* in balance, both internally and in response to seasonal and other changes in the environment, Ayurvedic physicians are able to treat the entire person in a manner that ensures health in body, mind, and spirit.

❧ IDENTIFYING YOUR DOSHA ❧

The following traits can help you determine which *dosha* primarily makes up your individual constitution. Determining the specific nature of your constitution may require the assistance of a trained Ayurvedic practitioner, however.

Vata physical traits include thin body frame; low body weight; skin that is dry, cool, rough, and dark; black, dry, kinky hair; small, dry, brown, or black eyes; and large teeth, that can also be crooked or protruding. *Vata* persons tend to be hyperactive, vivacious, moody, enthusiastic, and intuitive, and have a propensity for eating and sleeping at all hours of the day and night. They are predisposed to nervousness, anxiety, cramps, and constipation.

Pitta physical traits include a medium build and moderate weight; skin that is soft, oily, warm, and fair; soft, oily, blonde, reddish, or prematurely gray hair; moderate-sized, yellowish teeth and soft gums; and penetrating eyes that are green, gray, or yellow in color. *Pitta* people are perfectionists, orderly and efficient, have a short temper, are punctual by nature and "ruled by the clock," intense, loving, passionate, and articulate. They are prone to suffer from ulcers, heartburn, hemorrhoids, and acne.

Kapha physical traits include a thick, heavyset build; skin that is oily, cool, and pale; thick, wavy hair that can be dark or light; strong, white teeth; and eyes that are big, attractive, and blue, with thick eyelashes. *Kapha* people are slow to anger; tend to procrastinate; show affection easily; have a relaxed manner; are forgiving, compassionate, and tolerant; sleep long and deeply; and eat slowly. They are predisposed to obesity, high cholesterol, allergies, and sinus and respiratory conditions. 🔥

The Twenty Basic Attributes

In addition to the five elements and the three *doshas*, Ayurvedic theory emphasizes the importance of twenty fundamental attributes, or qualities, that are also found throughout creation. First codified by the physician-sage Charaka, each of these attributes is paired with its opposite, representing what Dr. Lad describes as "the extreme on a continuum." The twenty basic attributes are: heavy and light, soft and hard, oily and dry, stable and mobile, slimy and rough, gross and subtle, cold and hot, slow and sharp, dense and liquid, and cloudy and clear. "These attributes are present everywhere in the world around us, and within us, as well," Dr. Lad points out. "They can be observed in the weather, the foods we eat, the feel of our skin, and even our thoughts and moods. Moreover, we are constantly being affected by changes in these qualities."

According to Dr. Lad, each pair of attributes influences one another according to two basic Ayurvedic principles: *like increases like*, and *opposites decrease each other.* "These principles are part of the key to Ayurvedic healing," Dr. Lad says. "Whenever an imbalance occurs, successful treatment requires increasing the opposite qualites in order to restore harmony and balance. For instance, if too much heat is present, which is an excessive *pitta* attribute, a person will benefit from a cool drink or herbs with cooling properties, rather than staying in the sun or eating spicy foods. To a great extent, Ayurvedic treatment involves identifying a person's disease in terms of these basic attributes, and then setting right any imbalances that are present."

The Three Universal Qualities

According to Ayurveda, corresponding to the three *doshas* that make up each person's physical constitution are three universal qualities, or *gunas*, that serve as the basis for the differences in human temperament and psychological and moral dispositions. They are *satva, rajas,* and *tamas. Satva* is associated with stability, purity, wakefulness, understanding, clarity, and light. *Satva* also oversees the five senses and their corresponding organs, as well as the hands, mouth, feet, reproductive organs, and organs of excretion. *Rajas* is associated with dynamic movement, extroversion, aggressiveness, and emotions, and is said to govern the movements of the sensory and motor organs. *Tamas* is associated with inertia, dullness, confusion, and ignorance, and is said to give rise to the five elements.

According to Dr. Lad, these three subtle energies predispose a person's temperament, behavior, and life interests. "People of *satvic* temperament tend to have healthy bodies and their behavior and consciousness are very pure," he says. "They also tend to be very religious people. People of *rajas* temperament, on the other hand, are usually extroverted and interested in business, prosperity, power, and prestige. They can also be very political and enjoy wealth. People who are *tamasic* tend to be very egotistical and disrespectful of others, as well as being lazy and selfish. All three of these qualities can be modified to enhance well-being, which is one of the goals of Ayurvedic physicians. By carefully observing their patients, they can determine which *guna* is predominant and guide them toward a more balanced way of life, thereby improving their health."

Ayurvedic Theory of Disease

To fully understand how Ayurveda works, consideration must also be given to the Ayurvedic theory of the disease process. Like holistic medicine in general, Ayurveda does not view health as merely the absence of disease, but rather an optimal balance between body, mind, and spirit. For true health to occur there must be a balance among the *doshas,* the five elements, the basic attributes, and the *gunas* outlined above, as well as in the basic body tissues (*dhatus*), the three wastes (sweat, urine, and feces, referred to in Ayurveda as *malas*), and *agni* (digestive fire).

Ayurveda identifies seven *dhatus,* or basic body tissues: plasma and cytoplasm (*rasa*), blood (*rakta*), muscle (*mamsa*), fat (*meda*), bone and cartilage (*ashti*), bone marrow and nerves (*majja*), and the male and female reproductive tissues (*shukra* and *artava*). According to Dr. Lad, each *dhatu* is dependent on the one preceding it, and if there is a problem in any of them, those succeeding it will not receive proper nourishment and their respective tissues or organ systems may become impaired.

Proper production and elimination of the body's waste products are also vital to good health, as is healthy *agni*, the digestive fire that governs metabolism. "*Agni* maintains the nutrition of the body's tissues, as well as the strength of the body's immune system," Dr. Lad explains. "It destroys microorganisms, foreign bacteria, and toxins in the stomach and intestines. When *agni* is impaired due to an imbalance in the *doshas*, metabolism is adversely affected, lowering the body's resistance."

Recognizing that illness is not a random, sudden event, but the result of imbalances that occur over time, Ayurveda lists ten causative factors that contribute to disease. The first of these is the principle that "*like increases like*," meaning that each *dosha* can become aggravated by experiences and influences with qualities similar in nature to itself. For example, according to Dr. Lad, dry foods and fruit, excessive work, and being in a rush, which are all *vatic* in nature, aggravate *vata* in the system. In order to prevent and treat illness, therefore, Ayurvedic practitioners seek to balance each *dosha* with qualities that are its opposite.

Food and diet make up the second factor Ayurveda associates with health and disease. The underlying principle here is that following a diet that is appropriate to one's individual constitution helps to maintain health and vitality, while eating inappropriate foods over time can set the stage for disease.

The seasons play a role in health and disease, as well, and according to Ayurveda also have their predominant *dosha*. Autumn is considered to be primarily a *vata* period, while winter and early spring are considered *kapha*, and late spring and summer are times when *pitta* is predominant. "Each season brings its own challenges to health," Dr. Lad says. "The predominant *dosha* of each season tends to build up at that time and can cause aggravation, especially in someone of the same *doshic* nature."

Exercise is another factor that influences health and disease, with regular exercise that is appropriate for each person's specific constitution being advised for all people. Once again, balance is important, since too much exercise, like not enough exercise, can cause *doshic* imbalance. Dr. Lad recommends yoga stretches and aerobic exercise for all body types, but cautions that the amount and intensity of your exercise program should be based upon your individual constitution.

Age also plays a role in a person's health and illness. As mentioned above, Ayurveda divides the human life span into *kapha* (childhood), *pitta* (adulthood), and *vata* (old age) periods, with disease conditions with the same *doshic* qualities being most common for each life stage. Ayurveda teaches that awareness of the nature of each stage of life, as well as the diseases that are most common to it, can help keep the *doshas* in balance and maintain health.

Mental and emotional factors also influence health, as modern science is now confirming. "Both health and disease have psychological as well as physiological origins," Dr. Lad says. "Illness may begin in the mind and emotions and then affect the body, just as physical imbalances can generate mental disorders. Because of this, mind and body are never separated in Ayurveda."

Stress is another causal factor in the disease process. According to Ayurveda, stress disturbs the *doshas* and can lead to conditions associated with the particular *dosha* that is most aggravated.

Improper use of the senses can produce effects similar to stress. Ayurveda teaches that the senses can be overused, underused, or misused. "Overuse of the senses strains and stresses the nervous system," Dr. Lad explains, "while underuse, such as not paying attention or ignoring what we are perceiving, can lead to accidents. Misuse of the senses means using them in a wrong way, such as overeating or reading while lying down, which changes the angle of focus and builds up stress on the muscles of the eye."

Disregard of what we know can also cause disease, including failure to heed our intuition and inner wisdom. One example of this is ignoring the dietary recommendations for one's *doshic* body type. "For example," Dr. Lad says, "if a person who knows that her constitution is predominantly *pitta* decides to eat hot spicy food for lunch and then spends the rest of the summer afternoon working in the sun, she is disregarding her intelligence and asking for trouble."

Relationships are the final factor that influences both health and disease. "When clarity is lacking, feelings are repressed, or communication is absent in our relationships, stress builds up, disrupting our inner biochemistry and throwing the *doshas* out of balance, thus sowing the seeds of disease," Dr. Lad says. "When a negative emotion comes up in a relationship, pay attention to the feeling, without judging yourself or the other person. Or when someone close to you provokes feelings of hurt or anger, look inside to see what your thoughts and feelings are saying to you. By being honest, you achieve clarity, which will help you develop compassion and love."

Dr. Lad points out that contemplation of each of the ten factors above reveals that all of us have a great deal of choice and control over whether they will create a disease-producing imbalance in our lives. "This is true even of such apparently uncontrollable factors as the seasons and the weather," he says. "If it is cold, you can dress warmly. If it is hot, you can take it easy and stay out of the sun."

When these factors are ignored, however, disease will inevitably result, occurring over a six-stage process, which Ayurveda identifies as accumulation, aggravation, spread, infiltration, manifestation, and cellular deformity leading to structural distortion. According to Dr. Lad, due to the various factors outlined above, the *doshas* begin to accumulate in their respective body sites, with *vata* accumulating in the colon, *pitta* in the intestines, and *kapha* in the stomach. "This is the easiest stage at which to treat any incipient problem, since the person is still quite healthy," Dr. Lad says.

Aggravation occurs as the accumulated *doshas* keep building up within their respective body organs and attempt to move beyond them. In these two initial stages, according to Dr. Lad, one can often reverse this process simply by using common sense and applying the principle of opposite qualities. "But once the disease process has gone beyond the gastrointestinal tract and entered the third phase, it is no longer under one's own control, and trained medical help is needed," he says.

Once past the gastrointestinal tract, the process spreads into the bloodstream, searching for a place to take hold. "At this stage," Dr. Lad says, "the disease process has progressed to the point where eliminating the initial cause will not be enough. A *pancha karma* or similar purification program is needed in order to return the *doshas* to their respective sites in the GI tract so that they can be excreted from the body."

Failure to stop the the third stage of the disease process can result in the aggravated *dosha* entering an organ, tissue, or body system that is already weak or defective. "The newly arrived, aggravated *dosha* creates confusion within the cellular intelligence of the weaker tissue and overwhelms it, changing its normal qualities and functions as it combines with it to create an altered state," Dr. Lad explains. "If the condition is not interrupted at this stage, it will erupt as a full-blown disease."

During the fifth, or manifestation, stage, the seeds of disease have now sprouted and the person becomes sick, with symptoms that are far more pronounced and noticeable. If proper treatment is not provided at this stage, the final part of the process occurs as the disease fully develops. Now structural changes begin to appear, as well as complications to other tissues, organs, or body systems. "Function has already begun to be disturbed during the manifestation stage," Dr. Lad says, "but in this final stage, the structure of the tissue itself is affected, as well as surrounding tissues and systems. For example, in the fifth stage, aggravated *pitta* invading the stomach wall may manifest as an ulcer, but in the sixth stage, the *pitta* will perforate the ulcer and can cause hemorrhaging or provoke a tumor, making treatment far more difficult."

Because restoration of normal body function and balance is far easier during the earlier stages of this process, Ayurveda emphasizes prevention and awareness. "Awareness is the key," Dr. Lad points out. "The more you are alert to how your mind, body, and emotions are reacting to changing circumstances in your life, and the more aware you are of your specific constitution and your moment-to-moment health choices, the less opportunity you create for becoming sick."

CONDITIONS THAT BENEFIT FROM AYURVEDIC MEDICINE

Like a number of other therapies comprising the field of holistic medicine, Ayurveda's primary goal is to maintain harmony and balance in body, mind, and spirit, rather than treating specific disease conditions. Nonetheless, its ability to restore imbalances in the *doshas, gunas, dhatus,* and the other qualities and attributes outlined above theoretically makes Ayurvedic medicine a suitable primary or adjunctive treatment for the majority of illnesses. Although in recent years there have been a number of Western scientific studies involving Ayurvedic procedures and herbal formulas, additional research is needed before the full extent of Ayurveda's efficacy in treating illness can be known. In the meantime, preliminary findings indicate that there is much that this ancient healing system can contribute to modern-day treatment and prevention of disease. In *The Complete Book of Ayurvedic Home Remedies,* Dr. Lad lists over one hundred disease conditions that respond to Ayurvedic protocols, based on his own clinical experience. These conditions range from allergies, backache, colds and flu, and respiratory conditions, to gastrointestinal disorders, genitourinary conditions, PMS, stress, depression, and chronic fatigue. Other illnesses that research indicates Ayurvedic therapies can provide benefits for are aging, addiction, anxiety, asthma, cardiovascular disease, hypertension, hepatitis, vision problems, and scabies.

Aging

According to Dr. Lad, maintaining *doshic* balance and harmony is vital for ensuring cellular health and promoting longevity, making Ayurveda an effective therapy for slowing down the aging process. Meditation and mental/emotional self-observation, both essential components of Ayurveda (see "Therapies of Ayurvedic Medicine" earlier in this chapter), have also been shown to beneficially affect the aging process and extend longevity. One study of nursing home residents, for example, showed that patients who meditated regularly or practiced being aware of their emotions and daily actions lived longer and had better physiological and cognitive abilities than patients who received only conventional nursing home treatment. After three years, all patients in the meditation group were still alive, as were nearly 90 percent of those who practiced emotional awareness, compared to a lower percentage among the control group.

Addiction

Ayurveda recognizes that addiction is both psychological and physiological in nature, and its inherent mind-body approach to healing makes it effective for treating substance abuse. "Treatment depends on how serious and long-standing the addiction is," Dr. Lad says. For serious cases of addiction, a gradual dose reduction of the addictive substance is advised, rather than abrupt and complete cessation, in order to avoid the withdrawal symptoms that so often result in relapse. In conjunction with this approach, Ayurvedic physicians will usually prescribe a *pancha karma* program to cleanse and strengthen the affected organ systems, as well as diet therapy, appropriate herbal remedies, exercise, and meditation, which has also been shown to minimize the effects of stress during withdrawal, and to promote increased self-esteem.

Anxiety

According to Dr. Lad, anxiety is primarily due to aggravated *vata* in the nervous system. By employing massage, meditation, herbal teas, diet therapy, and yoga, most nonserious cases of anxiety can be successfully treated by Ayurvedic physicians, with the additional benefit that patients are empowered to continue these measures on their own, resulting in a lasting, effective self-care protocol.

Asthma

Pancha karma, diet therapy, yoga, and meditation are all useful components of Ayurveda for treating asthma and other respiratory conditions. Recent research also shows that *Boswellia serrata*, a commonly prescribed

Ayurvedic herbal remedy, is effective for treating bronchial asthma. In one double-blind, placebo-controlled study of forty patients who suffered with chronic bronchial asthma for between three to fifteen years, *Boswellia* was able to provide significant improvement in symptoms or complete relief in 70 percent of patients after only six weeks, compared to only 27 percent of subjects who experienced relief in the control group.

Cardiovascular Disease

A number of Ayurvedic remedies have shown potential as cardiovascular enhancers due to their antioxidant properties and ability to lower cholesterol levels. The Ayurvedic tonic *Amla* (Indian gooseberry), for instance, has been shown to reduce LDL cholesterol levels. A number of other Ayurvedic herbs, including *Terminalia arjuna, Inula racemosa,* and *Crataegus oxycantha,* have also been shown to promote cardiovascular health and to act as effective cardiacal tonics for angina, arrhythmia, ischemic heart disease, myocardial infarction, congestive heart failure, and high LDL levels. Two Maharishi Ayur-Veda herbal mixtures, MAK-4 and MAK-5, have also been shown to provide benefit for persons suffering from atherosclerosis (hardening of the arteries), due to their ability to prevent oxidation of LDL cholesterol.

Hypertension

According to Dr. Lad, hypertension, or high blood pressure, can be *vata, pitta,* or *kapha* in nature. "*Vata* is responsible for constriction of the blood vessels," Dr. Lad says. "*Pitta* is responsible for the rushing of the blood with more force, and *kapha* is related to increased blood viscosity." Ayurvedic physicians treat hypertension using diet therapy, botanical medicine, relaxation exercises, *pranayama,* meditation, and yoga, tailoring a treatment program to the condition's *doshic* qualities. Meditation alone has also been shown to be effective for significantly lowering blood pressure levels in persons with mild hypertension. One study of over one hundred older African American men and women found that regular practice of Transcendental Meditation (TM) resulted in far greater improvement in blood pressure levels than either progressive relaxation techniques or lifestyle modification. It has also been shown that people who meditate generally have lower blood pressure levels than the general population.

Hepatitis

In a preliminary study of sixty people carrying the hepatitis B virus, the Ayurvedic herbal remedy *Phyllanthus amarus* was shown to eliminate the virus completely in 59 percent of a test group of thirty-seven carriers, compared to only 4 percent within the control group. Thus far, however, additional studies have been unable to replicate such a result, suggesting a need for further research.

Vision

In a double-blind, placebo-controlled clinical trial 157 patients suffering from a variety of vision disorders, including cataract, dry eye syndrome, astigmatism, myopia, and allergic conjunctivitis, improved following treatment with an Ayurvedic herbal eye drop preparation, leading researchers who conducted the study to cite the preparation as "a useful drug in all conditions studied."

Scabies

Scabies is a highly contagious condition caused by mites beneath the skin, resulting in infection and itching. It is most commonly spread in schools, nursing homes, and barracks, and in the United States is primarily treated with lotions and shampoos that, although considered safe, contain ingredients similar in nature to DDT, a banned pesticide. As an alternative to such treatments, research has shown that a topical paste made from the traditional Ayurvedic remedies neem and turmeric is an effective alternative without risks of side effects or toxicity. One study in India, for instance, involving over eight hundred people with scabies, resulted in a complete cure in 97 percent of cases without any adverse effects.

Other studies have found that Ayurvedic medicine and its various components can be effective in treating diabetes, allergy, and kidney and liver disorders, and to provide antibacterial and antioxidant benefits, as well as stimulating immune enhancement, increased blood flow to the brain, and improved hormone-related neurological functioning.

DIAGNOSIS AND TREATMENT

"In the West, the term *diagnosis* generally refers to identification of disease after it has manifested," Dr. Lad says. "In Ayurveda, however, the concept of diagnosis implies a moment-to-moment monitoring of the interactions between order and disorder in the body. Symptoms of disease are always related to derangement of the balance of the *doshas*. Once the nature of the imbalance is understood, health can be reestablished through proper treatment."

A variety of Ayurvedic techniques enable skilled practitioners to detect early signs of imbalance before the disease process actually manifests. Through their use, Ayurvedic physicians are able to detect signs of disease early on, before they become overt, enabling them to prescribe preventive measures that can keep the illness from progressing. Among the techniques employed by practitioners of Ayurveda are diagnosis of the pulse, tongue, face, eyes, lips, nails, and urine.

Pulse Diagnosis

According to Dr. Lad, both a person's constitution and the status of his or her bodily organs can be determined through pulse diagnosis. "The beats of the pulse not only correspond to the heartbeat, they also indicate the status of the *pranic*, or vital energy, current circulating through the blood to each of the vital organs. By feeling the superficial and deep pulsations, skilled practitioners can determine the condition of these organs, including their *doshic* qualities."

While facing the patient, the practitioner will take the pulse of both wrists, using the index, middle, and ring fingers. The pulse may also be checked at the temporal artery, just above the temple on the side of the head; the carotid artery on the neck, just above the clavicle; the brachial artery, inside the arm and above the elbow; the femoral artery, inside the front of the leg where it meets the pelvis; the posterior tibial artery, just behind the ankle; and the dorsalis pedis artery, on the top of the foot.

"Each finger rests on a meridian (energetic pathway) of the element associated with the *dosha* of that part of the body," Dr. Lad explains. "For example, the index finger, which rests on the *vata dosha*, detects bodily air, while the middle finger, which rests on the *pitta dosha*, detects fire. The ring finger, which feels the *kapha* pulse, detects water. When *vata* is predominant in the patient's constitution, the index finger will feel the pulse strongly, indicating aggravated *vata*. Aggravated *pitta* will be felt in the middle finger, while aggravated *kapha* is felt by the ring finger."

Additionally, superficial, or light, touch on the right wrist allows the practitioner to determine the condition of the large intestine, gallbladder, and pericardium; while superficial touch of the left wrist reveals the status of the small intestine, stomach, and bladder. Deep touch of the right wrist reveals the status of the lung, liver, and the body's *vata-pitta-kapha* relationship. Deep touch of the left wrist reveals the condition of the heart, spleen, and kidney.

Dr. Lad advises that the pulse should not be checked after eating or consuming alcohol, hard physical labor, sex, massage, sunbathing, sitting close to a fire, during a bath, or while the patient is hungry, all of which can temporarily alter the pulse rate, making for an inaccurate reading.

Tongue Diagnosis

According to Ayurvedic theory, different parts of the tongue are related to different organs in the body, and the tongue's size, shape, contour, surface, margins, and color all provide indications of a person's health. "If there are discolorations, depressions, or elevations on certain areas of the tongue, the organs corresponding to those areas are defective," Dr. Lad explains. "For example, impressions of the teeth along the margin of the tongue indicate poor intestinal absorption, while a coating covering the tongue indicates toxins in the stomach or intestines." *Doshic* imbalances within the body's organs and bodily tissues can also be determined by tongue diagnosis, as can a person's mental/emotional state to a certain degree.

Facial Diagnosis

The face also reveals the condition of a person's health to skilled Ayurvedic practitioners. "The face is the mirror of the mind, and its lines and wrinkles are very revealing," Dr. Lad states. "Horizontal wrinkling on the forehead, for example, is an indication of deep-seated worries and anxieties, while vertical lines between the eyebrows reveals emotions that are being held by the liver and spleen. The status of the organs can also be revealed by observing the face. Lower eyelids that are full and puffy indicate that the kidneys are impaired, for instance."

Eye Diagnosis

Ayurveda holds that a person's eyes can also provide an indication of his or her health status and individual constitution. According to Dr. Lad, small eyes indicate a preponderance of *vata* in the body, as do frequent blinking, drooping eyelids, and dry or scanty eyelids. When *pitta* is dominant in the body, the eyes tend to be moderate in size, sharp, lustrous, and sensitive to light. The eyes of a person with a preponderance of *kapha*, by contrast, tend to be large, beautiful, and moist, with long, thick lashes. Examination of the color, size, and shape of the iris is also part of Ayurvedic eye diagnosis.

Lip Diagnosis

The lips are another indicator of health and personal constitution and are examined by Ayurvedic practitioners according to size, shape, surface, color, and contour. According to Dr. Lad, thin, dry lips are *vata*; red lips correspond with *pitta*; and lips that are thick and oily correspond with *kapha*. The condition of the lips can also provide clues to specific health conditions. For example, dry or cracked lips signify dehydration and likely *vata* imbalance, while pale lips are often a sign of anemia.

Nail Diagnosis

"According to Ayurveda, the nails are a waste product of the bones," Dr. Lad says. During diagnosis, Ayurvedic practitioners examine the size, shape, surface, and contour of the patient's nails, and note their condition. "If the nails are dry, crooked, rough, and break easily, *vata* predominates in the body," Dr. Lad says. "If they are soft, pink, tender, and easily bent, *pitta* predominates. When they are thick, strong, soft, and very shiny with a uniform contour, then *kapha* predominates."

Nail color and condition serve as indicators of particular disease conditions, as well. For example, pale nails indicate anemia, yellow nails are a sign of a possible liver disorder, while blue nails may signify a delicate heart or lungs. Longitudinal striations usually indicate malabsorption of nutrients, while a stepped surface running horizontally along the nails often denotes malnutrition.

Each nail and thumb also corresponds to an organ of the body, according to Dr. Lad. "The thumbnail is related to the brain and skull, the index finger corresponds to the lungs, the middle finger relates to the small intestines, the ring finger is associated with the kidneys, and the little finger relates to the heart," he says. "Thus, to an Ayurvedic physician, spots, striations, and other abnormalities in the nail of a specific finger can often reveal an imbalance in the organ the finger corresponds to."

Urine Diagnosis

Just as conventional medicine often employs urinalysis to determine a patient's health status, Ayurvedic physicians also diagnose urine to help determine the health of their patients. Dark yellow urine indicates a *pitta* disorder, according to Dr. Lad, whereas cloudy urine is a sign of aggravated *kapha*, and urine that is brownish-black signifies a *vata* imbalance. The odor of urine is also significant. "If urine has a foul odor, this indicates that there are toxins in the system," Dr. Lad says. "An overly sweet smell, on the other hand, could be a possible sign of diabetes, while urine that has an acidic odor and is accompanied by a burning sensation indicates excess *pitta*."

In addition to the above methods of diagnosis, Ayurvedic physicians at times also employ palpation, auscultation (listening for sounds within the body, as with a stethoscope), a patient interview or questionnaire, and diagnoses of saliva, sweat, and stool samples. Once a proper diagnosis has been made, an appropriate treatment plan is implemented based on the patient's constitution, the present condition of the *doshas* in the body, and the cause or causes of the illness, such as diet, lifestyle, mental/emotional patterns, or genetic predisposition.

"The first line of treatment is to remove the cause of the disease," Dr. Lad says. "In conjunction with that, the practitioner will prepare the proper regimen of treatment, which can include diet, exercise, *pranayama*, and so forth, according to the patient's specific needs, as well as the time of year, the climate, and the patient's age." The treatment protocol begins with a period of detoxification, then proceeds to a rejuvenation program, as outlined earlier in this chapter in "The Therapies of Ayurvedic Medicine."

HEALING CHRONIC ILLNESS: 🌾 A CASE HISTORY 🌾

The following case history illustrates Ayurveda's potential for treating chronic illness. A forty-two-year-old woman came to Ayurvedic practitioner and herbalist Candis Cantin Packard, of Placerville, California, suffering from a variety of chronic conditions that left her weak and debilitated. According to Packard, the woman's condition had begun three years earlier, following a knee operation, during which time she had received "dozens of anesthetics, gone into shock, and almost died." In addition, she had also lost twenty pounds and felt that she had never recovered from the trauma of her ordeal.

During her initial consultation, the woman revealed that she had once suffered from colitis and that it had begun to flare up again, although less severely than before. In addition, due to various drug therapies to help her mother's pregnancy, the woman had been born with a double uterus, a weak kidney, and an appendix on the wrong side of her body. "She also suffered from stomach bloating, arthritis in her left hand, anxiety attacks, shortness of breath, heart palpitations, allergies, eczema, and vaginal yeast infection," Packard says. "Prior to coming to me, she was taking birth control pills, antihistamines, and Motrin for her arthritis pain, and had recently begun a regimen of wheat grass juice and antioxidant vitamins."

As she examined her, Packard paid attention to the fact that the woman was of medium build, with fair skin, hair, and eyes, and observed that she seemed very driven, ambitious, and had a strong will. "Her pulse was quite weak, but had a slight 'jumping' quality to it," Packard explains. "The sides of her tongue were very red, indicating heat in her liver and gallbladder, and the back of her tongue was coated yellow, which indicated heat in her intestines or colon." Based on this diagnosis, Packard determined that the woman's basic constitution was predominantly *pitta*, with secondary *vata* and *kapha*, and that her current condition was due to aggravated *vata* and *pitta*. "Among the signs that pointed to *vata* were her anxiety, heart palpitations, bone problems, spasms in the colon, arthritis, and shortness of breath; while her *pitta*-provoked symptoms were her colitis, allergies, and vaginal infection," Packard says.

Packard put the woman on a diet that would pacify *pitta*, and suggested a *vata*-pacifying lifestyle. "Her meals were to be taken at regular hours and never skipped," Packard says. "And she was to go to bed no later than 10 P.M., and avoid watching the news or reading anything that might arouse turbulent emotions. I also had her massage her feet each night with a mixture of sesame and lavender oils to promote calm, as well as using a herbal pillow stuffed with calming herbs. In addition, I eliminated all alcohol from her diet, along with white sugar, all dairy products, and yeasted breads. In order to rebuild healthy flora in her intestinal tract and vaginal region, I recommended acidophilus supplements three times a day, and instructed her in the use of a herbal vaginal douche, followed by a second douche containing acidophilus whenever she experienced a yeast infection."

Packard also dealt with the woman's arthritic hand, which her physician had instructed her to ice daily. "All the ice was doing was stopping the flow of healing blood to the hand," Packard says. "Instead of this, I instructed her in the Chinese healing method of moxibustion (see Chapter 13) in order to warm the area and break down any blockages. This was followed by the application of warming liniment on the hand."

Lastly, Packard prepared specific herbal remedies in the form of capsules and teas, in order to detoxify and rejuvenate the woman's liver and gallbladder. "I also had her take two capsules of amalaki, one of the herbs in the triphala compound, each night before bed, which is excellent for bleeding disorders, colitis, palpitations, and general debility, and useful for regenerating *pitta*," Packard says. "She drank half a cup of aloe vera juice twice a day, as well. For her arthritis, she took a herbal formula three times a day, and before retiring drank a relaxing tea containing a mixture of nervine herbs."

One month after her session with Packard, the woman phoned to say that her arthritis was much improved and that she no longer suffered from anxiety attacks. She was also sleeping better, passing solid stools, and free of her vaginal infection. "By following my recommendations, she was able to return to work full-time," Packard reports. "This has been a strain on her, but she now rests during her times off and believes she now knows how to conduct her life in a way that allows her healing process to continue." 🌿

YOUR FIRST SESSION

Since the goal of Ayurveda is a tailor-made treatment plan that meets the needs of each patient's constitution and presenting condition, initial visits to Ayurvedic practitioners typically last an hour or more, so that a complete patient history and diagnosis can be made. During your first visit, expect to have your pulse taken, both at your wrists and possibly other areas of your body, as well as an examination of your tongue. Diagnoses of your eyes, face, lips, nails, and urine may also occur, as well as conventional diagnostic measures if the practitioner you select is also a holistic physician. A comprehensive questionnaire or interview regarding your dietary and sleeping habits, lifestyle, and the nature of your eliminations will also be part of your first visit, so that your practitioner can most accurately determine your predominant *dosha* as well as whatever *doshic* imbalances are contributing to your current condition.

Following the diagnosis process, your practitioner will most likely recommend specific dietary and lifestyle measures that are appropriate for you. These recommendations should be adhered to if you expect to fully benefit from your treatment. Botanical remedies or other supplements may also be prescribed, as well as specific yoga and *pranayama* exercises to stimulate immune function and improve vitality. In order to remove toxins and restore harmony to the *doshas*, a *pancha karma* program may also be advised, requiring several days of consecutive detoxification treatments overseen by your practitioner. (In some cities, you will also have the option of receiving *pancha karma* at a special facility or spa, although the cost of such stays can be expensive.)

Follow-up visits are generally scheduled weeks or months apart and typically last less than an hour. As your health improves and you become educated in the Ayurvedic protocols best suited to your health, you will be expected to take responsibility for your own well-being by making the protocols part of a daily self-care routine.

SELECTING AN AYURVEDIC PRACTITIONER

Currently there are not many qualified practitioners of Ayurveda in the United States, nor is there a national standard for certification. Because of the degree of variance among practitioners in terms of skill and competence, you should choose a practitioner who has been in practice for at least a few years and has completed training at a recognized Ayurvedic university in India or from the domestic Ayurvedic institutions listed in the "Resources" section on the following page. Look for a practitioner with a Bachelor or Doctor of Ayurvedic Medicine and Surgery (B.A.M.S. or D.A.M.S.) degree, and avoid practitioners with little clinical experience. As an alternative, seek a holistic M.D. with training in Ayurveda. To locate a practitioner, contact the organizations listed in the "Resources" section.

Ayurveda is usually not covered by health insurance companies in the United States, although you may be able to have your treatments paid for if your practitioner is also an M.D. In addition, fees for treatment can vary widely. Dr. Lad, for instance, charges $70 for an initial consultation and $50 for follow-ups, but it is not uncommon for fees to range as high as $200 or more for an initial consultation, with follow-ups costing anywhere from $75 to $150 or more. Fees for *pancha karma* treatments at an overnight spa or special facility also vary, ranging on the average from $850 to $3,000.

THE FUTURE OF AYURVEDIC MEDICINE

While Ayurveda remains still relatively unknown in the United States, the likelihood that it will become more widely available is high, given the increased coverage it is receiving in the media, and the proliferation of research that is now being conducted on it and its various subspecialties, such as Ayurvedic herbal formulas, yoga, and meditation. Currently, there are a number of studies under way examining Ayurveda's efficacy for treating various disease conditions, including studies by the National Cancer Institute and the National Institutes of Health's Office of Complementary and Alternative Medicine. Due to Ayurveda's emphasis on prevention and its many self-care protocols, it is also likely to grow in popularity among people looking to take more responsibility for their health care needs. And, as Dr. Lad points out, Ayurveda's benefits are not limited to health alone. "Ayurveda comprehensively illuminates the basic laws and principles governing life on earth," he says. "By understanding oneself according to Ayurvedic principles, by identifying one's own constitution, and by recognizing sources of *doshic* aggravation, one can not only follow the proper guidelines to cleanse, purify, and prevent disease, but also uplift oneself into a realm of awareness previously unknown."

RESOURCES

To learn more about Ayurvedic medicine, or to locate a practitioner, contact the following organizations:

The Ayurvedic Institute (founded by Dr. Lad)
11311 Menaul Blvd., NE
Albuquerque, New Mexico 87112
Phone: (505) 291-9698, Fax: (505) 294-7572
Web site: *www.ayurveda.com*

The American School of Ayurvedic Sciences
2115 112th Avenue, NE
Bellevue, Washington 98004
Phone: (425) 453-8022

New England Institute of Ayurvedic Medicine
1815 Massachusetts Avenue
Cambridge, Massachusetts 02140
Phone: (508) 755-3744, Fax: (508) 770-0618

The American Institute of Vedic Studies
PO Box 8357
Santa Fe, New Mexico 87504
Phone: (505) 983-9385, Fax: (505) 982-5807
Web site: *www.vedanet.com*

The National Institute of Ayurvedic Medicine
584 Milltown Road
Brewster, New York 10509
Phone: (888) 246-6426
Web site: *www.niam.com*

The Maharishi College of Vedic Medicine
2721 Arizona Street NE
Albuquerque, New Mexico 87110
Phone: (888) 895-2614
Web site: *www.maharishi-medical.com*

Additional Internet Resources:

www.ayurvedic.org
ayurvedahc.com

RECOMMENDED READING

Frawley, David. *Ayurvedic Healing.* Morson Publishing, 1990.
Lad, Vasant. *Ayurveda: The Science of Self-Healing.* Lotus Press, 1985.
———. *The Complete Book of Ayurvedic Home Remedies.* New York: Harmony Books, 1998.
Lad, Vasant, and David Frawley. *The Yoga of Herbs: An Ayurvedic Guide to Herbal Medicine.* Lotus Press, 1986.
Lad, Vasant, and Usha. *Ayurvedic Cooking for Self-Healing.* 2d ed. The Ayurvedic Press, 1997.
Packard, Candis Cantin. *Pocket Guide to Ayurvedic Healing.* The Crossing Press, 1996.

CHAPTER 13

Traditional Chinese Medicine and Acupuncture

Traditional Chinese medicine (TCM), also known as Oriental medicine, is one of the oldest medical systems in the world and is based on a philosophy very much in accord with the principles of holistic medicine. According to David Molony, Ph.D., Lisc. A.c, executive director of the American Association of Oriental Medicine (AAOM), "The healing disciplines of Oriental medicine promote the idea that ultimate wellness is the result of a healthy body, mind, and spirit. Health and illness, instead of being viewed as static, isolated conditions distinct from other aspects of a person's life, are considered dynamic states that are unique to that person and reflective of his or her whole being. To TCM practitioners, any illness in one part of the body is connected to a vulnerability or weakness in another part."

TCM's holistic nature can be more fully appreciated when one considers how many different healing methods it encompasses (see "The Therapies of Traditional Chinese Medicine" later in this chapter). Proper diet, physical exercise (especially Tai Chi Chuan and *Qigong*), breathing exercises, acupuncture (the best-known aspect of TCM in the West), meditation, lifestyle counseling, massage, Chinese herbal medicine, and *moxibustion* (heating acupuncture points with smoldering mugwort, also known as *moxa*), are all components of TCM. Separately or in conjunction with each other, they are used to integrate body, mind, and spirit to prevent illness and promote optimal health. Because of its holistic health care approach, TCM continues to grow in popularity within the United States, especially as increasing numbers of physicians, like those who are members of the American Academy of Medical Acupuncture (AAMA), become trained in its methods in order to more comprehensively care for their patients.

❦ FAST FACTS ❦

There are approximately ten thousand licensed practitioners of acupuncture/TCM in the United States, with an additional one thousand practitioners being certified each year. Over three thousand medical doctors and osteopaths (D.O.'s) also include acupuncture as part of their practice, as do a growing number of naturopathic physicians (N.D.'s) and chiropractors.

In 1995, twelve million Americans elected to receive acupuncture treatments for their health care needs. Since then, it is estimated that this number has increased during each successive year.

Over fifty schools and colleges of acupuncture and traditional Chinese medicine exist in the United States.

Thirty-nine states and the District of Columbia regulate the practice of acupuncture. Of these, twenty-five states license, register, certify, or otherwise set training standards for acupuncturists for independent practice.

The World Health Organization, the American Chiropractic Association, the American Osteopathic Association, and the American Veterinary Medical Association all endorse acupuncture.

Sources: American Academy of Medical Acupuncture, American Association of Oriental Medicine ❦

HISTORY AND ORIGINS
OF ACUPUNCTURE AND TCM

The roots of traditional Chinese medicine extend back to antiquity, originating with the study of the healing properties of plants and flowers. "During this time," Dr. Molony explains, "Chinese monks and holy men began to search for a magic elixir that would bestow eternal life. Though, as far as we know, they did not succeed, through their experiments they discovered that many plants and flowers had powerful preventive, healing, and strengthening properties. Out of these discoveries, the field of Chinese herbal medicine emerged, which soon spread from village to village as tribes traded with each other. Archaeologists have discovered ancient prescriptions etched on carved bones and shells dating as far back as 1500 B.C. that refer to herbs and illnesses, although written historical and scientific records did not occur until about 200 B.C."

Playing a crucial role in the discovery and systematic recording of the properties of various plants and flowers was the emperor Sheng Nung, whose reign began around 2800 B.C. Revered in China as "the patron saint of herbology," Sheng Nung is also attributed with formulating the principle of *yin-yang*, which holds that two opposite but equal energies are necessary for life to exist. Sheng Nung's formulation of this central TCM tenet was based on his observation that everything in nature was made up of two currents that manifested as light and dark, hot and cold, masculine and feminine, and so forth. When these currents are not in harmony with each other, imbalance occurs, setting the stage for disease to occur. If the imbalance is not corrected, ultimately it can lead to death. In addition, Sheng Nung also theorized that an energy force flowed throughout the body that was responsible for its health. This theory eventually evolved into the concept of *qi* ("chee"), another basic tenet of traditional Chinese medicine. Sheng Nung also documented the existing theories of his day regarding the heart, pulse, and circulation four thousand years before European medicine had any concept of them.

Pursuing his investigations, Sheng Nung, it is claimed, regularly went into the countryside to gather and test the healing properties of hundreds of plants, using himself as the test subject. The end result was *Sheng Nung's Herbal*, which was orally passed down for two thousand years among the royalty of the emperor's court and the villagers living in nearby towns. "*Sheng Nung's Herbal* is China's first comprehensive book about the healing power of herbs," Dr. Molony says. "It describes over 250 herbs by taste, functions, and health benefits, and lists over 150 conditions that the herbs can successfully treat. While the first written version of Sheng Nung's Herbal did not appear until about 100 B.C., the information attributed to the original version is nevertheless remarkable in its accuracy."

Of equal importance, Sheng Nung also formulated one of the main principles of Chinese herbology that remains valid today. Every herbal formula, he taught, must contain at least one herb that actively targets the condition being treated, while also containing a number of secondary herbs that enhance the primary herb's action and prevent side effects. Today, modern science has verified the actions and effects of many of the herbs Sheng Nung first discussed nearly five thousand years ago.

Sheng Nung's work was carried on by Huang Ti, known as the Yellow Emperor, and his court physician, Qi Bo. Together they developed the first detailed system for diagnosing a variety of disease conditions and cataloged the herbs that could treat them. From there, they went on to establish traditional Chinese medicine as a complete medical system, and in the process developed the earliest main source of acupuncture theory. Their work, known as the *Huang Ti Nei Jing (Yellow Emperor's Classic of Medicine)*, considered to be the oldest medical textbook in the world, was also orally passed down for two thousand years before being formally written down, and is still consulted today by TCM researchers and practitioners. According to Joseph Helms, M.D., founding president of the American Academy of Medical Acupuncture, the *Nei Jing* regards the body as a reflection of the universe, with the physician's primary role being to maintain its "harmonious balance," both internally and in relation to the patient's outer environment.

Following Huang Ti's reign, a number of royal court physicians continued to contribute to TCM. During the Shang dynasty (1600 B.C.), Yi Tuen invented the technique of herbal decoction, which enabled herbs to be liquefied and used as tonics and in soups. Five hundred years later, Zhou Li codified herbs according to their "five tastes" (sour, bitter, sweet or bland, spicy, and salty), a classification that is still employed by TCM practitioners today. Around 500 B.C. the art and science of pulse diagnosis (sphygmology), one of TCM's fundamental methods of diagnosis, was developed by the physician Pin Choi.

Between 400 B.C. and 200 B.C., the philosophy of traditional Chinese medicine underwent another shift, merging with the ideas about life and the universe that comprised the teachings of Confucius and Lao-tzu, the father of Taoism. Both of these great Chinese philosophers transformed Sheng Nung's theory of nature's two opposite, yet equal, life principles into a spiritual philosophy in which all aspects of life, including health, are dependent upon the harmonious interaction between the forces of yin and yang. According to Confucius, inherent harmony is the nature of the universe, but humans, because of their actions, both good and bad, can affect this universal harmony. The code of behavior that Confucius established was meant to assist people in acting in harmony with the universe, with "good action" resulting in a wide variety of benefits for mankind, including good health.

Lao-tzu personalized Confucius's concept of universal harmony, declaring, in essence, that man is a universe unto himself, and that our personal harmony and disharmony are a direct manifestation of the personal ebb and flow of the yin and yang energies within us. Health, therefore, is possible only when we follow the Tao (literally the "Way") so that both inner and outer harmony can be achieved. As Lao-tzu's Taoist principles began to infuse traditional Chinese medicine, illness and its treatment became viewed "as one part of the great cosmic interplay of opposites and the universal striving toward harmony."

Following Confucius and Lao-tzu, TCM continued to develop, beginning with the Han dynasty (206 B.C. to A.D. 265), during which time the *Nan Jing (Classic of Difficult Issues)* was written. Presenting TCM as a comprehensive system of medicine, the *Nan Jing* theorized that the body contains a system of points and pathways that can be used to diagnose and treat disease. During the middle of the second century A.D., Zhang Chong Jin, considered the Hippocrates of traditional Chinese medicine, became the first physician to categorize illnesses as either yin ("cold") or yang ("hot") conditions, recommending appropriate herbal formulations that are still employed today. Further refinement of the principles of TCM and the practice of acupuncture was carried on throughout the remainder of the Han dynasty, well into the Ming dynasty (A.D. 1368 to 1644). In A.D. 282, the *Zhen Jiu Jia Yi Jin (Comprehensive Manual of Acupuncture and Moxibustion)* was published. It is the oldest classical manuscript devoted entirely to acupuncture and moxibustion still in existence today. Nearly fourteen hundred years later, in 1601, the *Zhen Jiu Da Cheng (Great Compendium of Acupuncture and Moxibustion)* was published, becoming the first source of acupuncture information to reach Europe, thanks to Latin translations of the text by missionaries from Portugal, France, Holland, and Denmark between the seventeenth and nineteenth centuries. As a result, between 1800 and 1840, a variety of acupuncture experiments were conducted by physicians in France, Germany, Italy, England, Sweden, and the United States. Because of their rudimentary nature, however, such experiments eventually waned. (Even so, Sir William Osler, considered the father of modern Western medicine, advocated the use of acupuncture as a treatment for lower back pain in the first edition of his famous textbook *Principles and Practice of Medicine*.) In Europe, research was not renewed until the 1900s, while in the United States no meaningful research was conducted until the 1970s, largely as a result of a *New York Times* article written by James Reston on July 26, 1971, in which he described how acupuncture successfully treated his pain following an appendectomy. After the article's publication, interest in acupuncture rose, following reports from visiting Western physicians of Chinese acupuncturists capable of providing surgical pain relief using only acupuncture needles. Since that time, acupuncture in particular, and TCM in general, have continued to be studied in the United States, with guidelines for its training, education, and regulation being established on state and national levels. In France throughout the twentieth century, and in much of Europe since the 1950s, the clinical practice of acupuncture has developed alongside conventional medical science, due in large part to the work of scholar and diplomat George Soulie de Morant, who was stationed in China between 1901 and 1917. During his tenure there, he published a number of articles on, and translations of, Chinese and Japanese medical texts, and following his return to France, he taught acupuncture theory and its clinical applications to French and other European physicians. He also gave the West the term *meridian* to describe the acupuncture points and pathways that are part of TCM theory. Today, increasing numbers of U.S. and European physicians and nurses are studying and practicing acupuncture in order to integrate it into their conventional medical practice, while the number of students embarking upon full-time training in traditional Chinese medicine also continues to grow.

THE THERAPIES OF TRADITIONAL CHINESE MEDICINE

Traditional Chinese medicine incorporates a wide range of treatment methods to promote health and manage disease. Although each of these therapies can be effectively used alone, many TCM practitioners employ them in conjunction with each other in order to help their patients achieve optimal health in body, mind, and spirit. The treatment methods include diet therapy, Chinese herbal medicine, acupuncture, moxibustion, cupping, massage, and combination breathing and physical exercises known as Tai Chi Chuan and *Qigong.*

Diet Therapy (Chinese Nutrition)

Like other branches of holistic medicine, TCM stresses the importance of proper diet in order to achieve and maintain optimal health. Chinese nutrition has been an essential component of TCM for thousands of years. Unlike modern Western nutrition, which correlates diet with the nutrient composition of foods, TCM diet therapy is more concerned with the energetic and therapeutic properties foods contain, and classifies them according to their yin or yang nature. (See "How Acupuncture and TCM Work" later in this chapter.) As in all other aspects of traditional Chinese philosophy, the principles of balance and harmony play an important role in Chinese nutrition, as does the recognition that each person's dietary needs are specific and unique. For these reasons, practitioners of Chinese dietary therapy consider not only the energies contained in the foods they prescribe, but also their method of preparation, the time of year and geographical location in which they are to be eaten, and the body type of each patient. Emphasis is placed on adapting dietary protocols to each individual's needs and treating the whole person, not just his or her disease. Because food plays such an elemental role in health, Chinese nutrition by itself can often provide a significant improvement in one's overall health.

Chinese Herbal Medicine

According to Dr. Molony, Chinese herbal medicine is the world's oldest and most comprehensive form of internal medicine and, along with acupuncture, one of the primary components of TCM. "Some of the earliest written records ever discovered in China are about herbs and their use in treating a variety of illnesses and medical conditions," Dr. Molony says. "Some people go so far as to say that one of the chief reasons for the development of written language in China was to record herbal medical information for future generations." Supporting this notion is Huang Ti's *Classic of Internal Medicine*, which is believed to have originally been compiled as early as 2800 B.C. One of the most important texts on Chinese herbalism, a fifty-two-volume set known as the *Ben Cao Kong Mu (Compendium of Materia Medica)*, was compiled by the physician Li Shih-chen in the sixteenth century, and describes nearly two thousand herbs and over eleven thousand herbal remedies.

In TCM, herbs are classified into sixteen categories and further categorized according to their appearance and various properties, including "nature" (yin or yang), "action," "taste," "hot," or "cold." Most of the raw ingredients used in preparing Chinese herbal formulas are of plant origin, while a few are derived from mineral or animal sources. According to Dr. Molony, few Chinese herbs are used alone for medicinal purposes, with cinnamon, clove, and ginkgo biloba being among the exceptions. "The skillful combination of herbs, matching them according to their unique individual properties, is fundamental to the remarkable effectiveness of Chinese herbal formulas in treating a variety of illnesses in a safe and gentle fashion," Dr. Molony says. "In addition to their yin or yang nature, herbs also possess many other therapeutic properties that make each one unique. These properties dictate why certain herbs are combined to treat a specific ailment, as well as how the treatment itself will progress."

Chinese herbal formulas can be taken internally as decoctions (herbs boiled in water), or in the form of teas, pills, powders, tinctures, or syrups. Herbs can also be used as inhalants; applied to plasters, poultices, and salves; or be taken as suppositories, or in enemas and douches. Properly prescribed, Chinese herbs work to restore the body's harmony and balance by reestablishing the proper relationship between yin and yang and promoting the flow of *qi* energy throughout the body.

Acupuncture

The most popular form of traditional Chinese medicine in the West, acupuncture involves the application of various types of acupuncture needles into specific sites along the body, known as acupoints, in order to restore the flow and balance of *qi*, or "life force," energies throughout the body, and to improve internal organ function. Acupoints to be needled are selected according to a patient's specific needs, and needle insertion is quick and usually painless, often provoking feelings of calm and relaxation. Acupuncture needles are made of stainless steel, gold, or silver, and their length varies according to the effect the acupuncturist seeks to achieve (calm or stimulation), and the area of the body where they are inserted. After insertion, the depth of which also varies, the needles may be left in place or gently rotated, flicked, or raised in a stroking motion, depending on the condition being treated and the patient's diagnosis. After use, the needles are disposed of in accordance with medical biohazard regulations. Of all the subset therapies of TCM, in the United States acupuncture has been the most carefully researched and is also becoming popular among holistic veterinarians as an appropriate treatment for pet care. The animals' positive response rate contradicts the notion that the many benefits acupuncture provides for humans derives from a placebo response. As a veterinary procedure, it is primarily used to alleviate chronic pain and to provide pain relief during surgery.

In addition to traditional acupuncture, a variety of related procedures can also be employed by acupuncturists, including auriculotherapy, electroacupuncture, and sonopuncture. Auriculotherapy, also know as ear acupuncture, originated in France shortly after World War II. It was developed by Paul Nogier, M.D., who discovered that certain points along the *auricula*, or outer ear, formed a reflex system capable of affecting other body areas when they were properly stimulated. Nogier's original published research was subsequently supported by researchers in China and Japan, eventually leading to Nogier's recognition as the father of modern ear acupuncture by the Chinese government. Originally used to treat and control pain, dyslexia, and other functional disturbances, in the United States auriculotherapy is now well known as a successful therapy for treating alcohol, drug, and nicotine addiction.

Electroacupuncture uses small electrical impulses that are generated through acupuncture needles, and is primarily employed for general pain relief and, at higher frequencies, as an adjunct to surgical procedures, especially those related to the abdomen. It was first used in 1958 in China for a tonsillectomy, where today it is commonly prescribed as a method of surgical analgesia.

Sonopuncture, the least well-known method of acupuncture, involves the use of laser, sound, or sonar waves that are transmitted along various acupoints.

Moxibustion

This form of treatment consists of applying heated *moxa* (mugwort) to the acupoints. Moxa is placed placed either directly on the acupoints to be treated or atop a slice of gingerroot, and it is removed when it becomes too warm for the patient. Moxibustion is often used in conjunction with acupuncture as a means of enhancing the body's self-healing capacities.

Cupping

Cupping is a method of stimulating acupoints that has been in use in China since the third century B.C. It involves lighting a match in cups made of glass, pottery, metal, or bamboo, then quickly removing it as the cups are applied to the skin, causing a suction that keeps the cups tightly in place. As a result of this suction, blood circulation increases. Although cupping can be uncomfortable, it is not painful and is useful for treating painful muscles, low back pain, soft-tissue injuries, rheumatism, sprains, and bronchial conditions. It, too, is often used in conjunction with acupuncture.

Massage

A variety of massage therapies can be employed by TCM practitioners, the most common of which is acupressure, which essentially is acupuncture without needles. Instead, practitioners use their fingertips or fingernails to apply pressure to various acupoints to remove blockages and stimulate the flow of *qi*. It is a useful treatment option for patients with an aversion to needles. However, its application is less specific than that of acupuncture, and therefore its benefits may be slower to achieve. In Japan, a variation of acupressure, known as *shiatsu*, is widely popular as a health care treatment. Other variations include reflexology, or Zone Therapy (acupressure applied to specific points in the feet, hands, and around the ankles), and *Tui Na* (a combination of acupressure and physical manipulation). Acupressure can also be used as an effective self-care technique.

Tai Chi Chuan and Qigong

Tai Chi Chuan (also known as *Tai Chi* or *Taiji*) and *Qigong* are ancient systems of exercise incorporating breathwork, visualization, and movement designed to promote the cultivation of *qi* energy throughout the body's various organ systems. Historically, Tai Chi developed from *Qigong* itself, with both practices having their roots in the principles of Taoist philosophy. In China, both disciplines are practiced daily by hundreds of millions of people, and are also included (especially *Qigong*) as part of normal hospital therapy.

Of the two disciplines, Tai Chi Chuan is better known in the United States. Its gentle, flowing movements help promote health and prevent illness, reduce stress and muscular tension, and enhance flexibility and posture. It is also well known for its ability to promote relaxation. Because of its gentle nature, it is ideally suited for people of all ages, yet it also forms the basis of a potent martial art.

Practitioners of Tai Chi Chuan execute a sequence of movements known as a form. A short form usually takes five to ten minutes to perform, while longer forms can take half an hour or longer. When properly executed, the movements are precise and synchronized with the breath as the practitioner becomes aware of, and learns to "flow with," the *qi* energy in and around the body. For this reason, Tai Chi Chuan is often referred to as a type of moving meditation.

Qigong is a form of energy exercise geared toward creating balance and self-regulation within the body. Meaning "to cultivate *qi*," *Qigong* was once jealously hidden from most of Chinese society, but today enjoys widespread popularity and the official support of the Chinese Ministry of Health and is the subject of intensive research by the Chinese scientific community.

Recent research has shown that *Qigong* enhances respiration and metabolism, improves immune function, and aids in digestion and absorption, as well as being capable of restoring balance to disordered or overstimulated cells in the cerebral cortex. *Qigong* is also effective for normalizing blood pressure levels, reducing recovery times from surgery, and as a treatment for obesity, addiction, respiratory conditions, and allergies, among other disease conditions.

Unlike Tai Chi, *Qigong* places less emphasis on movement, focusing on learning how to feel and move energy inside the body. Many systems and traditions of *Qigong* exist, ranging from relatively simple calisthenic movements to complex autoregulatory exercises, which enable practitioners to intentionally alter their own brain-wave patterns, heart rate, and other organ functions. Research conducted with *Qigong* masters verified that they are also able to transmit *qi* energy to other people, manipulate limbs, and perform accurate diagnosis of patients' conditions without conversation or touch. Despite its subtlety, *Qigong* is easy to learn under the guidance of a competent instructor.

HOW ACUPUNCTURE AND TCM WORK

"The goal of TCM and each of the treatment methods it comprises is to integrate the patient's body, mind, and spirit in order to prevent illness and to promote the ultimate wellness that is every individual's natural right," Dr. Molony says. "Instead of defining patients only by their diseases, TCM practitioners are trained to look for the underlying, subtler origins of illness, while taking into consideration a patient's strengths and weaknesses. All illness, no matter how great or small, is an indication of a fundamental imbalance in the patient, resulting in a weakness that allowed his or her illness to occur. Knowing this, practitioners of Chinese medicine regard the symptoms of illness as clues to the underlying nature of their patient's imbalance, and understand that the real problem may actually be far removed from the more obvious ailment."

To illustrate his point, Dr. Molony uses the familiar example of a person beset with frequent colds throughout the winter. "Conventional treatment for such a person might involve using antihistamines, aspirin, and decongestants to relieve the acute cold symptoms," he explains, "but unless the underlying condition that left the patient vulnerable to respiratory infection is treated, then whatever quick relief may occur will only be temporary. Eventually, the cold will return, and because of the possible side effects of the drugs the patient was using, new and more serious problems might also arise."

According to Dr. Molony, a TCM practitioner, while still treating the acute cold symptoms, would also seek to discover the patient's deeper, more serious imbalance. "In such a case, short-term treatment might involve the use of cooling herbs to ease fever and congestion, but the long-term goal would be to eliminate the patient's susceptibility to respiratory viruses altogether, possibly by using a completely different group of warming herbs, for instance, in accordance with TCM's most basic principle, the yin-yang dynamic."

Along with the philosophy of yin and yang, TCM and the various treatment methods it includes are based on the following principles: *the five energies, the meridian system,* and *the twelve major organs.*

Yin and Yang

The principle of yin and yang has been a core tenet of not only TCM, but also Chinese philosophy, art, and science since the dawn of recorded history. "In the West, we tend to understand the yin-yang principle as referring to two separate, distinct energies that are the exact opposite of each other, one negative and one positive," Dr. Molony explains. "The Chinese view is more subtle, however, recognizing that yin and yang are not separate, static energies, but codependent and constantly in motion toward each other. Neither energy can exist without the other, and a bit of each is contained within the other."

According to Chinese medical theory, yin energy is characterized as cool, passive, feminine, and dark, and is associated with cold, heavy, moist, and negative states, as well as winter, rain, night, and the moon. Yang energy is said to be warm, active, masculine, and bright, and associated with states that are hot, light, dry, and positive. Summer, fire, day, and the sun are also associated with yang energy. From the perspective of traditional Chinese medicine, as long as these complementary energies remain in harmony with each other, health remains, but when disharmony occurs between them, illness results. The first symptom of illness is often a change in energy levels, according to Dr. Molony, indicating that a fundamental imbalance has occurred. "The imbalance may be either in the body, or between the patient and his or her environment. In TCM, such imbalances are usually viewed as either excesses or deficiencies of yin or yang energy that need to be restored to harmony."

"As in Nature, so in Man," the famous dictum of the great Taoist philosopher Lao-tzu, is also central to the theory of yin and yang. Essentially, it means that each human being is a microcosm of the larger, macrocosmic universe, and just as yin and yang energies are part of everything in nature, they also interact within each of us, and must be maintained in a fluid state of harmonious balance in order for optimal health to be achieved.

"This principle is at the heart of TCM treatment methods," Dr. Molony says. "In nature, yang conditions are necessary to restore balance to excessive or deficient yin conditions, and vice versa. Warm sunlight can ease the effects of flooding due to excessive cold rains, for example. This same principle holds true in treating illnesses, which in TCM are categorized as either excessive or deficient yang or yin conditions. In Chinese herbology, for instance, herbs that are classified as yin are generally used to treat yang conditions, while yang herbs are used to treat yin conditions. Understanding how yin and yang energies interact with each other in nature makes it easier for TCM practitioners and their patients to recognize how those same energies can be used to achieve a life of health and balance."

The Five Energies

Traditional Chinese medical theory holds that there are five elemental energies within our bodies that are essential for proper physical, mental, and emotional functioning, and for our further growth and development. These five energies are *Jing, Shen, qi, blood,* and the *Jin Ye* fluids. In some texts, these energies are sometimes called the body "humors," "essences," or "processes," according to Dr. Molony. "The difference in language is due to the fact that each of these five energies is difficult to define in conventional terms," he says. "Moreover, only two of them have a physical character. The other three are what we might think of as pure, or immaterial, energies. Each of them plays a unique role in the body, however, and all of them are the products of yin and yang."

Jing energy, or "essence," corresponds to the genetic material of DNA, and governs the body's developmental growth processes and the rate and degree of its deterioration. People with strong *Jing* at birth are said to be predisposed to a long, healthy life. Weak *Jing*, on the other hand, is an indication that the baby may grow up to be susceptible to chronic infections or immune disorders. TCM practitioners strengthen Jing with diet, herbs, acupuncture, and lifestyle counseling.

Shen, or "psyche" or "spirit," is most similar to the Western concept of the "soul" or "higher consciousness." "It is the driving energy behind mental, spiritual, and creative activity," Dr. Molony explains. "Mild depression, anxiety, and chronic restlessness are signs of moderately weak *Shen*, while clinical depression and psychosis indicate *Shen* is significantly weaker." Herbs, acupuncture, meditation, and physical exercises such as Tai Chi Chuan and *Qigong* can all be employed by TCM practitioners to strengthen Shen.

Qi, the most important of the five energies, is considered the most dynamic and immediate energy of the body, resulting from the interaction of yin and yang energies. Often referred to as "vital energy" or the "life force," *qi* is also the energy most familiar to Westerners. "The Chinese believe that everything in the universe is composed of *qi*, from the smallest object to the largest planet," Dr. Molony says. "According to Chinese theory, the body is a wellspring of *qi*, which acts much like an electrical current that constantly flows within, around, and in and out of the body, enriching the blood, *Jin Ye* fluids, and eventually the organs. Ultimately, all actions of the body depend on *qi* before they can occur or be maintained." *Qi* plays many roles in a person's health, including keeping the body warm, maintaining the proper function of the organs and tissues, protecting against external or environmental influences, and mixing and metabolizing the food and air we consume into vital substances such as blood. Because of its various roles, TCM further categorizes *qi* into distinct classifications. The most important of these are *Yuan*, or original *qi* (the *qi* we inherit from our parents and the universe); *Gu*, or food *qi* (received from our foods and liquids); *Kong* or air *qi* (received from the air we breathe); *Zheng*, or organ *qi* (the *qi* that circulates through the body's meridian systems, formed by the interaction of *Yuan*, *Gu*, and *Kong qi*); *Ying*, or nutritive *qi* (which helps transform food, air, and liquids into nourishment for the body); and *Wei*, or protective *qi* (also known as surface *qi* because it circulates outside of the body to protect it from external causes of imbalance and disease).

Four types of *qi* imbalances are believed to be responsible for illness, according to Dr. Molony. These are deficient *qi*, sinking *qi* (an extreme case of deficient *qi* in which a particular organ is no longer able to properly function), stagnant *qi* (caused when the normal flow of *qi* is slowed down or blocked, as in cases of bruising, swelling, sprains, or fractures), and rebellious *qi* (*qi* flowing in the wrong direction, as when stomach *qi* causes a gastric reflux). "Identifying these *qi* imbalances is one of the first things a TCM practitioner does before suggesting a treatment regimen," Molony says. "When balance is restored to the flow of *qi*, health soon follows."

Blood is the second most important of the five energies, according to Dr. Molony, and to TCM practitioners refers to more than just the body's circulatory fluid. "In TCM, blood is the physical manifestation of the *qi* energy itself and shares certain *qi* functions in the body," he says. "These include bringing nourishment to all of the body's organs, vessels, tissues, and muscles; lubricating them; and enhancing mental functioning."

Illness can occur as a result of any of the following three blood imbalances: *deficient blood*, which is caused when the spleen system is unable to produce a good supply of blood from food or nutritive *qi*; stagnant blood, which occurs when the flow of blood is slow or sluggish; and heat in the blood, which can be caused by many factors, especially internal imbalances of yin and yang energies.

The *Jin Ye fluids*, which are similar to blood in that they also have a physical property and provide lubrication and moistening for the organs, are the last of the five energies. "The difference between the *Jin Ye* fluids and blood is that they perform these functions in a very precise way, beginning with how they are processed in the spleen," Dr. Molony explains. "It is within the spleen that the foods and liquids we ingest are metabolized into two types of fluids, pure and impure. Impure fluids pass on to the intestines for further separation, while pure fluids are sent to the lungs, where they are further processed into light or heavy fluids. The light, watery fluids are called *Jin*, and the heavier, thicker fluids are known as *Ye*."

According to Dr. Molony, *Jin* fluids circulate from the lungs to the body's surface to moisten the skin and muscles, thereby enhancing the role of protective *qi*. *Ye* fluids, on the other hand, are circulated into the kidneys, where they undergo another separation process, resulting in pure and impure *Ye* fluids. Impure *Ye* is excreted as waste, while pure *Ye* assists the kidneys and spleen in working with the body's nutritive *qi*. "Maintaining a balance in the *Jin Ye* fluids is important for optimal health," Dr. Molony says. "When *Jin Ye* fluids become deficient, illnesses such as dehydration or constipation can occur, while when they are excessive or accumulate, a condition known in TCM as 'dampness,' congestion or edema frequently results."

The Meridian Systems

According to TCM theory, the body contains a series of energetic pathways, known as the meridian systems, through which *qi* and other life energies flow to nourish the body's organs and tissues. Twelve major meridian pathways are recognized by TCM. Running along the body's surface, connecting its exterior with its interior, each one of them is associated with a specific vital organ. "When *qi* circulates on the surface of the body, it flows from meridian to meridian, and then from organ to organ, delivering vital *qi* energy to every part of the body over the course of twenty-four hours," Dr. Molony says. Specific sites along these pathways, referred to as acupoints, allow access to the meridian systems, each of them corresponding to particular organs and their function. There are more than one thousand acupoints on the body, which are stimulated by TCM practitioners using acupuncture, moxibustion, or acupressure in order to ensure the unobstructed flow of *qi* throughout the body.

Chinese herbs can also play an important role in maintaining the overall vitality of *qi* as it travels along the meridian pathways. "Since herbs are essentially yin or yang in character, their inherent energy has a therapeutic relationship with the meridians," Dr. Molony explains. "According to Chinese medical theory, particular herbs and herbal formulas are said to have a unique affinity for particular meridians. Therefore, the correct use of Chinese herbs stimulates specific meridians, thus treating their corresponding organs in much the same way that acupuncture does."

While Western science has no direct parallel to the meridian system, research has shown that there is a definite relationship between meridians, acupoints, and the body's electrical currents. Numerous studies conducted since the 1950s employing electrical devices that measure galvanic skin response, have not only verified the existence of the meridian systems, but also suggest that acupoints have a higher level of electrical conductivity than other sites along the body. Researchers Robert O. Becker, M.D., and Maria Reihmanis, under a grant from the National

Institutes of Health, have also proved that electrical currents do, in fact, flow along the meridian pathways, and that the acupoints themselves act as amplifiers that boost the electrical signals as they move through the body. As a result of their research, they reasoned that the insertion of acupuncture needles into acupoint sites can reduce or eliminate pain by blocking or interfering with the flow of energy that would otherwise stimulate it. Such findings are all the more remarkable, Dr. Molony points out, when one considers that the Chinese body of knowledge regarding acupuncture and the meridian system extends back at least four thousand years.

MODERN SCIENTIFIC EXPLANATIONS ❦ OF THE MERIDIAN SYSTEM ❦

Recent research by Western scientists into acupuncture and the meridian system has uncovered a number of physiological mechanisms that help to explain how acupuncture works. Over the last decade, researchers have determined that stimulating acupuncture points along the meridians affects both the central and the peripheral nervous system, and triggers the production and release of endorphins and enkephalins, the body's natural pain-killers. Other research suggests that acupuncture also triggers the release of neural hormones such as serotonin, which is known for its sedative effects. One explanation of these effects may lie with the acupoints' own electrical properties, which when stimulated may alter the body's neurotransmitters. In addition, research conducted since the late 1970s has shown that acupuncture activates the body's opioid peptide system, thereby influencing normal nervous system pathways to alter the process and perception of pain. According to Joseph Helms, M.D., founding president of the American Academy of Medical Acupuncture, acupuncture also simultaneously activates multiple body systems, including the nervous system, the blood circulatory system, the lymphatic system, and the body's "electromagnetic bio-information system." While scientists are still seeking a definitive explanation as to how and why acupuncture works, its validity is no longer in question, given the mounting body of both clinical and anecdotal evidence supporting its effectiveness in treating pain and providing relief for many other chronic conditions. ❦

The Twelve Major Organs

Corresponding to the meridian system are the organ systems, known as *Zang Fu*, identified by traditional Chinese medicine. "The organs are both the manufacturers and storehouses of all the body's vital energies, fluids, and biological functions," Dr. Molony explains. "In TCM there are twelve major organs, each of which has a characteristic yin or yang nature. In addition, each yin organ is paired with its complementary yang organ, and together they perform their unique and critical functions in the body."

The body's yin organs are considered the most important, according to Dr. Molony. Known as solid, or *Zang*, organs because they are found deep in the body, the yin organs are the lungs, the heart, the liver, the spleen, and the kidneys. They are essential for manufacturing, storing, and regulating the Five Energies outlined above. While technically not an organ at all, the pericardium, the membrane surrounding the heart, is classified as the sixth yin organ. "The reason the pericardium is given organ status is because Chinese medicine views process as being far more important than structure, and the pericardium plays a crucial role both in protecting the heart and in enhancing many of its functions," Dr. Molony says.

The five yang organs, known as *Fu*, are hollow and found closer to the surface of the body. They are the large intestine, the small intestine, the gallbladder, the bladder, and the stomach. "The function of the yang organs is largely gastrointestinal and involved in receiving, metabolizing, and excreting various body fluids and wastes," Dr. Molony says. "Included with these organs is a sixth yang organ, known as the triple warmer. It has no anatomical equivalent in conventional Western medicine and is considered in TCM to be an energy system that enhances the process of ingesting, metabolizing, and eliminating nutrients and wastes. As such, it helps move *qi* energies throughout the body while regulating the other organ functions. It also plays a role in sexual and reproductive processes." Beginning at the tongue and ending at the anus, the triple warmer is divided into three parts. The upper part extends from the tongue to the diaphragm, the middle area covers the diaphragm to the navel, and the lower section is comprised of the section of the body between the navel and anus. Its yin counterpart is the pericardium.

Within the system of Chinese medical theory, the organs have more comprehensive functions than those commonly assigned to the same organs by conventional medicine. The lungs are said to control and regulate vital *qi* and respiration, along with water passage and metabolism. The lungs also house a person's original *qi*, and are associated with the hair and skin. Their complementary yang organ is the large intestine.

The heart is said to house the spirit and controls the blood and blood vessels. It is associated with the tongue and face, and its yang counterpart is the small intestine.

The liver stores and regulates blood and promotes the flow of *qi*. Considered the house of the soul, it is associated with the eyes, muscles, and tendons, and its complementary yang organ is the gallbladder.

The kidneys store *Jing* and control reproduction, growth and development, and water metabolism. They also oversee the production of bone and marrow, and regulate brain function. Considered the seat of willpower, the kidneys are associated with the ears, loins, and lower back, and their yang counterpart is the bladder.

Lastly, the spleen governs the transport and transformation of blood and vital fluids, moves *qi*, holds the organs in place, and controls muscles. The house of the mind, the spleen is associated with the mouth, skin, and limbs, and its complementary yang organ is the stomach.

All of the above concepts, taken together, enable TCM practitioners to determine not only what acute measures are required to provide relief from illness, but, just as important, to discover how a patient is functioning at the deeper levels of his or her being (body, mind, and spirit) in order to restore harmony and balance to the entire person.

CONDITIONS THAT BENEFIT FROM ACUPUNCTURE AND TCM

Traditional Chinese medicine's primary emphasis, like that of holistic medicine overall, is on preventive care, as expressed in the famous Chinese axiom "An ounce of prevention is worth a pound of cure." In China, this precept was illustrated by the fact that traditional Chinese doctors were paid by their patients to keep them well and were expected to work without pay should their patients become sick. As another famous Chinese dictum says, "It is foolish to wait to dig a well until a person is thirsty." In the United States, however, the majority of patients still continue to delay seeking medical attention until disease strikes. As a result, TCM treatment methods are often relegated in the United States to disease care, as well, leaving most patients who are experiencing TCM for the first time to wonder what conditions it provides benefit for.

A partial answer to that question was provided by the World Health Organization (WHO), the medical branch of the United Nations in 1979, when it issued a provisional list of over forty disease conditions for which traditional Chinese medicine can effectively serve as a primary or adjunctive treatment. Included in this list (see below) are conditions of the upper respiratory tract (including the common cold), the respiratory system, eye disorders, disorders of the gastrointestinal tract, neurological disorders, musculoskeletal disorders, and disorders of the mouth. WHO also reports that acupuncture is able to achieve relief of symptoms in "over 80 percent" of patients suffering from coronary heart disease, and is effective in controlling fever, inflammation, and pain.

THE WORLD HEALTH ORGANIZATION'S LIST OF CONDITIONS THAT BENEFIT ❧ FROM ACUPUNCTURE ❧

The following health conditions have been determined by the World Health Organization to respond beneficially to acupuncture treatment:

UPPER RESPIRATORY TRACT
Acute sinusitis
Acute rhinitis
Common cold
Acute tonsillitis

RESPIRATORY SYSTEM
Acute bronchitis
Bronchial asthma (most effective in children and patients without complicating diseases)

EYE DISORDERS
Acute conjunctivitis
Myopia (in children)
Cataract (without complications)
Central retinitis

GASTROINTESTINAL DISORDERS
Hiccough
Spasms of the esophagus and cardia
Gastroptosis
Acute and chronic gastritis

Gastric hyperacidity
Chronic duodenal ulcer
Acute duodenal ulcer (without complications)
Acute and chronic colitis
Acute bacillary dysentery
Constipation
Diarrhea
Paralytic ileus

NEUROLOGICAL AND MUSCULOSKELETAL DISORDERS
Headache and migraine
Trigeminal neuralgia
Facial (Bell's) palsy (within six months of onset)
Pareses following stroke
Peripheral neuropathies
Sequelae of poliomyelitis (within six months of onset)
Ménière's disease
Neurogenic bladder dysfunction
Nocturnal enuresis
Intercostal neuralgia
Cervicobrachial syndrome
"Tennis elbow"
"Frozen shoulder"
Sciatica
Low back pain
Osteoarthritis 🌿

In 1991, WHO further endorsed TCM by advocating its use as a system of medicine to be used worldwide in order to meet the health care needs of the twenty-first century. In 1995, acupuncture gained a further foothold within the mainstream of conventional medicine when the Food and Drug Administration approved acupuncture needles as safe and effective medical devices, for the first time sanctioning a medical device that was rooted in a tradition completely outside that of conventional mainstream medicine.

The list of conditions for which acupuncture has been scientifically verified to provide effective treatment or relief continues to grow. For instance, studies have found that acupuncture can be effective in treating a variety of rheumatoid arthritis conditions, providing relief in 80 percent of patients suffering from joint degeneration caused by the disease. Evidence also suggests that acupuncture can be useful in treating disease conditions caused by pesticide poisoning, radiation, air pollution, and other environmental toxins. In 1998, a panel of twenty-five experts, acting under the auspices of the National Institutes of Health, concluded that acupuncture showed "promising results" as an effective therapy for nausea and vomiting following chemotherapy and postoperative surgery and dental pain, and that it "may be useful as an adjunct treatment or an acceptable alternative, or be included in a comprehensive management program" for treating addiction, headache, menstrual cramps, tennis elbow, fibromyalgia, myofascial pain, osteoarthritis, low back pain, carpal tunnel syndrome, and asthma, as well as being useful in rehabilitation following stroke.

Research indicates that the diagnostic methods of traditional Chinese medicine are useful in accurately predicting survival rates of patients with primary liver cancer. In another study, Chinese herbal remedies were shown to prolong survival for primary liver cancer patients, allowing them to recuperate to the point where they could successfully undergo surgery and "complete regimens of chemotherapy." More recently, an Australian study found that Chinese herbal medicine offered "nearly three times more relief (roughly a 60 percent improvement in symptoms)" than conventional medicine in the treatment of irritable bowel syndrome, a chronic digestive condition that afflicts as much as 20 percent of the U.S. population.

Another study revealed the promise that moxibustion holds as an alternative to cesarean births. The study, conducted by researchers in Italy and China, involved 260 women experiencing first-time pregnancies whose babies were still in a breech position after thirty-three weeks. Half of the group received daily moxibustion treatments for one to two weeks, while the remaining control group received conventional care. The babies belonging to the mothers receiving moxibustion became "measurably more active," and 75 percent of them, versus less than half of those in the control group, were able to move into a proper position in time for a normal delivery. If further research confirms these findings, moxibustion could soon become an integral aspect of modern Western obstetric care, helping to reduce the United States' high rate of cesarean births. Recent research also suggests that auriculotherapy (ear acupuncture) used in conjunction with a high-protein diet can promote weight loss and reduce food cravings and a tendency for bingeing, enabling most patients (over 60 percent) to maintain weight loss and avoid a return to carbohydrates even after the treatment is completed. A variety of studies (double-blind, single-blind, and uncontrolled) also showed that acupuncture can provide "significant improvement of 'breathlessness'" in asthma patients and allow for a reduction in medication.

Since the 1980s, acupuncture, particularly in the form of auriculotherapy, has shown good success for treating alcohol, drug, and nicotine addiction, and for reducing the need for prescription painkillers. Usually no more than four or five acupoints on the ear are stimulated, resulting not only in diminished cravings for the addictive substance in question, but also a state of relaxation and clearer thinking that can enable addicts to regain control of their lives. An analysis of a residential drug treatment program in Miami where auriculotherapy is used found a better than 75 percent long-term (two years or longer) success rate among clinic graduates, compared to only 20 percent among graduates of standard drug treatment programs. Today there are hundreds of substance abuse programs in the United States that incorporate acupuncture as either a primary or adjunctive treatment, and acupuncture detoxification programs are also employed in a number of other countries as well, including Canada, Mexico, Great Britain, Germany, Sweden, Spain, Hungary, and Saudi Arabia.

Acupuncture's greatest level of acceptance in the United States thus far, however, has occurred primarily in the area of pain management, due to U.S. research focused on that issue. According to Dr. Helms, acupuncture is particularly effective as a primary therapy for acute musculoskeletal lesions such as soft-tissue contusions, acute muscle spasms, sprains and strains of muscles and tendons, and acute entrapped nerves. It can also alleviate chronic musculoskeletal pain, although usually in conjunction with one or more other approaches. Among the conditions in this category, Dr. Helms includes repetitive strain disorders, such as carpal tunnel syndrome; plantar fasciitis; muscle tension headaches; temporomandibular joint pain (TMJ); shoulder pain; degenerative disc disease; osteoarthritis; neuralgia; and pain following surgery.

Among the research findings that attest to acupuncture's ability to mitigate pain are the following:

Of fifty patients suffering from chronic low back pain, 83 percent of those receiving acupuncture treatment showed noticeable improvement and needed fewer pain medications, compared to only 30 percent among those who received conventional care.

Ninety-one percent of women receiving acupuncture to treat dysmenorrhea experienced pain relief, compared to only 36 percent of the
women in the control group, and also required 41 percent less pain
medication.

In a study of thirty patients with migraine, acupuncture reduced migraine
pain by as much as 43 percent, and achieved a similar reduction in
the need for pain medication.

Study subjects suffering from chronic neck pain lasting an average of
eight years experienced an 80 percent reduction of symptoms after
twelve weeks of treatment, compared to only 13 percent in the control group, while symptoms in 60 percent of the control group actually worsened.

Acupuncture was also found to be as effective as pain medication among
patients suffering from kidney stones, without the side effects.

Other categories of disease cited by Dr. Helms as being responsive to
acupuncture include the respiratory and gastrointestinal disorders listed
above; gynecological conditions, including infertility and dysmenorrhea;
genitourinary disorders, including prostatitis, male infertility, certain
forms of impotence, and irritable bladder; and acute mental and emotional disturbances, such as anxiety, worry, excitability, early-stage
depression, and fear. (Acupuncture has shown little or no value for deep-
seated or chronic mental and emotional conditions, however.)

For all of the conditions mentioned above, the best time to begin
acupuncture treatment is in the early stages, according to Dr. Helms,
although its flexibility and adaptability make it useful at almost any stage
of treatment.

DIAGNOSIS AND TREATMENT

"In TCM, diagnosis of the patients is a complicated process involving
considerable scientific skill and the ability to observe the patient's condition objectively and, as much as this is possible, subjectively," Dr. Molony
says. Although physicians who incorporate traditional Chinese medicine
into their practice may employ conventional diagnostic techniques, such
as X-rays and blood tests, to assess their patients' health, most practitioners of acupuncture and TCM rely on time-proven, noninvasive methods
of diagnosis that primarily fall into four categories—visual observation,
listening and smelling, patient interview, and touch (palpation and pulse
diagnosis). "TCM practitioners train for many years in these four

primary methods of patient assessment," Dr. Molony says. "In addition, they learn how to assess symptoms and illness in a variety of ways, based on how yin and yang, qi, blood, the *Jin Ye* fluids, and the organs are functioning in the body and interacting with each other."

According to Dr. Molony, symptoms and illness are primarily categorized as being essentially yin or yang in nature; as conditions associated with yin (cold, internal, damp, deficient), yang (heat, external, dry, excess), *Jing* (weak or deficient), or *Shen* (weak or agitated); or as imbalances of *qi* (deficient, sinking, stagnant, rebellious), blood (deficient, stagnant, heat), organs (deficient or excess yin, yang, or *qi*), or the *Jin Ye* fluids (deficient or excess).

Visual Observation

In this stage of diagnosis, the practitioner carefully notes the patient's appearance and physical characteristics, including body type and movement; the appearance of the eyes, lips, and complexion; and the condition of the hair, skin, and tongue. "When the results of these observations are considered in total, they provide the practitioner with a good idea of the nature of the patient's imbalance, and indicate whether there is an overall pattern of excess or deficiency," Dr. Molony explains. "For instance, a heavyset patient will generally be prone to yang conditions, while thin or fine-bonded people are more susceptible to yin conditions. If the patient has a pattern of rapid movement, he or she may suffer from conditions characterized by excess heat. People who move slowly or sluggishly, on the other hand, are more likely to have conditions of excess cold. By then noting the condition of the patients' hair, skin, and tongue, as well as the appearance of their eyes, lips, and complexion, the practitioner begins to get an accurate symptom and illness profile."

Listening and Smelling

Acupuncturists and TCM practitioners also listen carefully for any signs of cough, wheezing, or congestion, the tone of a patient's voice, and to how he or she breathes. "Rapid breathing and a loud voice can indicate excess heat conditions," Dr. Molony says, "while shallow breathing and a soft voice will usually indicate internal cold."

Some practitioners also note patients' body odor, and the smell of their breath and, if necessary, their saliva, urine, and feces. "The nature of these smells—for instance, are they foul or sour?—can also tell a lot about a patient's condition," Dr. Molony says.

Patient Interview

Unlike conventional physicians, who on average devote little time to their patients during office visits, TCM practitioners take an extensive medical history of their patients during the initial consultation, and continue follow-up inquiries throughout the course of treatment. "Besides obtaining as much information as possible about the patient's current symptoms, previous illnesses, and a history of illness in the patient's family, TCM practitioners also ask questions about a variety of physical, emotional, and lifestyle factors that to patients often seem unrelated to their specific ailment," Dr. Molony says. "Areas of questioning can include food and drink preferences, sensitivities to climate or other external conditions, sleep patterns, digestion and elimination habits, work and personal relationships, sex, emotions, and whether the patient is experiencing any pain or congestion in the nose, throat, chest, eyes, ears, or head."

Touch

This category of diagnosis consists of two distinct methods, palpation and pulse diagnosis. *Palpation* involves palpating or lightly massaging the skin and various acupoints along the meridian pathways. "Touching the skin allows the practitioner to make a general assessment of body and skin temperature and to determine if the skin is moist or dry," Dr. Molony explains.

"Palpating the meridian points that correspond to specific internal organs is done to make a determination about muscle tone, sensitivity, or pain, all of which can alert the practitioner to disharmonies in the corresponding internal organs."

Pulse diagnosis, or sphygmology, has been a part of traditional Chinese medicine for over two thousand years. "It is both a complex science and an art that takes years to properly master," Dr. Molony says. "Adept practitioners can detect six different pulses on each wrist, each of which corresponds to one of the twelve major organs. In addition, skillful practitioners can further distinguish over thirty pulse qualities in each of the twelve wrist pulses. By analyzing these qualities, they can identify not only current organ imbalances, but also past imbalances and latent imbalances that might manifest in the future."

After the practitioner has applied each of these four diagnostic methods, he or she then organizes the symptoms according to TCM's Eight Principles of diagnosis. "TCM practitioners categorize symptoms of illness in eight principal ways, starting with whether they are primarily yin or yang in nature," Dr. Molony says. "According to TCM theory, it is not enough to simply identify the general type of symptoms or illness a patient is experiencing, such as whether it is a heat, wind, or damp condition. It is also crucial to determine the specific nature of the illness, and to note how far it has progressed, and how the entire body is responding to it."

As we have seen, illnesses that are yin in nature are accompanied by internal, cold, and deficient symptoms, while yang conditions are characterized by symptoms that are external, hot, and excessive. Taken together, these eight states comprise the Eight Principles—Yin: Internal, Cold, Deficient; Yang: External, Hot, Excess. "Both yin and yang are fluid states, with each of them always containing a bit of their opposite," Dr. Molony says. "Symptoms are fluid, as well, and frequently occur in combination. Using the Eight Principles, a practitioner might categorize an illness as external-cold, internal-hot, and deficient-yang, for example, and then match it with the proper course of treatment, including follow-up visits to monitor recovery and adjust the treatment as needed."

HEALING ARTHRITIS: 🌿 A CASE HISTORY 🌿

In his *Complete Guide to Chinese Herbal Medicine*, Dr. Molony cites a case history that illustrates how the diagnostic system of traditional Chinese medicine can be used to create an effective treatment program. One of his patients, a thirty-eight-year-old man named John, came to him suffering from aching and swollen joints. Noticing that John was overweight, Dr. Molony assumed that his knees, particularly his right one, which hurt him the most, would be the area of his body most likely to first manifest arthritic symptoms.

During the interview process, John revealed that when his joint pain was at its worst, the joints themselves also became hot. Almost every movement John made was painful, and he admitted to constant sleep difficulties because he was unable to find a comfortable sleeping position. Previously, he had tried sleeping medications but abandoned their use because they left him even more tired in the morning. In order to get relief, John wrapped his right knee in ice each day after work, which helped to reduce the swelling and pain. His left knee and right hand occasionally required the same type of care.

In addition, John disclosed that he sometimes suffered from headaches and was always thirsty. Dr. Molony also observed that he perspired heavily, even after minor exertion, and that he had trouble sitting still, despite the pain that moving about caused him. Occasionally, he also suffered from skin rashes, and observation of his tongue revealed a thin, yellow coating.

Dr. Molony diagnosed John as suffering from early-stage arthritis and intermittent bouts of sciatica, along with high blood pressure that was exacerbated by his weight problem. "From the perspective of traditional Chinese medicine, John was experiencing symptoms of wind-damp and wind-chill, along with stagnant *qi* and blood, deficient yin, and rising heart fire," Dr. Molony explains. "I determined that he needed an herbal formula that would relieve his pain, while dispelling wind and damp, cooling the heart fire, invigorating and tonifying the blood, moving *qi*, and nourishing yin. I prescribed clematis and stephania, along with lifestyle and diet counseling as the treatment I felt John would best respond to. Over time, his symptoms noticeably improved."

YOUR FIRST SESSION

Your first visit to a TCM practitioner or acupuncturist who is not also a medical doctor will usually consist of an evaluation similar in scope to the diagnostic methods described above. Medical acupuncturists may employ conventional diagnosis, as well. Once your condition has been determined, your practitioner will then discuss with you an appropriate plan of treatment, which will usually commence during this same visit. In the majority of cases, acupuncture will be part of that treatment program. In some cases it will be used alone; in others, Chinese herbs, diet therapy, and lifestyle counseling will also be included.

One of the most common concerns of people considering acupuncture for the first time is whether the use of needles will hurt them. Although people experience acupuncture differently, the vast majority of them experience little or no pain when the needles are inserted, and no pain at all once the needles are in place. Since acupuncture needles are very thin and solid, and their points are smooth, their insertion is far less painful than injections of hypodermic needles or blood sampling, and there is far less risk of bruising or skin irritation. Many patients commonly experience feelings of deep relaxation shortly after the needles are inserted, as well, especially during the first few sessions.

Another common concern has to do with potential side effects. No harmful side effects have ever been attributed to acupuncture or TCM when properly administered by competent practitioners. In some cases, however, patients will experience what is sometimes referred to as a "healing crisis," a concept that is common to most of the therapies within the field of holistic medicine. Just as a stagnant pond may show clear water on its surface, but when stirred will become muddy before the stagnation clears up, so too can the body's symptoms sometimes worsen before healing occurs. In the case of acupuncture and TCM, such a worsening usually lasts for only a few days and stems from the body's energy (qi) being redirected as a result of treatment. Other changes can occur, as well, such as alterations in appetite, sleeping patterns, bowel and urinary functions, and mental and emotional states. Rather than being a cause for alarm, they are actually indications that the treatment is working. Be sure to let your practitioner know if you experience such symptoms so that he or she can monitor them and make any adjustments to your treatment that might be advisable.

The length of treatment is another concern, and treatment time can vary substantially from person to person. In general, one to two treatments each week over the course of several months may be recommended for serious, chronic conditions, while fewer visits are usually required for acute health problems. If your aim is to maintain your health before illness strikes, four to six visits per year may be all that is necessary, providing that you also follow a healthy lifestyle.

To enhance your treatment program, the American Academy of Medical Acupuncture (AAMA) recommends the following guidelines:

Let your practitioner know everything that you are doing so that he or she can help you get the most benefit from your treatments.
Avoid eating large meals immediately before or after treatment.
Don't overexercise, engage in sex, or consume alcohol for six hours before and after treatment. Substance abuse of either drugs or alco-

hol will also seriously interfere with your treatment, especially if indulged in during the week prior to each session.

Plan your activities so that you can rest after your treatment, especially during your first few visits.

If you are taking prescription medications, continue to do so according to your doctor's instructions.

Keep a written log of your response to your treatment and share it with your practitioner to ensure that follow-up treatment is appropriate for your particular problem.

To get the best results from your treatment, take a proactive role regarding your health. Be sure to follow any lifestyle and dietary suggestions that your practitioner makes, and don't be afraid to ask questions so that you can fully understand your treatment's progression. Passive reliance on your practitioner to "make you better" will pay far fewer dividends to your health than making an active commitment to become optimally healthy.

SELECTING AN ACUPUNCTURIST OR TCM PRACTITIONER

As in any new endeavor, it is important that you select an acupuncturist or TCM practitioner whom you can trust and who is competent. Be sure to check the credentials of your practitioner. Thirty-nine states, along with the District of Columbia, require state licensing for acupuncturists. Of these, the following twenty-five states, along with the District of Columbia, set rigorous training standards: Alaska, California, Colorado, Florida, Hawaii, Iowa, Louisiana, Maine, Maryland, Massachusetts, Montana, Nevada, New Jersey, New Mexico, New York, North Carolina, Oregon, Pennsylvania, Rhode Island, Texas, Utah, Vermont, Virginia, Washington, and Wisconsin. If you live in a state that doesn't require licensing, choose a practitioner who is certified by the National Commission for the Certification of Acupuncturists, or a member of the American Association of Oriental Medicine or the American Academy of Medical Acupuncture. (For contact information, see the "Resources" section at the end of this chapter.)

After you have assured yourself of your practitioner's competency, determine how much he or she charges per treatment. First-time visits to nonphysician acupuncturists and TCM practitioners average between $40 to $100 or more, while follow-up treatments normally range from

$35 to $75. Medical acupuncturists generally charge a bit more. Extra costs may also be incurred for any Chinese herbal formulas that may be recommended. Some insurance companies now cover acupuncture treatment costs. Examine your policy beforehand, and ask your practitioner if he or she accepts insurance payments.

Insist on disposable needles to prevent the risk of infection. Such needles are now used by nearly all acupuncturists in the United States, but it is still a good idea to make sure your practitioner is one of them.

Finally, be realistic about what your goals are in seeking treatment, and discuss them with your practitioner during your first session, and during the course of your treatment. Don't hesitate to voice any dissatisfaction you may have with the progress you are making. If your views are not honored, or an explanation is not offered that satisfies you, you may need to consider working with a different practitioner.

THE FUTURE OF ACUPUNCTURE AND TRADITIONAL CHINESE MEDICINE

In all likelihood, both acupuncture and traditional Chinese medicine as a whole will continue to gain broader acceptance in the United States and around the world as viable systems of health care. A 1994 sampling of Norwegian physicians, for example, found that over 80 percent of them felt that acupuncture should be integrated into Norway's national health care system, and the same percentage of physicians also said they "would not try to interfere with a patient's wish to try acupuncture treatment for cancer." Based on their findings, researchers who conducted the sampling postulate that acupuncture will become an integral part of Norway's health care system in the near future. In the United States, a survey of members of the American Academy of Medical Acupuncture found that over 80 percent of respondents used acupuncture in their practice to treat pain, particularly low back pain, myofascial conditions, simple headache, sciatica, shoulder pain, and tennis elbow. Nearly 70 percent of AAMA's members also used it to treat chronic sinusitis, and 65 percent found it useful for treating gastrointestinal disorders. When asked why they used acupuncture, the physicians' most common response (91 percent) was that "it works," while 76 percent of those surveyed used it "because the standard medical approach was inadequate." The results of such studies, coupled with ongoing research validating the efficacy of acupuncture and other disciplines of TCM, suggest that physicians are now joining the lay public in their willingness to explore China's ancient healing techniques.

"In the best of all worlds," Dr. Molony says, "traditional Chinese medicine will work hand in hand with conventional medicine to offer the finest possible holistic health care to all individuals. TCM's emphasis on preventive and holistic health, and on safe, natural, and affordable treatments that summon up the remarkable curative powers of the individual's body, mind, and spirit, will help more people to avoid needing emergency medical treatment. And when conventional medical intervention is called for, TCM will also be there to hasten and enhance recovery and revitalize patients, steering them toward a new and healthier life."

RESOURCES

To locate qualified acupuncturists and TCM practitioners, or to find out more about how acupuncture and TCM work, contact the following organizations:

American Association of Oriental Medicine (AAOM)
433 Front Street
Catasauqua, Pennsylvania 18032
Phone: (888) 500-7999
Fax: (610) 624-2768
Email: AAOM1@aol.com
Web site: *www.aaom.org*

American Academy of Medical Acupuncture (AAMA)
5820 Wilshire Blvd., Suite 500
Los Angeles, California 90036
Phone: (323) 937-5514
Fax: (323) 937-0959

National Certification Commission of Acupuncture and Oriental
    Medicine
P.O. Box 97075
Washington, D.C. 20090-7075
Phone: (202) 232-1404
Fax: (202) 462-6157

Accrediting Commission for Acupuncture and Oriental Medicine
1010 Wayne Avenue, Suite 1270
Silver Spring, Maryland 20910
Phone: (301) 608-9680
Fax: (301) 608-9576

Council of Colleges of Acupuncture and Oriental Medicine
1010 Wayne Avenue, Suite 1270
Silver Spring, Maryland 20910
Phone: (301) 608-9175

Internet Resources

Web site: *www.acupuncture.com*

RECOMMENDED READING

Kaptchuk, Ted. *The Web That Has No Weaver: Understanding Chinese Medicine*. Congdon and Weed, 1992.

Molony, David, with Ming Ming Pan Molony. The *American Association of Oriental Medicine's Complete Guide to Chinese Herbal Medicine*. Berkley Publishing Group, 1998.

Ni, Maoshing. *The Yellow Emperor's Classic of Medicine*. Shambhala Publications, 1995.

Worsley, J. R. *Acupuncture: Is It For You?* Harper & Row, 1973.

CHAPTER 14

Yoga

While yoga is not a medical therapy per se, holistic physicians often recommend it for its proven ability to diminish stress, increase flexibility and muscle tone, promote relaxation, and improve overall health. One of the earliest forms of mind-body medicine (see Chapter 5), yoga is also an integral part of Ayurvedic medicine (see Chapter 12) and has been practiced in India and other Asian countries for thousands of years. In the West, it gained scientific credibility in 1970, when early biofeedback experiments conducted at the Menninger Foundation in Topeka, Kansas, found that Indian yoga master Swami Rama was able to control various autonomic functions previously considered beyond the influence of conscious intent. These experiments revolutionized Western science's understanding about the relationship between the mind and the body, and how they interact to create both health and disease. Once learned, yoga is ideally suited as a daily self-care routine, and in the past decade its popularity as a fitness regimen has surged, with yoga schools and instructors now available in most communities across the United States, to meet the needs of the growing number of people interested in its benefits.

⚘ FAST FACTS ⚘

The word *yoga* means "union" or "to yoke," indicating its original purpose as a way of life intended to create both an integration of mankind's physical, mental, and spiritual energies, and to serve as a discipline that would ultimately result in unifying the *atman*, or individual self (soul) with the *Paramatman*, or Absolute Being (God).

In India, where it originated, yoga represents a complete way of life similar to the holistic lifestyle advocated by practitioners of holistic medicine. In addition to its many physiological benefits, in the East, yoga is traditionally practiced as a means of overall personal development (body, mind, and spirit) that integrates yogic breathing practices and physical postures with an ethical code of conduct, vegetarian diet, meditation, and the cultivation of spiritual awareness. By contrast, in the West, yoga is primarily practiced as a means of enhancing health and alleviating various disease conditions.

Male practitioners of yoga who are adept in its practice are often referred to as *yogis*, while female adepts are known as *yoginis*. ❧

HISTORY OF YOGA

Archaeological evidence indicates that yoga originated in India at least five thousand years ago, during the time of the Indus-Sarasvati civilization, a maritime people who traded their goods throughout Mesopotamia and parts of Africa. Today they are recognized as having developed one of the earliest sophisticated sewage systems, along with advanced multistory architecture, brick roadways, and public baths. The first recorded references to yoga occur in the Vedas, considered to be the oldest written spiritual scriptures in the world and which, along with the Upanishads, written centuries later, served as the philosophical basis for Hinduism, India's most popular religion. In the Vedas, yoga is portrayed as a ritual practice intended to lead beyond the dualities of the outer, temporal world into a state of transcendent union with God.

In the centuries following the appearance of the Vedic teachings, a variety of techniques and meditative exercises were developed to better enable yoga practitioners to still their minds and achieve deeper levels of awareness, during which time the great spiritual classics of Hinduism, such as the Bhagavad Gita (meaning "The Lord's Song") were also written. In the second century B.C., the practice of yoga was further codified by the yogic sage Patanjali in his *Yoga Sutras*, which are still referred to by yoga teachers and students alike today. Patanjali's teachings embodied what is known as *raja yoga*, also known as *asthanga yoga*, or the "eightfold path." The purpose of *raja yoga* is to bring about greater control and regulation of both the mind and body, which over time is said to lead to a refinement of the senses, both inner and outer, preparing them for the direct experience of the Divine. Its eight "limbs" are *yama, niyama, asana, pranayama, pratyahara, dharana, dhyana,* and *samadhi,* each of which is outlined more fully in "How Yoga Works" later in this chapter.

In subsequent centuries, yoga's focus on achieving union with God began to shift to include techniques designed to uncover the untapped potentials of the body itself. Rather than seeking to "leave the world behind" by merging with "the formless Beyond," during this time, a number of yogi masters devised yoga methods of physical rejuvenation and life extension, seeking to actually change the body's biochemistry and even make it immortal. From their explorations, a system of physical postures and breathing techniques known as *hatha yoga* was created. Over time, *hatha yoga* grew to include *kundalini yoga* and *tantra yoga* (see following page). Today, there are literally hundreds of *asanas* (postures) and their variations within the various *hatha yoga* systems, with yoga remaining an integral tradition in India. Yoga is popular in other regions of Asia, as well, where it sometimes appears under other names, such as Tibetan Buddhism, or Lamaism, of which the Dalai Lama is the world's foremost recognized authority.

In the United States, although the spiritual teachings of India influenced such famous Americans as Ralph Waldo Emerson and Henry David Thoreau, yoga and Hindu philosophy did not truly come to the public's awareness until 1893, when the Parliament of Religions convened in Chicago. There, Swami Vivekananda, sent to the United States by his teacher, the famed Indian saint Ramakrishna, made a lasting impression on the Parliament's primarily Western audience and went on to spend years traveling across the United States and other countries sharing the teachings of yoga and *Vedanta,* India's nondualistic philosophy. A few decades later, in 1920, Paramahansa Yogananda arrived in Boston, and within five years had established the Self-Realization Fellowship in Los Angeles. Best known in the West as the author of *Autobiography of a Yogi,* the first book to offer Western readers a vivid, behind-the-scenes account of the development of a yoga master and the true nature of yoga's scope, Yogananda remained an influential teacher in the West until his death in 1952. After he died, his body remained in a state of physical incorruptibility for twenty days, as attested to by a notarized letter provided to the Self-Realization Fellowship by the mortuary director of Los Angeles' Forest Lawn Memorial Park, where the body was temporarily interred.

Following the warm reception given to Vivekananda and Yogananda, numerous other Indian yoga masters traveled to the United States to train

Westerners in various yoga practices. For many Americans, yoga continued to be perceived as a fad practice (particularly in Hollywood, where it was embraced by many screen celebrities) steeped in pseudomysticism. But that perception was dramatically changed in 1970, when Elmer and Alyce Green (see Chapter 5), using biofeedback instrumentation, revolutionized Western science's understanding of the "mind-body connection" with their experiments involving Swami Rama, founder of the Himalayan International Institute of Yoga Science and Philosophy in Honesdale, Pennsylvania. Among the achievements Swami Rama demonstrated was the ability to voluntarily maintain different brain-wave rhythms, as well as altering his thyroid output and stopping his heart from pumping blood for a full seventeen seconds without any harmful effects. Since that time, numerous scientific studies have further validated yoga's benefits for a host of conditions, both physical and psychological.

✹ TYPES OF YOGA ✹

The form of yoga most familiar to Westerners is known as *hatha yoga*, which deals primarily with breathing exercises and physical postures that can improve overall health and provide greater control over various body functions such as heart and respiration rates. The ultimate goal of *hatha yoga*, however, is to make the mind and body fit instruments for perceiving greater levels of spiritual awareness.

A variety of other yoga practices exist, as well, although for the most part they are less well-known in the West. What follows is a brief overview of some of them.

Karma Yoga

Also known as "the yoga of action," *karma yoga* emphasizes a way of life in which individuals live their lives responsibly, using their talents in selfless service to humanity. While worldly success is not shunned by *karma yoga* practitioners, neither is it actively sought. Instead, practitioners learn to remain detached from the fruits of their actions, choosing instead to focus on the opportunities for growth in each present moment.

Bhakti Yoga

Known as "the yoga of devotion," *bhakti yoga* is considered a path of joyful self-surrender in which practitioners dedicate themselves to the worship of God in all of their thoughts and actions. In the process, *bhakti yogis* come to see "the Divine in all things," ultimately achieving a state of nondual consciousness, or *samadhi*, in which all of life is recognized as One Absolute Being. One of the most famous *bhakti* yogis was the Indian saint Ramakrishna, who would regularly enter into states of spiritual ecstasy in the course of his daily life experiences.

Jnana Yoga

"The yoga of knowledge," *jnana yoga* involves cultivating one's awareness in order to distinguish between what is real (eternal and everlasting) and what is illusory (temporal and finite). Practitioners of *jnana yoga* focus on a process of self-observation and meditation, seeking to detach themselves from the actions and desires of the ego in order to uncover their true spiritual nature.

Kundalini Yoga

This yoga practice concerns itself with the subtle life force energy known as *kundalini,* which in most people is said to lie as a "coiled serpent" at the base of the spine. Through various meditative, breathing, and physical exercises, practitioners of *kundalini yoga* seek to "awaken" this serpent energy so that it rises through each of the body's seven major chakras (energy centers), until it is able to flow freely along the spine to an area at the top of the head known as the crown chakra. As this process occurs, corresponding changes in consciousness occur. In the Eastern yoga traditions, *kundalini* is taught slowly by a teacher, or guru, to ensure that students proceed through the process safely, since the premature activation of *kundalini* energies is considered dangerous. In the West, this understanding is often ignored, however.

Mantra Yoga

Within the yoga tradition, certain sounds are said to contain frequencies capable of heightening consciousness, leading to improved powers of awareness and concentration, as well as spiritual purification. Such sounds are known as mantras, and *mantra yoga* involves chanting or meditating on them as part of a daily spiritual practice. The most famous mantra is *Om,* which is said to be one of the secret names for God. Regular practice of *mantra yoga* is said to focus the practitioner's mind on the Divine, leading to a refinement in thought and a detachment from the ego's worldly concerns. In the West, research by mind-body practitioners such as Herbert Benson, M.D. (see Chapter 5), has also shown that *mantra yoga* triggers the "relaxation response," a state of physiological equilibrium capable of counteracting the effects of stress and habitual tension. In the West, the most popular form of *mantra yoga* is Transcendental Meditation.

Tantra Yoga

Tantra yoga, which was first written about in India between A.D. 400 and 600, emphasizes acceptance of one's nature, including one's sexuality. The word *tantra* itself means "weaving" or "expansion," and practitioners of *tantra yoga* are concerned with weaving and expanding all aspects of themselves in order to more fully unite "the spirit with the flesh" while more deeply perceiving the divine joy in each moment. In India and other Eastern countries where it is practiced, *tantra* is considered a complete way of life that is intended to help practitioners fulfill their highest potential while simultaneously achieving transcendent states of awareness. In the West, however, emphasis has primarily been given to *tantra's* various exercises for achieving more potent sexual experiences, often without regard to *tantra's* true nature as another path to God.

All of the above forms of yoga are said to be superseded by *raja yoga*, outlined in the Yoga Sutras of Patanjali. Often referred to as "the royal path," *raja yoga* encompasses elements of most other forms of yoga, and therefore can be adapted to suit each practitioner's temperament and background. Its primary aim is complete transcendence of the sensory or "lower" self, in order to achieve *samadhi*, or total union with God. Through its practice, one learns how to control thoughts, emotions, and desires, while plumbing the depths of the unconscious to free oneself from conditioned responses and limited, egoic beliefs, ultimately attaining mastery over his or her threefold nature—physical, mental/emotional, and spiritual. ❦

HOW YOGA WORKS

Classical, or *raja yoga*, not only encompasses a complete system of health, but also offers a systematic approach for living an optimum lifestyle for overall personal development. The first four "limbs" of classical yoga, *yama*, *niyama*, *asana*, and *pranayama*, comprise the system of *hatha yoga*, while the remaining limbs, *pratyahara*, *dharana*, *dhyana*, and *samadhi* are more concerned with yoga's original purpose—transcendent union with the Divine.

Yama and *niyama* together comprise a system of ethics and moral restraints, all of which are also conducive to health. *Yama* includes the observance of truthfulness, continence, nonpossessiveness, nonstealing, and nonviolence (which traditionally includes a vegetarian diet); while *niyama* involves cleanliness, contemplation (study of sacred writings), *tapas* (practices designed to perfect the body and the senses), and the cultivation of contentment and surrender to one's "higher nature." Over time, regular adherence to the principles of *yama* and *niyama* leads to greater self-mastery and a refinement in personal habits and traits.

Asana and *pranayama* together comprise the two most commonly practiced elements of yoga in the West. *Asana*, which means "ease" in Sanskrit, refers to the various yoga postures and exercises designed to create greater levels of physical well-being. There are two types of *asanas*, which are often called meditative and therapeutic. Meditative *asanas* are primarily sitting and supine postures intended to align the body, neck, and spine in a manner that promotes relaxation and enhances concentration during meditation. Therapeutic *asanas*, such as the headstand and shoulder stand, are more active postures that improve flexibility, strengthen muscle tone, and lead to increased bodily awareness and greater control over various physiological processes. Therapeutic *asanas* have also been shown to have a variety of benefits for a number of disease conditions.

Often practiced in conjunction with *asana*, *pranayama*, which is sometimes called "the science of breathing," involves various breathing exercises that serve to control the flow of *prana*, or life force energy, throughout the body. According to yogic theory, a system of 72,000 subtle nerve pathways, known as *nadis*, runs parallel to the physical nervous system. Prana is said to flow through the nadis, regulating health and influencing consciousness. *Pranayama* exercises help keep the *nadi* pathways unblocked, while strengthening the nervous system. They are also conducive to calming and focusing the mind, which in turn results in a lessening of bodily tensions.

The fifth aspect of *raja yoga*, *pratyahara*, is concerned with the control and gradual withdrawal of the senses from the physical world in order to better perceive the greater reality which lies within. Regular practice of *pratyahara* prepares one for *dharana*, which involves the systematic cultivation of the mind's powers of concentration. Together, they result in *dhyana*, a prolonged, one-pointed meditative state of superconsciousness, which ultimately leads to the eighth and final transcendent state of *samadhi*.

The primary focus on yoga by holistic practitioners is usually on *asana*, *pranayama*, and meditation, since each of these aspects has been shown by research to improve health. All three practices, performed separately, result in a deeper connection between the body, mind, and breath, but best results are achieved when they are performed in conjunction with each other. The *asanas* work to tone muscles and align the spine, while increasing strength and flexibility and revitalizing the body's inner organs. Although they usually involve minimal movement, proper execution of yoga *asanas* can initially be difficult to achieve. The reason for this lies in the fact that, contrary to popular belief, *asanas* are not simply intended for achieving flexibility. Unlike other stretching exercises, *asanas* are meant to be performed with awareness while simultaneously breathing in a relaxed, yet focused manner. When a yoga posture is properly executed, it automatically stimulates the unobstructed flow of pranic energy in a manner that the practitioner can viscerally feel. Proper execution means that the *asana* is performed without straining, from a midway point between movement and stillness. In this way, students of yoga gain greater bodily awareness and become better able to dissipate physical tension, while improving their ability to regulate various body functions.

Pranayama, like *Qigong* (see Chapter 13), also helps practitioners become more aware of the flow of energy through their bodies, and to better control it by regulating respiration rates. In this way, practitioners learn how to use the breath to release stress and promote calm during times of tension, and to increase their energy levels when necessary. The improved breathing habits that result from regular *pranayama* practice also helps purify the lymphatic system, an essential component of the immune system, and enhances blood circulation to bring increased amounts of oxygen and nutrients to the cells. *Pranayama* also allows patients to more deeply appreciate the mind-body connection as they experience the beneficial effects that proper breathing can have on their thoughts and bodies. Most *pranayama* exercises focus on breathing slowly and fully from the abdomen, in contrast to the shallow, chest-centered breathing patterns so prevalent among Western adults. Alternate nostril breathing, in which the breath is inhaled and exhaled through one nostril at a time, is another common *pranayama* exercise. Known in India as *nadi shodhana*, alternate nostril breathing is performed by closing one nostril with the thumb or finger while inhaling and exhaling in a deep, relaxed manner through the other nostril. On the second inhalation, breathing occurs through the opposite nostril, while the first one is closed. Nostrils continued to be alternated throughout the course of the exercise. The purpose of alternate nostril breathing is to purify the *nadi* pathways while balancing the flow of pranic energy between the body's left and right hemispheres, resulting in improved physiological functioning.

Meditation, which is covered more fully in Chapter 5, is another effective mind-body technique, and is also useful for reducing stress levels, improving mental functioning, and optimizing blood flow and oxygen consumption. In addition, people who practice meditation daily over time commonly report heightened experiences of joy and peace, as well as greater levels of awareness.

Depending on each patient's specific needs, holistic practitioners might prescribe specific *asana*, *pranayama* and meditation exercises that are most appropriate for his or her condition. For further support, patients may also be referred to competent yoga trainers to ensure that they learn how to perform their exercises properly. With time and practice, patients can incorporate their yoga skills into a daily self-care protocol in order to maintain the health benefits they achieve.

CONDITIONS THAT BENEFIT FROM YOGA

While yoga was originally never intended as a treatment for illness, since the 1970s thousands of scientific studies have confirmed its ability to provide a wide range of both physiological and psychological benefits, due to the positive lifestyle changes that typically result from its regular practice. Among the range of body functions that yoga has been shown to improve are heart rate, metabolism, motor skills, respiration, and sensory perception. Yoga can also reduce stress and anxiety, help regulate blood pressure levels, and alleviate pain. With regular practice, students of yoga can better regulate functions such as body temperature, skin resistance, and brain-wave activity, as well as improving memory and intelligence skills.

One of the reasons for yoga's effectiveness in improving and maintaining health is its ability to positively influence the body's endocrine and nervous systems, something that distinguished it from most other forms of exercise and physical activity. As mentioned above, regular practice of *pranayama* breathing exercises has been shown to have a beneficial effect on the nervous system, which in turn leads to greater control over various autonomic processes. In addition, certain *asanas* help to increase circulation within various nerve centers throughout the body, as well as within the endocrine glands. The gravitational effects of the shoulder stand, for instance, help to stimulate the thyroid gland, while the cobra pose, in which the practitioner lies flat on the stomach and then slowly bends backward from the waist, improves circulation in the intervertebral discs along the lumbar and sacral regions.

The following are some of the many conditions for which yoga has been scientifically proven to be beneficial.

Asthma

Regular practice of yoga *asanas* and *pranayama* exercises has been shown to improve respiration rates, increase lung capacity, and help alleviate a variety of respiratory conditions, including asthma. In a sixteen-week study of asthmatics conducted in 1998, for example, patients who practiced *asanas*, *pranayama*, and meditation three times a week in yoga classes required less use of their inhalers, compared to a control group, despite no statistical changes in pulmonary functions between both groups. The yoga group also reported dramatic improvements in relaxation and positive mental attitude, leading researchers to conclude that yoga can serve as a beneficial adjunctive treatment for managing asthma.

Previous studies published in the *Journal of Asthma* revealed even more dramatic improvements among asthmatics who practiced yoga. In the first study, 74 percent of 255 asthmatics who practice yoga were either cured, or showed significant improvement. A similar study, conducted over a year, found that 76 percent of 114 asthma patients were either cured or significantly improved, and revealed that asthma attacks could usually be averted by practicing yoga instead of using medications. When combined with meditation, another study found that yoga improved asthma symptoms in 93 percent of 15 asthmatics after nine years of practice, along with substantially reducing anxiety levels and enhancing concentration skills. Other research conducted at the All India Institute of Medical Science in New Delhi found that asthmatics can achieve "significant improvement" in their symptoms after as little as seven days of yoga practice.

Addiction

Due to its ability to reduce anxiety levels, enhance self-esteem, and improve mental functioning, yoga has recently been shown to be effective as an aid in treating drug addiction. One study found that users of marijuana showed a decline in substance abuse after partaking of a yoga and meditation training, while another study, conducted by researchers at

Harvard Medical School, found that yoga was just as effective as traditional psychotherapy in helping patients successfully complete methadone treatment programs. In the study, participants were divided into two groups, with the first group practicing *hatha yoga*, and the second group receiving psychotherapy. After six months, both groups had nearly identical scores in a variety of psychological and physiological tests. Drug use and criminal activity by both groups was also significantly reduced.

Back Pain

Yoga postures and breathing exercises help both to prevent and alleviate back pain, due to their ability to ease muscle tension, restore spinal alignment, and increase flexibility, as well as reducing stress, which is often implicated in back problems. Regular yoga practice also tends to result in greater awareness of correct body use, and to strengthen the cervical and lumbar regions of the body, both of which are most susceptible to accidents, injury, and trauma. By following a yoga program that combines *asana, pranayama*, and meditation, people prone to back pain can minimize and prevent recurrence of their symptoms in a variety of ways. In addition to promoting greater overall flexibility, *asanas* help to correct faulty posture, while strengthening weak muscles. *Pranayama* not only helps ease musculoskeletal tension, but positively influences rib movement and chest pressure, both of which can affect the spine. Meditation promotes stress relief, as well, and leads to improved awareness, psychologically and physiologically, enabling yoga practitioners to lower the incidence of movements and postures that can trigger back pain.

One of the most revealing surveys on the benefits of yoga in relation to low back pain was conducted in 1983 by researchers led by Robin Munro, Ph.D., founder of England's Yoga Biomedical Trust. In the survey, approximately 3,000 students of yoga were asked to evaluate to what degree yoga had resulted in improvement in their various ailments. Of the study group, 1,142 respondents suffered from back pain prior to beginning yoga practice. Ninety-eight percent of them reported that yoga had alleviated or completely relieved their back pain symptoms.

Carpal Tunnel Syndrome

A study published in 1998 in the *Journal of the American Medical Association* (*JAMA*) found that a simple yoga sequence of eleven *asanas* was capable of reducing pain related to carpal tunnel syndrome and improving overall hand strength more effectively than drugs, surgery, or other conventional treatment methods. Conducted by researchers at the University of Pennsylvania Medical School, the randomized study involved two groups of subjects. The control group wore wrist splints, a standard conventional medical treatment, while the second group engaged in a ninety-minute yoga class twice a week. There, they performed basic yoga postures designed to take each joint of the upper body through its full range of motion, while simultaneously stretching, strengthening, and aligning the hands, wrists, arms, and shoulders. After two months, participants in the yoga class experienced significantly reduced pain and exhibited greater hand strength than before they began the class, compared to the control group, which showed no improvement in pain or strength scores.

Cognitive Skills

Pranayama, particularly alternate nostril breathing, has been shown to improve communication between the left and right hemispheres of the brain, as well as increasing cognition and spatial memory. Electroencephalogram (EEG) studies of the brain's electrical impulses have found that breathing through one nostril increases brain activity in the opposite brain hemisphere. In a study published in 1991 in the *International Journal of Neuromedicine*, twenty-three men who practiced alternate nostril breathing exhibited improved cognition and performance skills associated with the opposite side of the brain. Another study published in 1997 revealed that students between the ages of ten and seventeen demonstrated major improvement in spatial memory tests after practicing *pranayama* for ten days. In the study, the students were divided into five groups, with the first four groups each practicing a specific *pranayama* breathing exercise. At the conclusion of the study, all four groups showed an average improvement of 84 percent in scores of spatial memory, compared to the control group, which showed little or no improvement.

Epileptic Seizure

Practice of a meditation technique known as *Sahaja yoga*, developed in the 1970s by yoga adept Mataji Nirmala Devi, has been shown by researchers to reduce the incidence of epileptic seizure. Regular practice of *Sahaja yoga* is said to lead to increased "vibratory awareness" of the body's various energy systems. In one study published in 1996, thirty-two patients suffering from idiopathic (no clear cause) epilepsy were randomly divided into three groups. The first group practiced *Sahaja yoga*, the second group practiced exercises intended to mimic *Sahaja yoga*, and the third group served as the control. During the course of the study, all three groups were also monitored with EEG analysis.

By the end of three months, those who practiced *Sahaja yoga* had a 62 percent reduction in their frequency of epileptic seizures, along with corresponding positive changes in their EEG readings. At the end of six months, positive EEG alterations continued, and the group's seizure rate was 86 percent less than their rate prior to the start of the study. Neither of the other two groups exhibited improvements in any of the study's test parameters. Additional research has shown that Sahaja yoga may also benefit other conditions, including cardiovascular conditions, respiratory disease, migraine, and hypertension.

Grip Strength

Recent research in India has shown that *pranayama* can increase grip strength within ten days. In the study, children at a yoga camp between the ages of eleven and eighteen were divided into five groups, with each group instructed to practice a specific breathing practice in conjunction with their *asana* practice. The first group was told to practice breathing only through the right nostril; the second group practiced breathing solely through the left nostril; and the third practiced alternate nostril breathing. The fourth and fifth groups practiced either breath awareness or *mudras* (specific types of yoga postures intended to enhance the flow of vital energy). At the end of ten days, all of the first three groups exhibited a significant increase in the strength of both hands, compared to the other two groups, neither of which demonstrated any change.

Heart Disease

Recent research has shown that following a yogic lifestyle of regular practice of *asanas*, *pranayama*, and meditation can reduce dangerous lipid levels in patients with angina and healthy subjects with risk factors for coronary heart disease. In another study conducted by researchers at the All India Institute of Medical Sciences, subjects in both of the above categories were evaluated for a variety of risk factors, including weight, serum cholesterol, triglycerides, high- and low-density lipoprotein levels (HDL and LDL) and the cholesterol-HDL ratio. The subjects were then divided into two groups, both of which were supplied with lifestyle advice, with one of the groups also receiving four days of yoga instruction, which they then practiced at home. Further evaluations of both groups were made after four, ten, and fourteen weeks. During each evaluation, the researchers found that patients in the yoga group showed a regular reduction of all lipid parameters except HDL, which is often referred to as "healthy cholesterol." In contrast, the control group exhibited inconsistent patterns of change in all risk-factor categories, indicating that regular yoga practice can provide cardiovascular benefit.

In another study conducted by researchers at Germany's Hanover Medical University, participants at risk for heart disease underwent a comprehensive yoga and meditation program for three months, while also being placed on a low-fat vegetarian diet. As in the previous study, a range of cardiovascular risk factors were evaluated prior to the program, along with a variety of hormone levels. After the program ended, all of the participants had a lower body-mass index, as well as reduced fibrinogen, LDL, and total serum cholesterol levels. Their hormone profiles were also improved, as were their blood pressure levels.

Mood and Vitality

Among the benefits commonly reported by regular practitioners of yoga are improved mood and increased energy levels. This was confirmed by a British study conducted in 1993. The study involved seventy-one healthy participants between the ages of twenty-one and seventy-six, and compared the effects of yoga, relaxation exercises, and visualization. Participants who practiced a thirty-minute yoga routine of *asanas* and *pranayama* had a significantly greater increase in mental and physical energy, accompanied by feelings of greater alertness and enthusiasm, denoting an improvement in mood. In comparison, those who practiced either relaxation or visualization exercises felt sleepier after each session.

A different study conducted in Meriden, Connecticut, achieved similar results. The study involved bilingual patients (English- and Spanish-speaking) who were taught yoga and mindfulness meditation techniques. Regular practice of the techniques resulted in marked improvement in the patients' physical and mental health. Many of the patients also experienced dramatic positive changes in their levels of self-esteem, as evidence by a shift in their attitudes, beliefs, habits, and behaviors.

Obsessive-Compulsive Disorder

A study conducted by researchers at the University of California, San Diego, found that regular practice of *pranayama* can be effective as a treatment for obsessive-compulsive disorder (OCD), as well as for other anxiety-related disorders. In the study, eight adults suffering from OCD were taught a specific *pranayama* technique, which they then practiced for a year. Prior to and during the study, baseline evaluations of their condition were made based on the Yale-Brown Obsessive-Compulsive Scale (Y-BOCS), a traditional evaluation method for OCD. Evaluations were retaken at three and six months, with a final evaluation made at the end of the year.

Of the eight patients, five completed the entire study. When it was over, four of the participants showed improvements ranging between 61 and 83 percent, based on their Y-BOCS readings, while the fifth patient's status declined by 18 percent. All of the patients also showed improvements in their overall symptoms and Perceived Stress Scale scores, and three of them were able to completely eliminate the need for medication within seven months or less, while the other two were able to reduce their dosage range by 25 and 50 percent.

Rehabilitation

A scientific review of yoga as a means of rehabilitation found that it can be effective in a number of ways. The study's findings indicated that yoga can help people who are mentally handicapped by boosting their cognitive ability, as well as their social and motor skills. Yoga was also shown to be helpful for restoring some degree of functional ability to people who are physically handicapped, and for reducing anxiety levels related to visual impairment among children with poor vision. In addition, yoga was found to improve sleep, appetite and general well-being among socially disadvantaged children and adults, including prisoners and children remanded to detention homes. The review also confirmed that yoga and meditation can aid in treating substance abuse, and be effective in helping to rehabilitate the lives of patients with coronary heart disease.

HEALING BRONCHITIS:
🌿 A CASE HISTORY 🌿

The following case, involving Robin Munro, Ph.D., clearly demonstrates yoga's ability to improve health. From childhood, Dr. Munro suffered from chronic bronchial problems, which first manifested as asthma and led to chronic bronchitis in his adulthood. Following a severe bronchial attack when he was thirty-seven, his condition worsened to the point where it could only be controlled by medication and repeated antibiotic treatments, which negatively affected both his personal and professional life.

In his search for a cure to his condition, Dr. Munro began to explore a variety of holistic alternatives, including yoga, which he had practiced for over a decade. In the course of his investigations, he met a physician from India, who prescribed for him a new yogic routine consisting of a series of simple *asanas* and *pranayama* techniques, along with vigorous exercise. In addition, the physician also suggested acupressure as a means for resolving Dr. Munro's bronchial attacks without drugs. Within a year, Dr. Munro no longer needed acupressure to relieve his symptoms, and within three years, he was completely symptom-free and has remained so today, more than twenty years later. Because of the personal benefits he gained from his yoga practice, in 1983, Dr. Munro founded the Yoga Biomedical Trust in England, which conducts research into the full range of benefits yoga can provide for both acute and chronic illness. 🌿

YOUR FIRST SESSION

Despite the proliferation of yoga books and videotapes, people interested in learning yoga are advised to initially seek the assistance of a certified yoga trainer or therapist (see the "Resources" section at the end of this chapter). The reason for this rests in the subtleties that underlie the yoga *asanas* and *pranayama* techniques. Learning how to properly perform the postures and breathing execises is essential to receiving the full range of yoga's benefits, something that is best undertaken under the supervision of a trained yoga teacher who can guide you and correct improper approaches that can be difficult to discern when practicing alone. In addition, trainers can help you personalize your yoga routine once you understand how to properly perform the exercises, allowing you to more quickly and effectively get the benefits you are looking for.

In seeking yoga instruction, be aware that there are various schools and styles of *hatha yoga*, ranging from approaches that emphasize gentle, flowing movements, to those that are more vigorous and require certain levels of strength and stamina. While all approaches can be beneficial, the style you choose should be reflective of who you are, and address your personal goals and specific needs. Don't be afraid to explore various styles until you find the one that most appeals to you. In addition, inquire about your instructor's certification and level of training, to ensure that he or she is competent. Before beginning yoga practice, inform your instructor of any diseases you may be suffering from, as well as any weaknesses or injuries you might have, such as bad knees or a constricted back. You should also consult with your physician.

As you begin your practice of yoga, proceed gently, remembering to breathe naturally and without force, keeping your attention centered on each exercise as you perform it. Also be careful not to strain your muscles, especially if you have limited flexibility to begin with. Yoga is a process that deepens over time. As you become more attentive to your breathing and focus your attention on the postures, you will find your flexibility increasing with regular practice. It is not necessary to overdo it, and any sensation of pain should be heeded as an indication that you have exceeded your limits for that day.

When you practice, wear comfortable clothing that allows for a free range of movement, and perform your yoga routine in a room that is neither too hot or too cold. Avoid performing yoga right after eating, as doing so can interfere with digestion and cause discomfort. For best results, practice yoga regularly, at least three times a week, and ideally daily, once you have learned how to perform your yoga routine properly.

THE FUTURE OF YOGA

Yoga's recent surge in popularity as an alternative to more traditional exercise programs, coupled with ongoing research regarding its many physical and psychological health benefits, suggests that it will continue to receive serious consideration by holistic and conventional health practitioners alike as a safe and effective protocol for improving and maintaining overall well-being. With yoga instruction already becoming more widely available in health clubs, as well as being incorporated in wellness plans such as those developed by Dr. Dean Ornish to treat cardiovascular disease and obesity, it is also likely that in the near future yoga will become a part of the growing number of holistic health care clinics now appearing across the United States and abroad.

RESOURCES

To learn more about yoga, or to find a yoga practitioner in your area, contact the following organizations.

International Association of Yoga Therapists
a division of Yoga Research and Education Center
P.O. Box 2418
Sebastopol, California 95473
Phone: (707) 928-9898
Web site: *www.yrc.org/iayt.html*

Yoga Research and Education Center
P.O. Box 2418
Sebastopol, California 95473
Phone: (707) 928-9898
Email: mail@yrec.org
Web site: *www.yrec.org*

Yoga Biomedical Trust
Royal Homeopathic Hospital
60 Great Ormond Street
London, England
WC1N 3HR
Phone: 0171 419 7195
Fax: 0171 419 7911
E-mail: yogabio.med@virgin.net
Web site: *freespace.virgin.net/yogabio.med*

An annual directory of yoga schools and instructors is published by *Yoga Journal.*
Contact:

Yoga Journal
2054 University Avenue
Berkeley, California 94704
Phone: (510) 841-9200

Fax: (510) 644-3101
Web site: *www.yogajournal.com*

RECOMMENDED READING

Feuerstein, Georg. *The Yoga Tradition: Its History, Literature, Philosophy and Practice.* Hohm Press, 1998.

Groves, Dawn. *Yoga for Busy People.* New World Library, 1995.

Iyengar, B. *Light on Yoga.* Schocken Books, 1987.

Vishnudevananda, Swami. *The Complete Illustrated Book of Yoga.* Harmony Books, 1980.

CHAPTER 15

Additional Therapies of Holistic Medicine

The art and science of holistic medicine is inclusive and comprehensive, as demonstrated by the willingness of holistic physicians to employ a full range of therapeutic approaches in order to ensure that their patients receive the most effective treatment. In addition to the therapies discussed in the preceding chapters, holistic physicians may also employ a number of other professional care therapies to help restore their patients to health. What follows is an overview of those that are also commonly used by members of the American Holistic Medical Association.

Allopathic Medicine

Practiced by M.D.'s and many D.O.'s, allopathic medicine is the primary system of medicine practiced in the United States. It is unrivaled when it comes to treating acute, life-threatening emergencies and is also well suited for trauma care. Allopathic medicine can be an integral part of an overall holistic treatment plan, depending on the nature of a patient's disease. Its primary limitations lie in its philosophy that the cause of disease is physical and ultimately visible, and its reliance on surgery and pharmaceutical medications, both of which can be invasive and fraught with potentially debilitating side effects. For a comparison between holistic and allopathic medicine, see Chapter 1.

Aromatherapy

Aromatherapy, a term coined by French chemist and perfumer René-Maurice Gattefosse in 1928, involves the use of plant extracts known as essential oils to promote and maintain overall health. While the historical roots of aromatherapy extend back thousands of years, with plants and their essential oils having been used therapeutically in ancient Egypt, Greece, India, and Rome, Gattefosse is considered the modern-day founder of aromatherapy. His work in the field began accidentally, when he burned his hand while at work in his laboratory. Knowing that lavender was used to soothe burns and inflammation, he placed his hand in a nearby vat of lavender oil, which caused his burn to heal quickly. Curious, Gattefosse began experimenting with the essential oils of other plants, and cataloging their healing properties. Today, aromatherapy is becoming increasingly popular in the United States, Europe, and elsewhere as both a primary and adjunctive healing aid, depending on the disease it is used to treat.

The benefits of aromatherapy can be gained by inhaling essential oils added to steaming water or through diffusion methods. The oils can also be absorbed through the skin through topical applications, hot and cold compresses, and massage or when added to a hot bath. In certain cases they can also be ingested, but only under the direction of a physician or aromatherapist skilled in their use.

Although more commonly used in the United States for cosmetic reasons and to improve the mood of home and work environments, research shows that aromatherapy offers many therapeutic benefits, as well, due to the pharmacological properties of essential oils and the fact that their small molecular size allows them to quickly and easily penetrate the tissues of the body. In addition, studies have shown that as essential oil molecules travel through the nasal cavity, they interact with, and influence, the brain's limbic system, thereby physiologically and psychologically influencing the various mechanisms the limbic system controls. These include heart and respiration rates, blood pressure, memory, hormone balance, and stress levels.

Depending on the type of oil used, aromatherapy is also effective at inducing brain-wave patterns associated with both calm and a heightened sense of energy. Certain essential oils also contain powerful antimicrobial properties, making them effective aids against viral and bacterial infections, and as immune function enhancers. Other oils promote the elimination of toxins, relieve pain, help regulate the central nervous system, reduce inflammation, and improve skin conditions. Among the conditions for which aromatherapy has been shown to have benefit are acne, anxiety, arthritis, burns, cystitis, colds and flu, digestive disorders, headache, muscle spasm, nausea, respiratory conditions, shingles, toenail fungus, and vaginitis.

Note: Overall, aromatherapy is safe and nontoxic and in many ways is also well suited as a self-care therapy. Certain essential oils, however, can cause skin irritation when applied directly in undiluted form. Pregnant women and people suffering from hypertension should first consult a skilled aromatherapist before using essential oils, and no essential oil should be taken internally without proper medical supervision.

Biological Dentistry

Biological dentistry utilizes nontoxic materials in place of conventional amalgam dental fillings that contain mercury, tin, silver, and other metals that can be harmful to overall health and cause hidden allergies and infections. Proponents of biological dentistry also maintain that dental problems such as cavities, infections, and temporomandibular joint syndrome (TMJ), along with the potential bio-incompatibility of conventional dental fillings, can cause or exacerbate dysfunction and illness throughout the body and in many cases contribute to chronic disease. Ironically, though the views held by practitioners of biological dentistry have so far been rejected by the American Dental Association (ADA), in the mid-1900s, it was one of the ADA's former directors of research, Weston Price, D.D.S., M.S., who made the discovery that toxins leaking from root canals can cause dysfunctions of the endocrine and nervous systems, cardiovascular disorders, and diseases of the kidneys and uterus. Moreover, Dr. Price discovered that when patients with root canals who also suffered from heart or kidney disease had their teeth with root canals removed, the majority experienced a complete resolution of their diseases without the need for any other form of treatment. The late Theron Randolph, M.D., founder of environmental medicine (see Chapter 4), also felt that the toxicity of conventional dental materials could negatively affect health.

Despite the ADA's dismissal of biological dentistry's claims, increasing numbers of holistic physicians now recognize the potential health hazards of amalgam fillings and infection due to root canal and are having their patients screened accordingly, especially those whose conditions are chronic and for which other types of therapy have proven ineffective. The principles of biological dentistry are also widely accepted in Europe, in part due to studies by the World Health Organization, which found that a single amalgam filling can release up to seventeen micrograms of mercury into the body per day. Since the early 1990s, both the sale and manufacture of amalgams have been banned in Germany, and in Sweden, amalgams have officially been discouraged by the Social Welfare and Health Administration for use in dental treatments of women who are pregnant. Here in the United States, since 1988 scrap dental amalgam has been listed as a hazardous waste product by the Environmental Protection Agency due to its high mercury content. And in 1993 a symptom analysis of 1,569 patients from the United States, Canada, Denmark, and Sweden who had their amalgam fillings removed was submitted to the Food and Drug Administration. Prior to the removal, the patients suffered from one or more of the following conditions: allergy, anxiety, bad temper, bloating, chest pain, concentration problems, depression, dizziness, fatigue, gastrointestinal disorders, gum problems, headache, high or low blood pressure, insomnia, irregular heartbeat, irritability, lack of energy, memory loss, multiple sclerosis, and muscle tremor. Once the amalgams were removed, improvement or complete cure rates were between 82 and 97 percent, depending on the condition.

One of the most dramatic cases of recovery following removal of dental amalgams was recounted by Tom Warren in his book, *Beating Alzheimer's*. In 1983, at the age of fifty, Warren was diagnosed with Alzheimer's disease after undergoing a CAT scan due to increasing symptoms of fatigue, memory loss, and difficulties concentrating and making conversation. Based primarily on his own research, Warren eventually determined that his condition was due to toxic metals and chemicals in his dental fillings and within his home environment. After having his amalgams replaced, eliminating his exposure to household chemicals, and adopting a lifestyle of regular exercise, a healthy diet, and nutritional supplementation, in 1987 a follow-up CAT scan revealed that his condition had reversed, and he was able to return to work after an eleven-year absence.

Note: While removal of amalgam fillings and root canals has been shown anecdotally to improve a variety of disease conditions, biological dentists stress that the removal process needs to follow an established protocol in conjunction with an appropriate detoxification and nutritional program.

It should also be noted that no evidence suggests that either amalgams or root canals are unhealthy for all people who have them.

To locate a competent biological dentist, see the "Resources" section at the end of this chapter.

Chelation Therapy

Chelation therapy is the practice of injecting EDTA (ethylene diamine tetracetic acid, also called edetic acid) into the veins, where the EDTA attaches itself to harmful plaque, lead, and other heavy metals, enabling them to be excreted from the body via the urine. At the physician's discretion, vitamins and other supplements can also be included in the EDTA solution. Chelation therapy was originally found to be effective in treating heavy-metal poisoning in the 1940s, but in recent decades, growing numbers of physicians have recommended it as an effective option in place of bypass surgery and angioplasty in treating coronary artery disease. In a 1988 study of 2,870 subjects suffering from ischemic heart disease (coronary artery blockage), researchers Efrain Olszwewer, M.D., and James Carter, M.D., head of nutrition at Tulane University's School of Public Health and Tropical Medicine, found that EDTA chelation resulted in significant improvement in 93.9 percent of all cases. In 1989, a double-blind study of patients suffering from peripheral vascular disease showed that every subject experienced statistical improvement after only ten chelation treatments. Other studies indicate that chelation therapy can help normalize cardiac arrhythmias, protect against iron poisoning, and improve cerebrovascular arterial occlusion, memory and concentration problems due to diminished circulation, and vascular-related vision problems.

Despite such research, chelation therapy is still considered a controversial treatment by most conventional physicians, and at best it remains a form of care that does not address the causes of coronary heart disease, but only relieves their symptoms. Typically a course of chelation therapy ranges from twenty to thirty visits, with each session lasting approximately three and a half hours. The procedure itself is painless and performed on an outpatient basis, with total treatment costs averaging around $3,000 to $4,000.

Note: Patients who elect to receive chelation therapy are advised to receive the following tests prior to, during, and after treatment: blood pressure and circulation, cholesterol and other blood component levels, blood sugar and nutritional status, kidney and organ function, and pre- and post-vascular tests. To locate a physician who is properly trained in the application of chelation therapy, contact the organizations listed in the "Resources" section at the end of this chapter.

Craniosacral Therapy (CST)

Craniosacral therapy is a gentle form of manipulation that focuses on detecting and rebalancing misalignments in the cranium, spine, and sacrum. The origins of craniosacral therapy date back to the early 1900s and the work of William Garner Sutherland, D.O., an osteopathic physician (see Chapter 6). Dr. Sutherland theorized that the bones of the skull, instead of becoming ossified by the time of adulthood, as was commonly believed, were instead designed to move against each other in accordance with the cranial rhythm of the cerebrospinal fluid. After two decades of experimentation, in which he discovered that compressing and otherwise manipulating the skull could both disturb or enhance cranial rhythms, Dr. Sutherland developed cranial osteopathy in the 1930s, only to see it branded as quackery due to the entrenched beliefs of the conventional medical community.

In the late 1970s, however, John Upledger, D.O., O.M.M., leading a team of Michigan State University anatomists, physiologists, biophysicists, and bioengineers, was able to scientifically verify Dr. Sutherland's hypothesis that the bones of the cranium do remain capable of motion throughout adulthood. Dr. Upledger's work served to establish the modern scientific model of the craniosacral system and led to his development of craniosacral therapy, which has since gained rapid recognition and acceptance by holistic practitioners worldwide.

Craniosacral therapy works by releasing tension and restriction in the meninges, the underlying membranes of the craniosacral system. This, in turn, helps to normalize and enhance the functioning of the central nervous system, which is encased and protected by the craniosacral system and its cerebrospinal fluid. Rather than treating symptoms, the primary goal of CST practitioners is to improve the functioning of the craniosacral system itself and to free it from the debilitating effects of stress. As this occurs, proper nerve function is restored, contributing to the reversal of stress-related conditions, particularly those associated with the head, neck, and back. Among the conditions that craniosacral therapy can benefit are anxiety, digestive problems, eye problems, fatigue, headache and migraine, injuries due to accidents, low back pain, sciatica, sinus problems, temporomandibular joint syndrome (TMJ), and tinnitus. In addition, craniosacral therapy has been shown to be highly effective for treating a variety of conditions common to infants and children, including birth trauma, colic, hyperactivity, learning difficulties, and otitis media. Emotional trauma, including post-traumatic stress disorder, can also favorably respond to CST, as can certain sensory disorders, such as dyslexia, impaired sense of taste or smell, and motor skill problems.

Craniosacral treatment sessions usually take place with the client lying comfortably on a bodywork table, wearing loose clothing and no shoes. During each session, which typically lasts from forty-five to sixty minutes, the practitioner employs light touch and palpation techniques along the craniosacral system, and sometimes will manually support the client's limbs and spine as stored tension is spontaneously released. CST is practiced by a growing number of M.D.'s and osteopathic physicians, along with chiropractors, dentists, and bodyworkers. Depending on the type of practitioner you choose, treatments can range from $35 to $250 per session.

Detoxification Therapy

In addition to being an integral part of other holistic therapies such as Ayurveda, environmental medicine, naturopathic medicine, and traditional Chinese medicine, detoxification therapy is often employed by practitioners of holistic medicine to help their patients eliminate stored body toxins that can negatively impact health. A variety of detoxification methods can be suggested for patients, depending on individual need. These include modified diets, fasting, hyperthermia (see Chapter 10), and bowel cleansing programs, such as colonics and enemas.

Note: Detoxification programs should be undertaken only after consultation with a qualified health professional, followed by his or her medical supervision.

Energy Medicine

Used to describe a wide range of subtle bioenergetic techniques and the use of both conventional and experimental microcurrent and magnetic energy devices, energy medicine may well become one of the most important aspects of holistic medicine in the twenty-first century, due to its ability to diagnose and treat disease in the human bioenergy field, often before it manifests physically in the body. Bioenergetic therapies within the field of energy medicine include *Qigong*, Therapeutic Touch, healing touch, and *jin shin jyutsu* (see Chapters 13 and 9). Distance healing, prayer, and meditation are other aspects of energy medicine (see Chapter 5), as are light, color, and sound therapies, and microcurrent therapies, which use devices such as the Acuscope, EAV, MORA, TENS unit, and cranial electrical stimulation tools. A variety of conventional diagnostic devices, such as the electrocardiogram (EKG), electroencephalogram (EEG), and magnetic resonance imaging (MRI) are also based on principles of energy medicine.

The concept of a bioenergy field, or "subtle energy body," surrounding the physical body has been a central tenet of both Ayurvedic and traditional Chinese medicine for thousands of years. This concept was also accepted by Samuel Hahnemann, the developer of homeopathy (see Chapter 11), as well as being part of the belief systems of most religious and spiritual teachings. According to practitioners of energy medicine, the bioenergy field consists of a series of pathways (meridians) and energy centers (chakras) through which vital, life force energies are absorbed and carried throughout the body, governing both physical and mental/emotional health. Optimal wellness depends on the free and unimpeded flow of this life force energy, while energy blockages or imbalances result in illness and impaired psychophysiological functioning. Practitioners of energy medicine employ diagnostic screening devices to measure the various bioenergetic frequencies emitted by the body and the body's organs in order to detect such blockages and imbalances. Through the use of electromagnetic signals, they can also unblock impeded bioenergy pathways, restoring the body's normal energy balance. They also work to protect against and counteract the effects of harmful electromagnetic frequencies in the environment, which many researchers believe are contributing to today's rising trend in chronic illness.

While the efficacy of energy medicine and how it works has yet to be fully understood, indications are that it will become an increasingly important, and perhaps dominant, form of health care in the years ahead, as researchers continue to bridge the gap between science and spirituality and unlock the secrets of mankind's multidimensional nature.

Enzyme Therapy

Enzyme therapy involves the use of plant and pancreatic enzymes taken as supplements to enhance health by improving digestion and the absorption of essential nutrients. Enzymes are protein molecules that are integral to every biochemical reaction that occurs in the body. Digestive enzymes are responsible for the digestion of proteins, carbohydrates, sugars, and fats, and are produced in the saliva glands, the stomach, the pancreas, and the small intestine. Pancreatic enzymes, by contrast, are present in the blood and intestines, and while they do not aid in the processes of digestion and predigestion in the stomach, they do assist in later stages of the digestion and assimilation of nutrients and help maintain the defense mechanisms of the immune system.

Due to poor diet and improper cooking and chewing habits, many people are deficient in the enzymes necessary for good digestion. These include protease, which digests proteins; amylase, which digests carbohydrates; lipase, which digests fats; and cellulase, which digests fiber and is available only in plant foods since the body does not produce it. By combining supplements of these enzymes with good eating habits and a diet rich in fruits, seeds, nuts, and raw or slightly steamed vegetables, many gastrointestinal conditions can be substantially improved, often to the benefit of other health complaints, due to the improved digestion and absorption of essential nutrients.

The use of plant enzymes in the United States was first pioneered by Edward Howell, M.D., beginning in the 1920s. Dr. Howell stressed the fact that diminished enzyme supplies interfered with the ability of vitamins, minerals, and body hormones to function properly in the body, and he was a staunch advocate of a diet rich in unprocessed, whole foods that included lots of raw fruits and vegetables. He also believed that an abundant supply of plant enzymes in the diet enabled the body's own internal enzyme supply to more efficiently support and maintain overall metabolic function, strengthening other body systems in the process. His research showed that plant enzymes are sensitive to heat and are destroyed when foods are cooked in temperatures above 118 degrees Fahrenheit. Canning, pasteurization, preservatives, and microwaves can also destroy or deactivate plant enzymes and negatively impact the digestive process. Today, Dr. Howell's findings are supported by an increasing number of holistic practitioners, who report improvement in numerous chronic conditions once their patients begin enzyme supplementation and adopt healthier eating habits.

The use of pancreatic enzymes to improve health extends even further back than Dr. Howell's research, beginning with the work of John Beard, a British embryologist who in 1902 was able to achieve therapeutic improvement in patients with cancerous tumors by injecting pancreatic enzymes directly into the tumors themselves. Later in the century, German researchers Max Wolf, M.D., and Karl Ransberger, Ph.D., built on Beard's work by using pancreatic enzymes to successfully treat cancer, multiple sclerosis, and various viral infections, as well as conditions due to inflammation of body tissues. Despite their research, pancreatic enzyme therapy today remains much more widely available in Europe and Mexico than in the United States. Overall, while conventional U.S. physicians now sometimes use enzymes to treat illness such as cystic fibrosis and celiac disease, they have exhibited little acceptance for enzyme therapy as a whole. Nonetheless, its use among holistic practitioners continues to grow.

Note: While numerous plant enzyme formulas are now available over the counter in most health food stores, they are best taken under the supervision of a health practitioner trained in their use.

Magnetic Therapy

The use of magnets as tools for enhancing health dates back to antiquity, as evidenced by records from ancient China, Egypt, Greece, and India. Today, magnetic therapy is an accepted medical treatment in China, Japan, Korea, Germany, Switzerland, Russia, and many nations in Eastern Europe and the former Soviet Union. In the United States, the use of magnets is becoming increasingly popular among holistic physicians, as well, and by many athletes, who use them to enhance their performance and speed recovery from pain and injury. Many racehorse trainers also use magnetic blankets in caring for their horses.

A variety of theories have been proposed to explain how magnet therapy works, based on ongoing experimentation. Current research indicates that magnets and magnetic pads and devices are able to block pain signals to the brain, increase endorphin levels, accelerate healing by increasing blood flow, restore blood pH levels, positively affect calcium ions (moving calcium to where it is needed in the body, and away from where it can cause damage, such as in arthritic joints), increase the rate of electron transfer in the cells (thereby improving overall physiological functioning), enhance enzyme function, and increase serotonin levels.

Among the conditions for which research shows magnetic therapy to be helpful are arthritis (both rheumatoid and osteo); back, neck, and shoulder pain; carpal tunnel syndrome; depression; dysmenorrhea (painful menstruation); eczema; endometriosis; epilepsy; fatigue; fibromyalgia;

headache and migraine; heel spurs; hypertension; insomnia; neuropathy caused by diabetes; pelvic inflammatory disease; psoriasis; shingles; soft tissue injuries; and urinary incontinence. The use of magnets has also been shown to speed recovery from surgery and increase the healing time for wounds and fractures. Magnets and magnetized water have also been shown to be useful in reducing tartar and dental plaque and for improving gum health.

Note: There are a variety of methods within the field of magnetic therapy, including the application of magnets over pain sites and specific acupuncture meridians (see Chapter 13), sleeping on magnetic pads and mattresses, wearing magnetic shoe insoles, and drinking magnetized water. All of these methods can be adopted as self-care measures, although initial consultation with a physician or other health practitioner familiar with the use of magnets is advised. In addition, magnet therapy should be avoided immediately after meals, and by pregnant women, people taking blood thinning medication, and people with implanted devices (such as pacemakers or insulin pumps) and metal plates and screws. Epileptics and people suffering from internal bleeding should also avoid using magnets without proper medical supervision.

Nambudripad Allergy Elimination Technique (NAET)

Developed by Devi Nambudripad, D.C., Ph.D., who first used it to cure herself of a lifelong pattern of serious food and environmental allergies, since the late 1980s, NAET has become increasingly popular among holistic and environmental physicians, as well as many other types of health practitioners as an aid in detecting and eliminating a broad spectrum of hidden allergies. Moreover, Dr. Nambudripad's clinical research has shown that NAET is effective in permanently eliminating both food and environmental allergic reactions in approximately 85 percent of all cases. Once the allergies have been eliminated, patients can then resume eating otherwise harmless foods and be exposed to other innocuous substances and environments without further reaction.

According to Dr. Nambudripad, the key to NAET's success lies in its ability to retrain the brain and nervous system not to react to allergenic substances that are otherwise harmless. Her research suggests that harmless substances that the body interprets as allergens cause blockages in the body's meridian system (see Chapter 13), which over time create further imbalances and lead to disease. At the root of many disease conditions,

Dr. Nambudripad believes, are undetected allergies that can trigger a wide variety of symptoms. In her own case, Dr. Nambudripad's multiple illness symptoms, which included arthritis, bronchitis, chronic exhaustion, eczema, migraine headaches, insomnia, and sinusitis, all vanished once she was able to detect and eliminate the allergies they were masking.

NAET practitioners use kinesiological muscle testing (see Chapter 9) to determine which substances their patients are allergic to, with suspected substances being held by the patient as the practitioner checks for muscle weakness, a sign that a particular substance is an allergen. Once allergens have been identified, practitioners then test various meridian points to determine which ones the substances are causing blockages in. Acupuncture is then used to treat the affected meridians while the offending substance is still held by the patient. This process, Dr. Nambudripad claims, serves to reprogram the patient's nervous system to no longer react to the substance in question. Once the treatment is completed, patients are instructed to avoid the substance for twenty-five to thirty hours, after which they can safely be exposed to it.

Dr. Nambudripad estimates that most allergic responses can be identified and successfully treated within fifteen to twenty treatments, usually spaced a week apart. Some patients require a longer series of treatments before full benefits are achieved, while others improve more quickly, depending on the nature of their condition. Due to its success, NAET practitioners are available in most states in the United States, and NAET is now spreading to Canada and Europe.

Note: Dr. Nambudripad cautions that anyone interested in NAET should contact a practitioner certified as having undergone her training (see the "Resources" section at the end of this chapter). According to her, a number of other practitioners who have not trained with her are claiming that they, too, are providing NAET, and although she cannot comment directly on the efficacy of their work, she states emphatically that their claims to be NAET practitioners are misleading.

Prolotherapy

Also known as reconstructive therapy or sclerotherapy, prolotherapy (*prolo* meaning "proliferation") is a nonsurgical technique that has an excellent track record for permanently relieving chronic musculoskeletal pain. Prolotherapy involves injections of saline-based solutions into ligaments and tendons where they attach to the bone. Ligaments serve to hold bones to bones in the joints, and when they become injured or weakened, they are slow to heal, resulting in pain that is exacerbated due to their many nerve endings and the fact that their blood supply is naturally limited. Tendons are the tissues that connect muscles to bones, and can be painful due to the same causes of joint pain. Prolotherapy is also effective for repairing injured discs and cartilage.

Prolotherapy works by causing a localized inflammation in the injected site, thereby stimulating increased blood supply and an increased flow of nutrients into areas of weakened tissue, causing them to repair themselves. The earliest historical version of prolotherapy dates back to ancient Greece and the time of Hippocrates, who was able to heal torn and dislocated shoulder joints by sticking them with heated poker irons, after which they would rapidly and seemingly miraculously heal. At present, one of the most famous proponents of prolotherapy is former U.S. surgeon general C. Everett Koop, M.D., who used prolotherapy in his medical practice after it successfully healed his own long-standing case of back pain, which had failed to respond to conventional medical treatments.

During a prolotherapy session, physicians use thin needles to inject saline solutions into the damaged ligaments and tendons around the affected joints. The solutions act as both an anesthetic and a natural irritant that stimulates the body's own healing mechanisms. Published studies performed by the Department of Orthopedic Surgery at the University of Iowa showed that both ligament and tendon strength and size can increase by as much as 40 percent following prolotherapy, providing for greater overall joint support and diminishing the likelihood of future injury. Other double-blind studies published in the prestigious medical journal *Lancet*, revealed that 88 percent of patients who receive prolotherapy experience significant improvement in their conditions, and that when patients do not improve, typically it is due to other factors inhibiting the body's healing process, including hidden infection or the use of cortisone treatments.

In general, prolotherapy requires between ten and thirty treatments to work, depending on the person and the severity of his or her joint damage, but some people respond much more quickly. Among the conditions for which prolotherapy has been shown to be effective, in many cases providing permanent relief, are arthritis (including degenerative arthritis), back pain, carpal tunnel syndrome, cluster and tension headaches, degenerative disc disease, fibromyalgia, general pain and deep muscle ache, heel spurs, hip degeneration, knee injuries, migraine, multiple sclerosis, muscular dystrophy, osteoporosis, polio, rotator cuff tears, sciatica, scoliosis, slipped disc, spinal defects, tennis elbow, temporo-mandibular joint syndrome (TMJ), and whiplash.

Note: Currently approximately only three hundred physicians use pro-lotherapy in the United States, although their number is growing due to continued research and the growing acceptance of prolotherapy on the part of medical schools, as well as its growing popularity among athletes suffering from sports injuries.

RESOURCES

To find out more about the therapies in this chapter, contact the following organizations.

Allopathic Medicine

American Medical Association
515 North State Street
Chicago, Illinois 60610
Phone: (312) 464-5000
Web site: *www.ama-assn.org*

Aromatherapy

National Association for Holistic Aromatherapy
P.O. Box 17622
Boulder, Colorado 80308
Phone: (800) 566-6735
Web site: *www.naha.org*

Pacific Institute of Aromatherapy
P.O. Box 6723
San Rafael, California 94903
Phone: (415) 479-9121
Fax: (415) 479-0119

Biological Dentistry

American Academy of Oral Medicine
2910 Lightfoot Drive

Baltimore, Maryland 21209
(410) 602-8585
Web site: *www.aaom.com*

Holistic Dental Association
P.O. Box 5007
Durango, Colorado 81301
Web site: *www.holisticdental.org*

Chelation Therapy

American College for Advancement in Medicine (ACAM)
23121 Verdugo Drive, Suite 204
Laguna Hills, California 92653
(800) 532-3688
Web site: *www.acam.org*

American Board of Chelation Therapy
1407-B North Wells Street
Chicago, Illinois 60610
(800) 356-2228

Craniosacral Therapy

Upledger Institute
11211 Prosperity Farms Road
Palm Beach Gardens, Florida 33410
Phone: (561) 622-4706
Fax: (561) 622-4771
Web site: *www.upledger.com*

Cranial Academy
8606 Allisonville Road, Suite 130
Idianapolis, Indiana 46268
Phone: (317) 594-0411
Fax: (317) 594-9299

Energy Medicine

International Society for the Study of Subtle Energies and Energy Medicine

11005 Ralston Road
Arvada, Colorado 80004
Phone: (303) 425-4625
Fax: (303) 425-4685
Email: issseem@compuserve.com
Web site: *www.issseem.org*

Magnetic Therapy

Bio-Electric-Magnetics Institute (BEMI)
2940 W. Moana Lane
Reno, Nevada 89509
Phone: (775) 827-9099

Bioelectromagnetics Society
P.O. Box 3651
Arlington, Virginia 22203
Phone: (703) 524-2367

North American Academy of Magnetic Therapy
28420 W. Agoura Road, Suite 202
Agoura, California 91301
Phone: (888) 457-1853

NAET

NAET Pain Clinic
6732 Beach Blvd.
Buena Park, California 90621
Phone: (714) 523-8900
Fax: (714) 523-3068
Email: naet@earthlink.net
Web site: *www.naet.com*

Prolotherapy

American Association of Orthopaedic Medicine
90 S. Cascade Avenue, Suite 1230
Colorado Springs, Colorado 80903
Phone: (800) 992-2063
Fax: (719) 475-8748

Web site: *www.aaomed.org*
Prolotherapy.com
Web site: *www.prolotherapy.com*

RECOMMENDED READING

Aromatherapy

Fisher-Rizzi, Suzanne, *The Complete Aromatherapy Handbook: Essential Oils for Radiant Health*. Sterling Press, 1991.
Tisserand, Robert B. *The Art of Aromatherapy*. Destiny Books, 1987.

Biological Dentistry

Huggins, Hal. *It's All in Your Head*. Life Science Press, 1986.
Ziff, Sam and Michael. *The Missing Link*. Bio-Probe, Inc., 1992.

Chelation Therapy

Cranton, Elmer. *Bypassing Bypass*. Hampton Roads, 1990.
Walker, Morton. *The Chelation Way*. Avery Publishing Group, Inc., 1990.

Craniosacral Therapy

Upledger, John. *Your Inner Physician and You*. North Atlantic Books, 1992.

Energy Medicine

Eden, Donna. *Energy Medicine*. Tarcher/Putnam, 1998.
Gerber, Richard. *Vibrational Medicine*. Bear & Company, 1988.

Magnetic Therapy

Philpott, William, and Sharon Taplin. *Biomagnetic Handbook*. Enviro-Tech Products, 1990.

NAET

Nambudripad, Devi. *Living Pain Free*. Delta Publishing Company, 1997.

Nambudripad, Devi. *Say Goodbye to Illness.* Delta Publishing Company, 1995.

Prolotherapy

Faber, William J., and Morton Walker. *Pain, Pain Go Away.* Ishi Press International, 1990.

About the American Holistic Medical Association

The American Holistic Medical Association (AHMA) is a national organization of physicians and other licensed health care practitioners who share a common vision of creating a primary medical care system that addresses the whole person—body, mind, and spirit. It was founded in 1978 by C. Norman Shealy, M.D., Ph.D., and a group of like-minded physicians in order to unite licensed medical doctors and osteopathic physicians (M.D.'s and D.O.'s) who practice holistic medicine, and to provide them with an organized forum in which they could further explore and promote holistic health care. Since its inception, the AHMA has grown to include an international membership of M.D.'s and D.O.'s representing nearly every medical specialty, as well as medical students studying for those degrees. In addition, the AHMA offers associate membership to other health care practitioners who are licensed, certified, or registered in the state in which they practice. Associate members of the AHMA include naturopathic physicians (N.D.'s), chiropractors (D.C.'s), practitioners of traditional Chinese medicine (O.M.D.'s), homeopathic physicians, nurses, dentists, podiatrists, psychologists, physical therapists, dieticians and clinical nutritionists, optometrists, social workers, pharmacists, and physician assistants.

The AHMA defines its vision as follows: "To transform health care so that it addresses physical, environmental, mental, emotional, spiritual, and social health, thereby contributing to the healing of the planet. As holistic physicians, we are committed to the health of all whom we serve, including ourselves. The essence of our vision is unconditional love." To further its mission, the AHMA holds an annual conference that provides a comprehensive presentation of the art, science, and practice of holistic medicine, and also sponsors or cosponsors numerous regional conferences and meetings nationwide. Since 1997 the AHMA, in conjunction with the American Board of Holistic Medicine (see below), has also presented a comprehensive continuing medical education course entitled "The Scientific Basis for Using Holistic Medicine to Treat Chronic Disease" to family practice medical schools and physicians and other health care practitioners throughout the United States.

In 1996, the AHMA's sister organization, the American Board of Holistic Medicine (ABHM), was formed by AHMA founding member Robert A. Anderson, M.D., and other AHMA member physicians. The stated purposes of the American Board of Holistic Medicine are to:

1. Evaluate the candidacy of applicants desiring certification as specialists in holistic medicine
2. Establish and maintain high standards of excellence in the specialty of holistic medicine
3. Improve the quality of medical care provided to the public
4. Serve the public, physicians, health practitioners, hospitals, therapists, educators, state medical boards, and third-party insurance carriers, by having available a roster of the diplomates certified by the Board

In December 2000 the ABHM, for the first time, established board certification for M.D.'s and D.O.'s in holistic medicine, effectively setting a new standard for quality health care in the United States. An additional goal of the ABHM is the establishment of these standards for the benefit of the public, the profession, state medical disciplinary boards, the courts, and third-party insurance carriers. ABHM certification is now helping to establish leadership and maintain quality as the art and science of holistic medicine are integrated into the nation's overall health care system, while also meeting the growing public demand and professional interest in holistic and alternative medical approaches.

For further information about the AHMA, or for referrals to AHMA physician members in your area, contact:

American Holistic Medical Association
6728 Old McLean Village Drive
McLean, Virginia 22101
Phone: (703) 556-9245
Fax: (703) 556-8729
Web site: *www.holisticmedicine.org*

To learn more about the American Board of Holistic Medicine, contact:

American Board of Holistic Medicine
Larry Hulbert, Executive Director
P.O. Box 5388
Lynnwood, WA 98043
Phone: (425) 741-2996
Fax: (425) 745-8040
E-mail: blh@halcyon.com

Bibliography

Chapter 1: The History and Philosophy of Holistic Medicine

"69% of Americans use alternative medicine." *Alternative Medicine Digest* 28 (Mar. 1999): 89.

Chung, M. K. "Why alternative medicine?" *American Family Physician* 54 (Nov. 15, 1996): 2184–85.

Goodman, M. et al. "Hostility predicts restenosis after percutaneous transluminal coronary angioplasty." *Mayo Clinic Proceedings* 71, no. 8 (1996): 729–34.

Ironson, G. et al. "Effects on anger on left ventricular ejection fraction in coronary artery disease." *American Journal of Cardiology* 70 (Aug. 1, 1992): 281.

Novack, D. H., et al. "Calibrating the physician: Personal awareness and effective patient care." *JAMA* 278 (Aug. 13, 1997): 502.

Ornish, Dean. "Can lifestyle changes reverse coronary heart disease? The Lifestyle Heart Program." *Lancet* 336 (July 21, 1990): 129–33.

Pizzorno, Joseph. *Total Wellness*. Prima Publishing, 1996.

Pizzorno, Joseph. Personal interview with the author, May 1998.

Quillin, Patrick. "Adjuvant Nutrition in Cancer Treatment." *Journal of Advancement in Medicine* 8 (Dec. 1995): 87.

Ramirez, A. J. "Stress and relapse of breast cancer." *British Medical Journal* 298 (Feb. 4, 1989): 291.

Shealy, C. Norman, M. D., Ph.D. "The Wellness Movement." *Bulletin of the Greene County Medical Society* (Aug. 1996): 27–28.

Stamler, R., et al. "Nutritional therapy for high blood pressure. Final report of a four-year randomized controlled study—the Hypertension Control Program." *JAMA* 257 (Mar. 20, 1987): 1484.

Chapter 2: The Holistic Self-Care Program

"Understanding your body's healing systems: An interview with Joseph Pizzorno, N.D." *The Healthy Edge Letter* 1, no. 5 (Dec. 1998): 8.

Chapter 3: Nutritional Medicine

Abraham, A., et al. "The effects of chromium supplementation on serum glucose and lipids in patients with and without non-insulin-dependent diabetes." *Metabolism* 41, 1992: 768–771.

Berr, C., et al. "Selenium and oxygen-metabolizing enzymes in elderly community residents: A pilot epidemiologic study." *Journal of the American Geriatric Society,* 41 (1993): 143–48.

Block, G., et al. "Epidemiologic evidence regarding vitamin C and cancer." *American Journal of Clinical Nutrition* 54, no. 6, suppl. (1991): 1310S–1314S.

Chen, M. F., et al. "Effect of ascorbic acid on plasma alcohol clearance." *Journal of the American College of Nutrition* 9, no. 3 (1990): 185–89.

Cheraskin, E. "Chronologic versus biological age." *Journal of Advancement in Medicine* 7, no. 1 (1994): 31–41.

———. "Vitamin C, cancer and aging." *Age* 16 (1993): 55–58.

Davis, R. H. et al. "Vitamin C influence of localized adjuvant arthritis." *Journal of the American Podiatry Medical Association* 80, no. 8 (1990): 414–18.

Diplock, A. "Indexes of selenium status in human populations." *American Journal of Clinical Nutrition* 57, suppl. (1993): 256S–258S.

DiSilvestro, R., et al. "Effects of copper supplementation on ceruloplasmin and copper-zinc superoxide dismutase in free-living rheumatoid arthritis patients." *Journal of the American College of Nutrition* 11 (1992): 177–80.

Gaby, Alan R. *Reversing and Preventing Osteoporosis.* Prima Publishing, 1994.

Garrison, Robert, and Elizabeth Somer. *The Nutrition Desk Reference.* 3d ed. Keats Publishing, 1995.

Hatch, G. E. "Asthma, inhaled oxidants and dietary antioxidants." *American Journal of Clinical Nutrition* 61, no. 3, suppl. (1995): 625S–630S.

Holford, Patrick. *The Optimum Nutrition Bible.* The Crossing Press, 1999.

Kunin, R. A. "Orthomolecular Psychiatry." In *The Roots of Molecular Medicine: A Tribute to Linus Pauling,* R. P. Heumer, ed. William Freeman & Company, 1986.

———. "Principles that identify orthomolecular medicine: A unique medical specialty." *Journal of Orthomolecular Medicine* 2, no. 4 (1987): 203–6.

Morris, B., et al. "The trace element chromium: A role in glucose homeostasis." *American Journal of Clinical Nutrition* 55 (1992): 989–91.

Null, Gary. *Gary Null's Ultimate Anti-Aging Program.* Broadway Books, 1999.

Oski, F. "Iron deficiency in infancy and childhood." *New England Journal of Medicine* 329 (1993): 190–93.

Pauling, Linus. "Orthomolecular psychiatry: Varying the concentrations of substances normally present in the human body may control mental disease." *Science* 160 (1968): 265–71.

Pfeiffer, Carl C. *Mental and Elemental Nutrients: A Physician's Guide to Nutrition and Health Care.* Keats Publishing, 1975.

Salonen, J., et al. "Serum copper and the risk of acute myocardial infarction: A prospective population study in men in eastern Finland." *American Journal of Epidemiology* 134 (1991): 268–76.

Stahelin, H. B., et al. "Plasma antioxidant vitamins and subsequent cancer mortality in the 12-year follow-up of the prospective Basel study. *American Journal of Epidemiology* 133, no. 8 (1992): 766–75.

Street, D. A. "A population-based case control study of the association of serum antioxidants and myocardial infarction." *American Journal of Epidemiology* 131, (1991): 719–20.

Tucker, D. M., et al. "Nutritional status and brain function in aging." *American Journal of Clinical Nutrition* 52 (1990): 93–102.

Wright, Jonathan V., and Alan R. Gaby. *The Patient's Book of Natural Healing.* Prima Publishing, 1999.

Chapter 4: Environmental Medicine

"Chemicals identified in human biological media: A data base." *United States Environmental Protection Agency. EPA* 560/13-80-036B (Oct. 1980) U.S. EPA.

Crook, William. "Food allergy: The great masquerader." *Pediatric Clinic of North America* 22, no. 1 (1975): 227–38.

Keon, Joseph. *The Truth about Breast Cancer: A 7-Step Prevention Plan.* Parissound Publishing, 1999.

Practice Guidelines for the Field of Environmental Medicine. American Academy of Environmental Medicine, 7701 East Kellogg Avenue, Wichita, Kans. 67207.

Rea, William J., et al. "Pesticides and brain function changes in a controlled environment." *Clinical Ecology* 2, no. 3 (1984): 145–50.

Schnare, D. W., et al. "Body burden reductions of PCBs, PBBs and chlorinated pesticides in human subjects." *Ambio: A Journal of the Human Environment* 13, nos. 5–6 (1984): 378–80.

What Is Environmental Medicine? American Academy of Environmental Medicine, 7701 East Kellogg Avenue, Wichita, KS 67207.

Chapter 5: Mind-Body Medicine

Achterberg, J., et al. "Behavioral strategies for the reduction of pain and anxiety associated with orthopedic trauma." *Biofeedback and Self-Regulation* 14, no. 2 (1989): 101–14.

Bach, Edward, and F. J. Wheeler. *The Bach Flower Remedies.* Keats Publishing, 1979.

Benson, Herbert. "Stress, anxiety and the Relaxation Response." *Behavioral Biological Medicine* 3 (1985): 1–50.

Benson, Herbert, and R. L. Allen. "How much stress is too much?" *Harvard Business Review* 58 (1980): 86–92.

Blanchard, E. B., and F. Andrasik. "Biofeedback Treatment of Vascular Headache." In *Biofeedback: Studies in Clinical Efficacy,* John P. Hatch, J. G. Fisher and John D. Rugh, eds.) Plenum Publishing Corp.

Blanchard, E. B. et al. "The prediction by psychological tests of headache patients' response to treatment with relaxation and biofeedback." *Self-Regulation Strategies: Efficacy and Mechanisms.* Biofeedback Society of America, 13th Annual Meeting, Chicago, Ill., Mar. 1982.

Bridge, L. R., et al. "Relaxation and imagery in the treatment of breast cancer." *British Medical Journal* 297, no. 5 (1988): 1169–72.

Caldwell, Christine. *Getting in Touch: The Guide to New Body-Centered Therapies.* Quest Books, 1997.

Callahan, Roger, and Joanne Callahan. "More Scientific Support-Psychotherapy and Deep Biological Change." *The Thought Field* 4, no. 2 (1998): 5–6.

———. *Thought Field Therapy and Trauma: Treatment and Theory.* Thought Field Therapy Training Center, Indian Wells, Calif. 1996.

Callahan, R., et al. Callahan Techniques Thought Field Therapy, Reference Material. *www.tftrx.com.*

Colchrane, G., and J. Freisen. "Hypnotherapy in weight loss treatment." *Journal of Consulting and Clinical Psychology* 54 (1986): 489–92.

Cox, D. J., et al. "Simple electromyographic biofeedback treatment for chronic pediatric constipation/encopresis: Preliminary report." *Biofeedback and Self-Regulation* 19 (1994): 41–50.

Dossey, Larry. *Healing Words.* HarperSanFrancisco, 1993.

Edelson, E. "Hopelessness begets hypertension." *HealthScout*, Feb. 21, 2000. *www.healthscout.com.*

Fahrion, Steven L. "Human potential and personal transformation." *Subtle Energies* 6, no. 1 (1995): 55–87.

Flaherty, G., and J. Fitzpatrick. "Relaxation technique to increase comfort level of postoperative patients: A preliminary study." *Nursing Research* 27, no. 6 (1978): 352–55.

Hahn, Y. B., et al. "The effect of thermal biofeedback and progressive muscle relaxation in reducing blood pressure of patients with essential hypertension." *Image—The Journal of Nursing Scholarship* 25 (1993): 204–7.

Holroyd, J. "Hypnosis treatment for smoking: An evaluative review." *International Journal of Clinical and Experimental Hypnosis* 4 (1980): 341–57.

Ivker, Robert, Robert Anderson, and Larry Trivieri. *The Complete Self-Care Guide to Holistic Medicine.* Tarcher/Putnam, 1999.

Kabat-Zinn, J., et al. "Four year follow-up of a meditation-based program for the self-regulation of chronic pain: Treatment outcomes and compliance." *Clinical Journal of Pain* 2 (1986): 159–73.

Kasloff, Leslie J. *The Bach Remedies: A Self-Help Guide.* Keats Publishing, 1988.

Kiecolt-Glaser, J. K., et al. "Psychosocial enhancement of immunocompetence in a geriatric population." *Health Psychology* 4, no. 1 (1985), 25–41.

Lambreau, Peter, and George Pratt. *Instant Emotional Healing.* Broadway Books, 2000.

Lawlis, G. F., et al. "Reduction of postoperative pain parameters by presurgical relaxation instructions for spinal pain patients." *Spine* 10, no. 7 (1985): 649–51.

Murphy, Michael. *The Future of the Body.* J. P. Tarcher, 1992.

Ornish, Dean. *Dr. Dean Ornish's Program for Reversing Heart Disease.* Random House, 1990.

Pert, Candace B. *Molecules of Emotion.* Scribners, 1997.

Pert, Candace B., and S. H. Snyder. "Opiate receptor: Demonstration in the nervous tissue." *Science* 179 (1973).

Pert, Candace B., et al. "Neuropeptides and their receptors: A psychosomatic network." *Journal of Immunology* 135 (1985): 820–26.

Rider, M. S., et al. "Effect of immune system imagery on secretory IgA." *Biofeedback and Self-Regulation* 15 (1990): 317–33.

Shapiro, Francine. "Efficacy of the Eye Movement Desensitization Procedure in the treatment of traumatic memories." *Journal of Traumatic Stress* 2 (1989): 199–223.

———. *EMDR.* Basic Books, 1997.

———. "Eye Movement Desensitization: A new treatment for post-traumatic stress disorder." *Journal of Behavior Therapy and Experimental Psychiatry* 20 (1989b): 211–17.

Shealy, C. Norman. *90 Days to Self-Health.* Brindabella Books, 1987.

———. *Sacred Healing.* Element, 1999.

Simonton, O. Carl. *Getting Well Again.* J. P. Tarcher, 1978.

Tinterow, M. "Hypnotherapy for chronic pain." *Kansas Medicine* 88, no. 6 (1987): 190–92, 204.

———. "The use of hypnotic anesthesia for major surgical procedure." *American Surgeon* 26 (1960): 732–37.

Trivieri, Larry. "Brain wave therapy: A breakthrough addiction therapy." *The Healthy Edge Letter* 1, no. 2 (1998): 1–4.

Chapter 6: Osteopathic Medicine

AOA Facts: About Osteopathic Physicians. Fact Sheet, 1998: American Osteopathic Association (AOA), 142 E. Ontario Street, Chicago, IL 60611.

Bezilla, T. A. "OMT and diffuse musculoskeletal complaints following a motor vehicle accident." *AOA Journal* 9, no. 4 (winter 1999): 16–18.

Brault, J. S., et al. "Counterstrain-induced tight hamstring release determined by palpatory diagnosis correlated with electromyography." 38th Annual AOA Research Conference Abstracts, 1994.

Degenhardt, B. F., et al. "Efficacy of osteopathic evaluation and manipulative treatment in reducing the morbidity of otitis media in children." 38th Annual AOA Research Conference Abstracts, 1994.

Fryman, V. M., et al. "Effect of osteopathic medical management on neurological development in children." Journal of the American Osteopathic Association 92 (1992): 729–44.

Fulford, Robert, with Gene Stone. *Dr. Fulford's Touch of Life*. Pocket Books, 1996.

Gamber, R. G., et al. "Treatment of fibromyalgia with osteopathic manipulation and self-learned techniques." 37th Annual AOA Research Conference Abstracts, 1993.

Heinking, K., et al. "Effect of osteopathic manipulative treatment on reflex sympathetic dystrophy in children." 37th Annual AOA Research Conference Abstracts, 1993.

Knebl, J. A., et al. "Improving functional ability in the elderly by osteopathic manipulative treatment." 37th Annual AOA Research Conference Abstracts, 1993.

Krpan, M. S., et al. "Low-back (LBP) treatment by high velocity low amplitude (HVLA) osteopathic manipulative treatment (OMT) and effectiveness measured by electromyography (EMG)." 36th Annual AOA research Conference Abstracts, 1992.

McKay-Hart, C., et al. "Incidence of somatic dysfunction in the general population." 36th Annual AOA Research Conference Abstracts, 1992.

OMT: Hands-On-Care. Fact Sheet, 1999: American Osteopathic Association (AOA), 142 E. Ontario Street, Chicago, IL 60611.

Osteopathic Manipulative Treatment Shown to Improve Gait in Parkinson's Patients. Press Release, Jan. 29, 1999: American Osteopathic Association (AOA), 142 E. Ontario Street, Chicago, IL 60611. (*www.am-osteo-assn.org/MediaCenter/Press%20Releases/parkinsons.htm*)

Osteopathic Medical Education. Fact Sheet, 1995: American Osteopathic Association (AOA), 142 E. Ontario Street, Chicago, IL 60611

Osteopathic Medicine. Fact Sheet, 1998: American Osteopathic Association (AOA), 142 E. Ontario Street, Chicago, IL 60611.

The People and Events That Shaped Our History: A Centennial Perspective, 1897–1997. American Osteopathic Association (AOA), 142 E. Ontario Street, Chicago, IL 60611.

Ragucci, M. V., et al. "The management of restless legs syndrome using the pedal lymphatic pump." 40th Annual AOA Research Conference Abstracts, 1996.

Stock, A. D., et al. "The effects of OMT on the tender points associated with fibromyalgia." 37th Annual AOA Research Conference Abstracts, 1993.

Sttle, T. F., et al. "The effect of osteopathic manipulative treatment on the antibody response to hepatitis B vaccine." 40th Annual AOA Research Conference Abstracts, 1996.

Sucher, B. M. "Myofascial manipulative release of carpal tunnel syndrome: documentation with magnetic resonance imaging." *Journal of the American Osteopathic Association* 93 (1993): 1273–78.

————. "Myofascial release of carpal tunnel syndrome." *Journal of the American Osteopathic Association* 93 (1993): 92–94, 100–101.

"Study by NEJM Shows OMT as an Effective, Low-Cost Therapy for Back Pain." Press Release, Nov. 3, 1999. American Osteopathic Association (AOA), 142 E. Ontario Street, Chicago, IL 60611. (*www.am-osteo-assn.org/MediaCenter/Press%20Releases/nejmback.htm*)

What Is a D.O.? Fact Sheet, 1999: American Osteopathic Association (AOA), 142 E. Ontario Street, Chicago, IL 60611.

Chapter 7: Chiropractic

"About Chiropractic: Benefits." American Chiropractic Association, 1701 Clarendon Blvd., Arlington, VA 22209.

"About Chiropractic: Research." American Chiropractic Association, 1701 Clarendon Blvd., Arlington, VA 22209.

"Americans' Perceptions of Practitioners and Treatment for Back Problems: A Comprehensive Summary of Survey Findings." American Chiropractic Association, 1701 Clarendon Blvd., Arlington, VA 22209. 1995.

"Beating Addiction." *Alternative Medicine* No. 29 (1999): 36–40.

Bigos, S. et al. "Acute Low Back Problems in Adults." Clinical Practice Guideline, No. 14, AHCPR Publication No. 95-0642, Rockville, Md. Agency for Health Care Policy and Research, Public Health Service, U.S. Dept. of Health and Human Services, Dec. 1994.

Boline, P., et al. "Spinal manipulation vs. amitriptyline for the treatment of chronic tension-type headaches: A randomized clinical trial." *Journal of Manipulative and Physiological Therapeutics* 18, no. 3 (1995): 148–54.

Chiropractic: State of the Art. American Chiropractic Association, 1701 Clarendon Blvd., Arlington, VA 22209, 1998.

Coulter, Ian. "Efficacy and risks of chiropractic manipulation: What does the evidence suggest?" *Integrative Medicine* 1, no. 1 (1998): 61–66.

Coulter, Ian, et al. "A comparative study of chiropractic and medical education." *Alternative Therapies* 4, no. 5 (Sept. 1998): 64–75.

"Doctors of Chiropractic: Part of Your Health Care Team." American Chiropractic Association, 1701 Clarendon Blvd., Arlington, VA 22209.

"Fact Sheet on Chiropractic." American Chiropractic Association, 1701 Clarendon Blvd., Arlington, VA 22209.

Goertz, C. M. H., et al. "The chiropractic report card: Patient satisfaction study." *Journal of the American Chiropractic Association* 34, no. 10 (1997): 40–47.

Herzog, W., et al. "Electromyographic responses of back and limb muscles associated with spinal manipulative therapy." *Spine* 24 (1999): 146–53.

Jensen, G. A., et al. "Employer-sponsored health insurance for chiropractic services." *Medical Care* 36, no. 4 (1998): 544–53.

Klougart, N., et al. "Infantile colic treated by chiropractors: a prospective study of 316 cases." *Journal of Manipulative and Physiological Therapeutics* 12, no. 4 (1989): 281–88.

Koes, B., et al. "Randomised clinical trial of manipulative therapy and physiotherapy for persistent back and neck complaint." *British Medical Journal* 304 (1992): 601–5.

Manga, P., et al. *A Study to Examine the Effectiveness and Cost-Effectiveness of Chiropractic Management of Low-Back Pain.* Kenilworth Publishing, Richmond Hill, Ontario, 1993.

Meade, T. et al. "Randomised comparison of chiropractic and hospital outpatient management for low back pain: Results from an extended follow up." *British Medical Journal* 311 (1995): 349–51.

Reed, W. R., et al. "Chiropractic management of primary nocturnal enuresis." *Journal of Manipulative and Physiological Therapeutics* 17, no. 5 (1994): 596–600.

Rondberg, Terry. *Chiropractic First.* The Chiropractic Journal, 1998.

Rosomoff, H. "Do herniated discs produce pain?" *Clinical Journal of Pain* 1, no. 1 (1985): 91–93.

Shekelle, P. G., et al. "The Appropriateness of Spinal Manipulation for Low Back Pain: Project Overview and Literature Overview." RAND Corporation, Santa Monica, Calif., 1991.

Stano, Miron. "The economic role of chiropractic: Further analysis of relative insurance costs for low back care." *Journal of the Neuromusculoskeletal System* 3, no. 3 (fall 1995): 139–44.

Whiplash Debilitating, Yet Often Ignored. PRNewswire, Feb. 9, 2000, *www. prnewswire.com.*

Chapter 8: Botanical Medicine

Bordia, A. "Effect of garlic on blood lipids in patients with coronary heart disease." *American Journal of Clinical Nutrition* 34 (1981): 2100–2103.

Brevoort, Peggy. "The booming U.S. botanical market: A new overview." HerbalGram 44 (1998): 33.

Brown, Donald. *Herbal Prescriptions for Better Health.* Prima Publishing, 1996.

Capsaicin Study Group. "Treatment of painful diabetic neuropathy with topical capsaicin: A multicenter, double-blind vehicle-controlled study." *Archives of Internal Medicine* 151 (1991): 2225–29.

Cassileth, Barrie. *The Alternative Medicine Handbook.* W. W. Norton & Company, 1998.

Diamond, W. John, and W. Lee Cowden. *Definitive Guide to Cancer.* Future Medicine Publishing, 1997.

Farnsworth, N. R., et al. "Medicinal Plants in Therapy." *Bulletin of the World Health Organization* 63, no. 6 (1985): 965–81.

Ford, Norman. *Eighteen Natural Ways to Beat a Headache.* Keats Publishing, Inc. 1990.

Ghannoum, M. A. "Studies on the anticandidal mode of action of allium sativum (garlic)." *Journal of General Microbiology* 134 (1988): 2917–24.

Johnson, M. G., and R. H. Vaughn. "Death of Salmonella typhimurium and Escherichia coli in the presence of freshly reconstituted garlic and onion." *Applied Microbiology* 17 (1969): 903–5.

Kandil, O. M., et al. "Garlic and the immune system in humans: Its effect on natural killer cells." *Fed. Proc.* 46 (1987): 441.

Lau, B. H., et al. "Garlic compounds modulate macrophage and T-lymphocyte functions." *Mol. Biother.* 3 (1991): 103–7.

McCaleb, Rob. "Boosting immunity with herbs." Herb Information Green-paper. Herb Research Foundation, Boulder, Colo., 1997. (*www.herbs.org /greenpapers/immune.html*).

———. "Controversial Products in the Natural Foods Market." Herb Research Foundation. Boulder, Colo., 1997. (*www.herbs.org/greenpapers/controv.html*) 1997.

McCarthy, D. J., et al. "Treatment of pain due to fibromyalgia with topical cap-saicin: A pilot study." *Seminars in Arthritis and Rheumatism* 23 (1994): 41–47.

Molony, David. *Complete Guide to Chinese Herbal Medicine.* Berkeley Books, 1998.

Mose, J. "Effect of echinacea on phagocytosis and natural killer cells." Med Welt 34 (1983): 1463–67.

Murray, Michael, and Joseph Pizzorno. *Encyclopedia of Natural Medicine.* 2d ed., rev. Prima Publishing, 1998.

Pizzorno, Joseph. *Total Wellness.* Prima Publishing, 1996.

"Supermarkets experience fastest rate of growth in mainstream dietary supple-ment market." Herb Research Foundation, Boulder, Colo., 1999.

Wacker, A., and W. Hilbig. "Virus-inhibition by Echinacea purpurea." *Planta Medica* 33 (1978): 89–102.

Warshafsky, S., et al. "Effect of garlic on total serum cholesterol: A meta-analysis." *Annals of Internal Medicine* 1119 (1993): 599–605.

Watson, C. P., et al. "Post-herpetic neuralgia and topical capsaicin." *Pain* 33 (1988): 333–40.

Weil, Andrew. "A new look at botanical medicine." *Whole Earth Review* 64 (1989): 3–8.

Weiner, Michael A., and Janet Weiner. *Herbs That Heal.* Quantum Books, 1994.

Chapter 9: Bodywork

1998 Massage Therapy Consumer Survey. American Massage Therapy Associa-tion, 802 Davis Street, Suite 100, Evanston, IL 60201.

Austin, J., and P. Aesubel. "Enhanced respiratory muscular function in normal adults after lessons in proprioceptive musculoskeletal education with exercises." *Chest* 102 (1992): 486–90.

Avis, Pauline, and David McNab. *Healing Disease with Rebirthing*. Mrtenjai Press, 1999.

Beard, Gertrude. *Beard's Massage*. 3d ed. W. B. Saunders Company, 1981.

Burton Goldberg Group. *Alternative Medicine: The Definitive Guide*. Future Medicine Publishing, 1993.

Byers, D. C. *Better Health with Foot Reflexology: The Original Ingham Method*, 4th ed. Ingham Publishing, 1983.

Bzdek, V., et al. "Effects of Therapeutic Touch on tension headache pain." *Nursing Research* 35 (1986): 101–6.

Caldwell, Christine. *Getting in Touch: The Guide to New Body-Centered Therapies*. Quest Books, 1997.

Claire, Thomas. *Bodywork*. Quill/William Morrow, 1995.

Connolly, L. "Ida Rolf." *Human Behavior* 6, no. 5 (May 1977): 17–23.

Cottingham, J., et al. "Shifts in pelvic inclination angle and parasympathetic tone produced by Rolfing soft tissue manipulation." *Physical Therapy* 68, no. 9 (Sept. 1988): 1364–70.

Dennis, R. J. "Functional reach improvement in normal older women after Alexander Technique instruction." *Journal of Gerontology: Medical Sciences* 54 (1999): M8–11.

Fact Sheet: "Demand for Massage Therapy." American Massage Therapy Association, 802 Davis Street, Suite 100, Evanston, IL 60201.

Feldenkrais, Moshe. *Awareness through Movement*. Harper and Row, 1972.

Ferrell-Torry, A. T., and O. J. Glick. "The use of therapeutic massage as a nursing intervention to modify anxiety and the perception of cancer pain." *Cancer Nursing* 16, no. 2 (1992): 93–101.

Field, Tiffany, et al. "Juvenile rheumatoid arthritis: Benefits from massage therapy." *Journal of Pediatric Psychology Proceedings* 22 (1997): 607–17.

Field, Tiffany, et al. "Massage therapy reduces anxiety and enhances EEG pattern of alertness and math computations." *International Journal of Neuroscience* 86 (1996): 197–205.

Field, Tiffany, et al. "Massage reduces anxiety in child and psychiatric patients." *Journal of the American Academy of Child and Adolescent Psychiatry* 3, no. 1 (1992): 125–31.

Field, Tiffany, et al. "Massage therapy effects on depression and somatic symptoms of chronic fatigue syndrome." *Journal of Chronic Fatigue Syndrome* 3 (1997): 43–51.

Field, Tiffany, et al. "Tactile kinesthetic stimulation effects on preterm neonates." *Pediatrics* 77 (1986): 654–58.

Fisher, K. "Early experiences of a multidisciplinary pain management programme." *Holistic Medicine* 3 (1988): 47–56.

Gordon, Richard. *Quantum-Touch: The Power to Heal.* North Atlantic Books, 1999.

Gutman, G., et al. "Feldenkrais versus conventional exercises for the elderly." *Journal of Gerontology* 32 (1977): 562–72.

Heidt, P. "Effect of Therapeutic Touch in anxiety levels of hospitalized patients." *Nursing Research* 30 (1981): 32.

Hellerwork Pearlsoft Research Study, Oct. 1982–Mar. 1983. Conducted by Body of Knowledge, Inc, 406 Berry Street, Mt. Shasta, CA 96067.

Krieger, Dolores. "The relationship of touch, with intent to help or heal, to subjects' in-vivo hemoglobin values: A study in personalized interaction." Proceedings, American Nurses Association 9th Nursing Research Conference, San Antonio, Texas, March 21–23, 1973, 39–78.

———. *The Therapeutic Touch.* Prentice-Hall, 1979.

———. "Therapeutic Touch During Childbirth Preparation by the Lamaze Method and Its Relation to Marital Satisfaction and State of Anxiety in the Married Couple." *Nursing Research Emphasis Grant for Doctoral Programs, U.S. Public Health Service #NU-00833-02.* Proceedings of the Research Day of Sigma Theta Tau, Epsilon Chapter. New York University, Nov. 7, 1984.

Lake, B. "Acute back pain: Treatment by the application of Feldenkrais principles." *Australian Family Physician* 14 (1985): 318–22.

"The Magic of Touch." *Life*, Aug. 1997, 52–62.

McKechnie, A. A., et al. "Anxiety states: A preliminary report on the value of connective tissue massage." *Journal of Psychosomatic Research* 26 (1983): 125–29.

Oleson, T., and W. Flocco. "Randomized controlled study of premenstrual symptoms treated with ear, hand, and foot reflexology." *Obstetrics & Gynecology* 83 (1993): 906–11.

Richardson, N. "Aston-Patterning." *Physical Therapy Forum* 6, no. 43 (1987): 1–3.

Samerel, N. "The experience of receiving Therapeutic Touch." *Journal of Advances in Nursing* 17, no. 6 (1992): 651–57.

Shealy, C. Norman. *Sacred Healing.* Element Books, 1999.

Smith, M. J. "Enzymes are activated by the laying-on of hands." *Human Dimensions* (Feb. 1973): 46–48.

Sunshine, W., et al. "Fibromyalgia benefits from massage therapy and transcutaneous electrical stimulation." *Journal of Clinical Rheumatology* 2, (1996): 18–22.

Touch Training Directory. Associated Bodywork & Massage Professionals, 28677 Buffalo Park Road, Evergreen, CO 80439, 1998.

Trivieri, L. "The lymphatic system: The overlooked key to vibrant health: An interview with Samuel West, D.N, N.D." *The Healthy Edge Letter* 1, no. 2, (April 1998): 5.

———. "Therapeutic touch and the dimensions of healing: An interview with Dr. Dolores Krieger." *The Healthy Edge Letter* 1, no. 3 (April 1998): 8.

Van Why, Richard. *The Bodywork Knowledge Base.* Available from the American Massage Therapy Association.

Wetzel, W. "Reiki healing: A physiologic perspective." *Journal of Holistic Nursing* 7, no. 1 (1989): 37–42.

Weil, Andrew. "The Power of Therapeutic Touch." *Dr. Andrew Weil's Self-Healing,* Jan. 1997, 4.

Weinberg, R. S., and V. Hunt, "Effects of structural integration on state-trait anxiety." *Journal of Clinical Psychology* 35 (1979): 319–22.

Wheeden, A., et al. "Massage effects on cocaine-exposed preterm neonates." *Developmental and Behavioral Pediatrics* 14 (1993): 318–22.

Wirth, D. "The effect of non-contact Therapeutic Touch on the healing of full thickness dermal wounds." *Subtle Energies* 1, no. 1 (1990): 1–20.

Witt, P. L., and J. MacKinnon. "Trager psychophysical integration: A method to improve chest mobility of patients with chronic lung disease." *Physical Therapy* 66, no. 2 (1986): 214–17.

Yates, John. *A Physician's Guide to Therapeutic Massage.* Massage Therapists Association of British Columbia, 1990.

Chapter 10: Naturopathic Medicine

Badger, Lane. "Moving to Center Court in Health Care: Interview with Joseph Pizzorno, Jr., N.D." Health World Online, *www.healthy.net/library/articles /lillipoh/naturopath.htm.*

Banneman, R., et al. *Traditional Medicine and Health Care Coverage.* World Health Organization, Geneva, Switzerland, 1983.

Bergner, Paul. *Safety, Effectiveness and Cost Effectiveness in Naturopathic Medicine.* American Association of Naturopathic Physicians (AANP), 601 Valley Street, Suite 105, Seattle, WA 98109, 1991.

"Congressional Testimony on Naturopathic Medicine." Press Release, Sept. 24, 1999. American Association of Naturopathic Physicians (AANP), 601 Valley Street, Suite 105, Seattle, WA 98109.

Murray, Michael, and Joseph Pizzorno. *Encyclopedia of Natural Medicine.* 2nd ed., rev. Prima Publishing, 1998.

Naturopathic Medical Education. Fact Sheet: American Association of Naturopathic Physicians (AANP), 601 Valley Street, Suite 105, Seattle, WA 98109.

"Nature Healing: Sebastian Kneipp." *German News: The Magazine* (May 1998) *www.germanembassy-india.org/news/98may/gn09.htm.*

Pizzorno, Joseph. *Total Wellness.* Prima Publishing, 1996.

Standish, L., et al. "One year open trial of naturopathic treatment of HIV infection Class IV-A in men." *Journal of Naturopathic Medicine* 3, No. 1, 1992, 42–64.

Trivieri, Larry. "Understanding your body's healing systems: An interview with Joseph Pizzorno, N.D." *The Healthy Edge Letter* 1, no. 5 (1998): 5–9.

"Two Naturopathic Physicians Appointed to Top Federal Advisory Panel." Press Release, July, 1999. American Association of Naturopathic Physicians (AANP), 601 Valley Street, Suite 105, Seattle, WA 98109.

Chapter 11: Homeopathy

Bellavite, Paulo, and Andrea Signorini. *Homeopathy: A Frontier in Medical Science.* North Atlantic Books, 1995.

Brigo, B., and G. Serelloni, G. "Homeopathic treatment of migraines: A randomized double-blind controlled study of sixty cases." *Berlin Journal on Research in Homeopathy* 1, no. 2 (1991): 98–105.

Callinan, Paul. "Homeopathy: How does it work?" Homeopathic House, 3/115 Kirkland Avenue, Coorparoo, Australia, QLD 4151. *www.ozemail.com.au /~daood/paulc.htm.*

Day, C. "Control of stillbirths in pigs using homeopathy." *Veterinary Record* 114 (1984): 216.

De Lange de Klerke, E., et al. "Effect of homeopathic medicines on daily burden of symptoms in children with recurrent upper respiratory tract infections." *British Medical Journal* 309 (1994): 1329–32.

Elia, V., and N. Marcella. "Thermodynamics of extremely diluted aqueous solutions." *Annals of the New York Academy of Sciences* 827 (1999): 241–48.

Fisher, P., et al. "Effect of homeopathic treatment on fibrositis (primary fibromyalgia)." *British Medical Journal* 299 (1989): 365–66.

Gibson, R. G., et al. "Homeopathic therapy in rheumatoid arthritis: Evaluation by double-blind clinical therapeutic trial." *British Journal of Clinical Pharmacology* 9 (1980): 453.

Jacobs, J. et al. "Treatment of acute childhood diarrhea with homeopathic medicine: A randomized clinical trial in Nicaragua." *Pediatrics* 93, no. 5 (1994): 719–25.

Kleijnen, P., et al. "Clinical trials of homeopathy." *British Medical Journal* 302 (1991): 316–23.

Linde, K., et al. "Are the clinical effects of homeopathy placebo effects? A meta-analysis of placebo-controlled trials." *Lancet* 350 (1997): 834–43.

Reilly, M., et al. "Is homeopathy a placebo response? Controlled trial of homeopathic potency with pollen in hayfever as model." *Lancet* (Oct. 18, 1986): 881–86.

Shealy, C. N. et al. "Osteoarthritic pain: A comparison of homeopathy and acetaminophen." *American Journal of Pain Management* 8 (1998): 89–91.

Shui-Yin Lo. "Anomalous state of ice." *Modern Physics Letters B* 10, no. 19 (1996): 909–919.

Ullman, Dana. "The thermodynamics of extremely diluted solutions: New scientific evidence for homeopathic microdoses." Homeopathic Educational Services, 1999. *www.homeopathic.com/articles/thermodynamics.htm*

Chapter 12: Ayurveda

Agnijotri, S, and A. D. Vaidya. "A novel approach to study antibacterial properties of volatile components of selected Indian medicinal herbs." *Indian Journal of Experimental Biology* 34, no. 7 (July 1996): 712–15.

Alexander, C. N., et al. "Transcendental Meditation, mindfulness, and longevity: An experimental study with the elderly." *Journal of Personal and Social Psychology* 57 (1989): 950–64.

Biswas, N. R., et al. "Comparative double blind multicentric randomised placebo controlled clinical trial of a herbal preparation of eye drops in some ocular ailments." *Journal of the Indian Medical Association* 94, no. 3 (Mar. 1996), 101–2.

Charles, V., and S. Charles. The use and efficacy of Azadirachta indica ADR ("neem") and Curcuma longa ("turmeric") in scabies. *Tropical Geographic Medicine* 44 (1992): 178–81.

Frawley, David. "Ayurveda, the World's Medicine for the Next Millennium." *India Post*, June 25, 1999.

Gupta, I., et al. "Effects of Boswellia serrata gum resin in patients with bronchial asthma: Results of a double-blind, placebo-controlled, 6-week clinical study." *European Journal of Medical Research* 3, no. 11 (Nov. 17, 1998): 511–14.

Jacob, A., et al. "Effect of Indian gooseberry (AMLA) on serum cholesterol levels in men aged 35–55 years." *European Journal of Clinical Nutrition* 42 (1988): 939–44.

Jevning, R., et al. "The physiology of meditation: A review: A wakeful hypometabolic integrated response." *Neuroscience and Biobehavior Review* 16 (1992): 415–24.

Kanase, A., et al. "Curative effects of mandur bhasma on liver and kidney of albino rats after induction of acute hepatitis by CCl(4)." *Indian Journal of Experimental Biology* 35, no. 7 (July 1997): 754–64.

Lad, Vasant. *The Complete Book of Ayurvedic Home Remedies*. Harmony Books, 1998.

Miller, A. L. "Botanical influences on cardiovascular disease." *Alternative Medicine Journal* 3, no. 6 (Dec. 1998): 122–31.

Packard, Candis Cantin. *Pocket Guide to Ayurvedic Healing*. The Crossing Press, 1996.

Schneider, R. H. "A randomised controlled trial of stress reduction for hypertension in older African Americans." *Hypertension* 26 (1995): 820–27.

Srivastava, S., et al. "Evaluation of antiallergic activity (type I hypersensitivity) of Inula racemosa in rats." *Indian Journal of Physiological Pharmacology* 43, no. 2 (April 1999): 235–41.

Sundaram, V., H. M. Sharma, et al. "Inhibition of low density lipoprotein oxidation by oral herbal mixtures Maharishi Amrit Kalash-4 and Maharishi Amrit Kalash-5 in hyperlipidemic patients." *American Journal of Medical Science* 314, no. 5 (Nov. 1997): 303–10.

Thyagarajan, S. P., et al. "Effect of phyllanthus amarus on chronic carriers of hepatitus B virus." Lancet 2, no. 8614 (1988): 764–766.

"Traditional Medicine." *New Grolier Multimedia Encyclopedia.* Grolier, Inc. 1993.

Tripathi, Y. B., et al. "Bacopa monniera Linn. as an antioxidant mechanism of action." *Indian Journal of Experimental Biology* 34, no. 6 (June 1996): 523–26.

Wallace, R. K., et al. "Systolic blood pressure and long-term practice of the Transcendental Meditation and Transcendental-Sidhi program: Effects of TM on systolic blood pressure." *Psychosomatic Medicine* 45 (1983): 41–46.

Werner, O. R., et al. "Long-term endocrinologic changes in subjects practicing the Transcendental Meditation and TM-Sidhi program." *Psychosomatic Medicine* 48 (1986): 59–66.

Yadav, P., et al. "Action of capparis decidua against alloxan-induced oxidative stress and diabetes in rats." *Pharmacology Research* 36, no. 3 (Sept. 1997): 221–28.

Ziauddin, M., et al. "Studies on the immunomodulatory effects of Ashwagandha." *Journal of Ethnopharmacology* 50, no. 2 (Feb. 1996): 69–76.

Chapter 13:
Traditional Chinese Medicine and Acupuncture

A Proposed Standard International Acupuncture Nomenclature: Report of a World Health Organization Scientific Group. World Health Organization, Geneva, Switzerland, 1991.

Bannerman, R. H., M.D. The *World Health Organization Viewpoint on Acupuncture.* World Health Organization, Geneva, Switzerland, 1979.

Becker, Robert, M.D. *Cross Currents: The Promise of Electro-Medicine, the Perils of Electropollution.* Jeremy P. Tarcher, 1990.

Burton Goldberg Group. *Alternative Medicine: The Definitive Guide.* Future Medicine Publishing, 1993.

Chatfield, K. B. "The treatment of pesticide poisoning with traditional acupuncture." *American Journal of Acupuncture* 13 (1985): 339–45.

Coan, R. M., et al. "The acupuncture treatment of low back pain: A randomized controlled study." *American Journal of Chinese Medicine* 8 (1980): 181–89.

Coan, R. M., et al. "The acupuncture treatment of neck pain: A randomized controlled study." *American Journal of Chinese Medicine* 9 (1982): 326–32.

Cowley, Geoffrey, and Anne Underwood. "What's 'Alternative'?" *Newsweek*, Nov. 23, 1998, 68.

Diehl, David L., Gary Kaplan, et al. "Use of acupuncture by American physicians." *Journal of Alternative and Complementary Medicine* 3, no. 2 (1997): 119–26.

"Doctor, What's This Acupuncture All About?" The American Academy of Medical Acupuncture, 5820 Wilshire Blvd., Suite 500, Los Angeles, California 90036.

Hau, D. M. "Effects of electroacupuncture on leukocytes and plasma protein in X-irradiated rats." *American Journal of Chinese Medicine?* (1980): 354–66.

Helms, Joseph, M.D. *Acupuncture Energetics: A Clinical Approach for Physicians.* Medical Acupuncture Publishers, 1995.

———. "Acupuncture for the management of primary dysmenorrhea." *Obstetrics & Gynecology* 69 (1987): 51–56.

———. "An overview of medical acupuncture." *Alternative Therapies* 4, no. 3 (May 1998): 35, 36, 42, 43.

Huard, P., and M. Wong. *Chinese Medicine.* World University Library, McGraw-Hill, 1968.

Jahnke, Roger, O. M. D. *The Most Profound Medicine.* Health Action Publishing, 1991.

Jobst, K. A. "A critical analysis of acupuncture in pulmonary disease: Efficacy and safety of the acupuncture needle." *Journal of Alternative and Complementary Medicine* 1, no. 1 (1995): 57–85.

Lee, Y-H, et al. "Acupuncture in the treatment of renal colic." *Journal of Urology* 147 (1992): 16–18.

Liu, F. "Application of traditional Chinese drugs in comprehensive treatment of primary liver cancer." *Journal of Traditional Chinese Medicine* 10, no. 1 (Mar. 1990): 54–60.

Molony, David, and Ming Ming Pan Molony. *Complete Guide to Chinese Herbal Medicine.* Berkley Books, 1998.

Niemtzow, Richard C. "A high-protein regimen and auriculomedicine for the treatment of obesity: A clinical observation." *Medical Acupuncture* 9, no. 2 (fall/winter 1997/1998).

Niemtzow, Richard C. "A high-protein regimen and auriculomedicine for the treatment of obesity: A second clinical observation." *Medical Acupuncture* 10, no. 2 (fall/winter 1998/1999).

Norhein, A.J. and V. Fonnebo. "Doctors' attitudes to acupuncture—a Norwegian study." *Soc. Sci. Med.* 47, no. 4 (Aug. 1998): 519–23.

"NIH Consensus Conference on Acupuncture." *Journal of the American Medical Association* 280, no. 17 (Nov. 4, 1998): 1518–24.

Vincent, C. A. "A controlled trial of the treatment of migraine by acupuncture." *Clinical Journal of Pain* 5 (1989): 305–12.

Weiss, Rick. "Medicine's latest miracle." *Health*, Jan./Feb. 1995.

Zhu Zhong-xiang. "Research advances in the electrical specificity of meridians and acupuncture points." *American Journal of Acupuncture* 9, no. 3 (July–Sept. 1981): 203–15.

Chapter 14: Yoga

Burton Goldberg Group. *Alternative Medicine: The Definitive Guide.* Future Medicine Publishing, 1994.

Feuerstein, Georg. *A Short History of Yoga.* Yoga Research and Education Center, P.O. Box 2418, Sebastopol, CA 95473, 1998.

Garfinkel, M., et al. "Yoga-based intervention for carpal tunnel syndrome: A randomized trial." *JAMA (Journal of the American Medical Association)* 280, no. 18 (1998): 1601–3

Health Conditions Benefited by Yoga, 1983–1984 Survey, Yoga Biomedical Trust, Royal Homeopathic hospital, 60 Great Ormond Street, London, England, WCIN 3HR.

Mahajan, A. S., et al. "Lipid profile of coronary risk subjects following yogic lifestyle intervention." *Indian Heart Journal* 51, no. 1 (1999): 37–40.

Murphy, Michael. *The Future of the Body.* J. P. Tarcher, 1992.

Naveen, K. V., et al. "Yoga breathing through a particular nostril increases spatial memory scores without lateralized effects." *Psychol Rep* 81, no. 2 (1997): 555–61.

Panjwani, U., et al. "Effect of Sahaja yoga practice on seizure control & EEG changes in patients of epilepsy." *Indian Journal of Medical Research* 103 (1996): 165–72.

Raghuraj, R., et al. "Pranayama increases grip strength without latenalization." Vivekananda Kendra Yoga Research Foundation, Bangalore, India, April, 1997.

Roth, B., and T. Creaser, T. "Mindfulness meditation-based stress reduction: Experience with a bilingual inner-city program." *Nurse Practitioner* 22, no. 3 (1997): 150–52, 154, 157.

Shaffer, H. J., et al. "Comparing Hatha yoga with dynamic group psychotherapy for enhancing methadone maintenance treatment: A randomized clinical trial." *Alternative Therapies Health Medicine* 3, no. 4 (1997): 57–66.

Shannahoff-Khalsa, D.S., and L. R. Beckett. "Clinical case report: Efficacy of yogic techniques in the treatment of obsessive compulsive disorders." *International Journal of Neuroscience* 85, no. 1–2 (1996): 1–17.

Schmidt, T., et al. "Changes in cardiovascular risk factors and hormones during a comprehensive residential three month kriya yoga training and vegetarian nutrition." *Acta Physiol Scand Suppl.* 640 (1997): 158–62.

Telles, S., and K. V. Naveen. *Yoga for rehabilitation: An overview.* Vivekananda Kendra Yoga Research Foundation, Bangalore, India, April 1997.

Uma, K. et al. "The integrated approach of yoga: A therapeutic tool for mentally retarded children: A one-year controlled study." *Journal of Mental Deficiency Research* 33, no. 5 (1989): 415–21.

Wood, C. "Mood change and perceptions of vitality: A comparison of the effects of relaxation, visualization, and yoga." *Journal of the Royal Society of Medicine* 86 (1993): 254–58.

Chapter 15: Additional Therapies of Holistic Medicine

Basset, I. B., et al. "A comparative study of tea-tree oil versus benzoyl peroxide in the treatment of acne." *Medical Journal of Australia* 153 (1990): 455–58.

Buck, D. S., et al. "Comparison of two topical preparations for the onychomycosis: Melaleuca alternifolia (tea tree) oil and clotrimazole." *Journal of Family Practice* 38 (1994): 601–5.

Buckle, J. "Aromatherapy." *Nursing Times* 89 (1993): 32–35.

Cranton, E. "Protocol of the American College of Advancement in Medicine for the safe and effective administration of intravenous EDTA chelation therapy." *Journal of Advancement in Medicine* 2, no. 1–2 (1989): 269–305.

Dental Amalgam: A Scientific Review and Recommended Public Health Service Strategy for Research, Education and Regulation. Final Report of the Subcommittee on Risk Management of the Committee to Coordinate Environmental Health and Related Programs. Public Health Service, Jan. 1993.

Environmental Health Criteria for Inorganic Mercury. World Health Organization, Geneva, Switzerland, 1991.

Faber, W. J. "Biological Reconstruction—Alternative to Hip Prosthesis." *www.prolotherapy.com.*

———. "Non-surgical tendon, ligament and joint reconstruction." *www.prolotherapy.com.*

———. "Resolve joint pain without surgery: Reconstructive therapy prevents injury and increases endurance." *www.prolotherapy.com.*

Gobel, H. et al. "Effect of peppermint and eucalyptus oil preparations on neurophysiological and experimental algesimetric headache parameters." *Cephalagia* 14 (1994): 228–34.

Grier, M., and Meyers, D. "So much writing, so little science: A review of 37 years of literature on edetate sodium chelation therapy." *Annals of Pharmacotherapy* 27 (1993): 1504–9.

Howell, Edward. *Food Enzymes for Health and Longevity.* Omangod Press, 1980.

Kahn, Sherry. *Healing Magnets.* Three Rivers Press, 2000.

Olszewer E., and J. Carter. "EDTA chelation therapy in chronic degenerative disease." *Medical Hypotheses* 27, no. 1 (1988): 41–49.

Price, W. *Dental Infections, Vol. 1: Oral and Systemic.* Benton Publishing, 1973.

Stevenson, C. "Measuring the effects of aromatherapy." *Nursing Times* 88 (1992): 62–63.

Trivieri, Larry. "NAET: A revolutionary approach for eliminating allergies." *The Healthy Edge Letter* 1, no. 1 (1998): 1–4.

Warren, Tom. *Beating Alzheimer's*. Avery Publishing, 1991.

Wolf, Max, and Kurt Ransberger. *Enzyme Therapy*. Vantage Press, 1972.

Ziff, S. "Consolidated symptom analysis of 1569 patients." *Bio-Probe Newsletter* 9, no. 2 (1993): 7–8.

Index